MODERN HEMATOLOGY

SECOND EDITION

CONTEMPORARY HEMATOLOGY

Gary J. Schiller, MD, SERIES EDITOR

MODERN HEMATOLOGY

Biology and Clinical Management, Second Edition

Edited by

REINHOLD MUNKER, MD
Louisiana State University, Shreveport, LA

ERHARD HILLER, MD
Ludwigs-Maximilians Universität, Munich, Germany

JONATHAN GLASS, MD
Feist Weiller Cancer Center, Louisiana State University, Shreveport, LA

RONALD PAQUETTE, MD
University of California Los Angeles, Los Angeles, CA

Foreword by

H. PHILLIP KOEFFLER, MD
Cedars-Sinai Medical Center, Los Angeles, CA

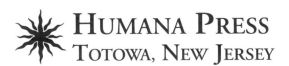 HUMANA PRESS
TOTOWA, NEW JERSEY

Library of Congress Cataloging-in-Publication Data

Modern hematology : biology and clinical management / edited by
Reinhold Munker ... [et al.]. -- 2nd ed.
    p. ; cm. -- (Contemporary hematology)
  Rev. ed. of: Modern hematology / Reinhold Munker, Erhard Hiller, Ronald Paquette. c2000.
  Includes bibliographical references and index.
  ISBN-13: 978-1-58829-557-6 (alk. paper);
  ISBN-10: 1-58829-557-5 (alk. paper)
  1. Blood--Diseases. 2. Hematology. I. Munker, Reinhold. II. Munker, Reinhold. Modern hematology.
III. Series.
  [DNLM: 1. Hematologic Diseases. 2. Hematologic Neoplasms. WH 120 M689 2006]
  RC633.M866 2006
  616.1'5--dc22
                                                                                    2006015501

FOREWORD

Technological advances have quickly propelled hematology forward; for example: microarray expression analyses; single-nucleotide polymorphism (SNP) chips (platforms to look at genomic changes); sophisticated fluorescent *in situ* hybridization; newly identified cell surface antigens associated with various diseases and cell types; understanding of transcription factors (engines of proliferation and differentiation of hematopoietic cells); and more complete knowledge of chromosomal changes, mutations and amplifications associated with various hematological malignancies. These advances have been the engines for better diagnosis and classification of hematopoietic disorders. Furthermore, a variety of new therapeutic approaches have come to the forefront, such as targeted therapies (thyrosine kinase inhibitors) for myeloproliferative disorders; lenalidomide for myelodysplastic syndrome (MDS) and multiple myeloma; demethylating agents for MDS and myeloid leukemia, as well as, humanized monoclonal antibodies for lymphomas. Many of these advancements have occurred since the first edition of *Modern Hematology: Biology and Clinical Management* by Dr. Rienhold Munker and colleagues was published 6 years ago.

This new edition, edited by Drs. Reinhold Munker, Erhard Hiller, Jonathan Glass, and Ronald Paquette, provides in clear terms an understanding of the cellular physiology, immunology, and molecular biology of hematopoietic disorders. It gives new diagnostic methodologies and guides the health care worker to practical approaches to the diagnoses and management of these blood disorders. The book covers all of the major hematopoietic diseases and a number of the rare diseases as they interface with new scientific knowledge. It has excellent "how to" tables providing dosage and time schedules of different chemotherapeutic agents, as well as clearly defined tables to aid in diagnosis and prognosis.

Modern Hematology: Biology and Clinical Management, Second Edition is a fine montage of applied research and practical approaches to diagnosis and management of our patients. The book is ideal for the house officers, fellows in training, interested scientists, as well as the practicing hematologist.

H. Phillip Koeffler, MD

PREFACE

In the 6 years since the publication of *Modern Hematology: Biology and Clinical Management*, major advances in the understanding, diagnosis, and treatment of blood disorders have again been made. Molecular studies are now used on a daily basis to diagnose a variety of hematological disorders and to guide their treatment. Targeted therapies, such as kinase inhibitors in myeloproliferative disorders and humanized monoclonal antibodies for lymphomas, have transformed the treatment approach to these diseases. Peripheral blood and even umbilical cord blood are now routinely used as sources of stem cells for transplantation. The growing use of nonmyeloablative transplantation emphasizes immunotherapy over cytotoxic chemotherapy. These advances motivated us to update *Modern Hematology: Biology and Clinical Management* with the latest clinical and scientific developments in hematology. We welcome the contributions of new authors. The growing use of databases prompted us to add an overview of printed and electronic resources for hematologists.

Modern Hematology: Biology and Clinical Management, Second Edition brings together facts, concepts, and protocols important for the practice of hematology. In 23 concise chapters, all major blood diseases are covered; rarer diseases are discussed if they are of scientific interest. The first two chapters introduce the reader to the scientific basis of blood disorders. As in the previous edition, each chapter is illustrated by tables, figures, and a selection of color plates. Our text is ideal for residents or fellows in training. However, students, physicians in other specialties, and even pure scientists may take advantage of our book both as a reference and a study guide. We hope that ultimately, all patients with benign and malignant blood disorders will benefit from the publication of *Modern Hematology: Biology and Clinical Management, Second Edition.*

Reinhold Munker, MD
Erhard Hiller, MD
Jonathan Glass, MD
Ronald Paquette, MD

CONTENTS

CONTRIBUTORS

MICHAEL COCKERHAM, PharmD • *Associate Professor of Clinical Pharmacy, Louisiana State University, Shreveport, LA*

MARTIN H. DREYLING, MD • *Associate Professor of Medicine, Ludwigs-Maximilians Universität, Munich, Germany*

JONATHAN GLASS, MD • *Professor of Medicine and Chief, Feist Weiller Cancer Center, Louisiana State University, Shreveport, LA*

SNEHALATA C. GUPTE, PhD • *Director, Surat Blood Transfusion Center, Surat, India*

JOHN HIEMENZ, MD • *Professor of Medicine, Louisiana State University, Shreveport, LA*

ERHARD HILLER, MD • *Professor of Medicine, Ludwigs-Maximilians Universität, Munich, Germany*

H. PHILLIP KOEFFLER, MD • *Division of Hematology/Oncology, Cedars Sinai Medical Center, Los Angeles, CA*

ALI MANSOURI, MD • *Professor of Medicine, Louisiana State University and Chief, Division of Hematology/Oncology, VA Medical Center, Shreveport, LA*

JAY MARION, MD • *Associate Professor of Medicine, Louisiana State University, Shreveport, LA*

REINHOLD MUNKER, MD • *Associate Professor of Medicine, Louisiana State University, Shreveport, LA*

RONALD PAQUETTE, MD • *Associate Professor of Medicine, University of California Los Angeles, Los Angeles, CA*

VISHWAS SAKHALKAR, MD • *Assistant Professor of Pediatrics, Louisiana State University, Shreveport, LA*

AMANDA SUN, MD, PhD • *Assistant Professor of Medicine, Louisiana State University, Shreveport, LA*

GRACE C. TENORIO, MD • *Assistant Professor of Pathology, Louisiana State University, Shreveport, LA*

GANG YE, MD • *Louisiana State University, Shreveport, LA*

Color Plates

1 Basic Biology of Hemopoiesis

Reinhold Munker, MD

1. INTRODUCTION

The formation of blood cells (hemopoiesis) is determined by the interaction of multiple genes and involves cytokines and other protein factors. The relative ease with which hematopoietic cells can be studied and the development of new techniques in cell biology have enabled us to understand many of the factors determining cell renewal and differentiation. Based on this knowledge, major progress has been made in the last 15 yr in the treatment and diagnosis of many hematological disorders. In this chapter, we describe the cell types involved in normal hematopoiesis and their interactions with one another. Furthermore, the basic techniques necessary for the study of hematopoietic cells in the normal and pathological state are outlined.

From: *Contemporary Hematology: Modern Hematology, Second Edition*
Edited by: R. Munker, E. Hiller, J. Glass, and R. Paquette © Humana Press Inc., Totowa, NJ

2. COMPONENTS OF BLOOD AND BONE MARROW

2.1. Sites of Hematopoiesis

During the first few weeks of embryonic life, the formation of blood cells takes place in the yolk sac. Later, until the sixth or seventh month of fetal development, the liver and spleen are the major hematopoietic organs. By the time of birth, more than 90% of all new blood cells are formed in the bone marrow. Here, the progenitor cells are found, in various stages of development, situated in anatomical niches in the bone marrow from where they are then released into the marrow sinuses, the marrow circulation, and further on into the systemic circulation.

During infancy and childhood, the marrow of all bones contributes to hematopoiesis. During adult life, hematopoietic marrow is restricted to certain bones (e.g., pelvic bones, vertebral column, proximal ends of the femur, skull, ribs, and sternum). Even in these areas, a proportion of the marrow cavity consists of fat. During periods of hematopoietic stress (e.g., in severe hemolytic anemias and in some myeloproliferative disorders), the fatty marrow as well as the spleen and liver can resume the production of blood cells. This situation is called extramedullary hematopoiesis.

2.2. Stromal Cells

Growth and differentiation of hematopoietic cells in the bone marrow is regulated by the extracellular matrix and microenvironment provided by stromal cells. These cells, including macrophages, fibroblasts in various stages of differentiation, endothelial cells, fat cells, and reticulum cells, nurture hematopoietic stem cells and progenitor cells by producing growth factors like granulocyte/macrophage colony-stimulating factor (GM-CSF), granulocyte colony-stimulating factor (G-CSF), interleukin (IL)-6, or stem cell factor. Other cytokines secreted by stromal cells regulate the adhesion molecules present on hematopoietic cells, allowing them to remain in the bone marrow or migrate to an area where the respective cell type is needed.

2.3. Hematopoietic Stem Cells

All hematopoietic cells of the organism derive from pluripotent stem cells that are capable of both self-renewal and differentiation into all hematopoietic lineages. As Fig. 1.1 shows, one stem cell provides progenitor cells for myelo- and monopoiesis, erythropoiesis, megakaryopoiesis, and lymphopoiesis. Other cell types such as stromal cells or dendritic cells also derive from the pluripotent hematopoietic stem cell. It has been estimated that one stem cell gives rise to at least 10^6 mature hematopoietic cells. Under normal conditions, the stem cells provide hematopoietic cells for the entire life span. Each day, a healthy adult organism produces more than 10^{12} hematopoietic cells. Many blood disorders

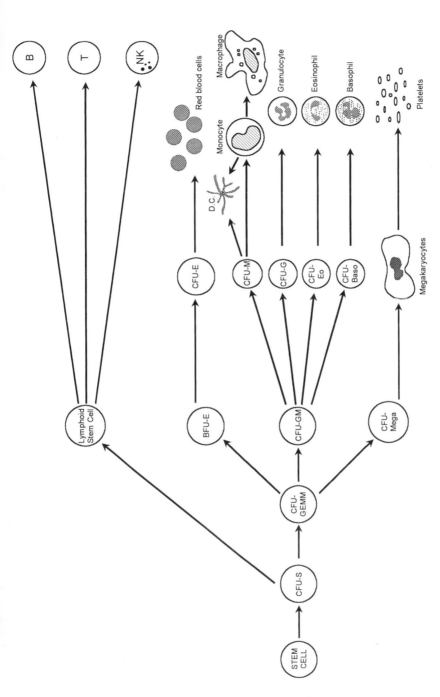

Fig. 1.1. Scheme of hematopoietic differentiation (for abbreviations, *see* text).

(e.g., leukemias, aplastic anemias, or myelodysplastic syndromes) are disorders of stem cells.

Stem cells are very rare, representing less than 0.01% of all nucleated cells in the normal bone marrow. Based on animal experiments, the morphology of stem cells is thought to be similar to that of small lymphoid cells. In recent years, the marker expression of human stem cells has been studied. Human stem cells express the surface proteins CD34 and c-kit and are negative for CD38 and lineage-specific markers. In animal systems, stem cells can be assayed as spleen colony-forming units (CFU) in irradiated hosts. Only the more differentiated progenitors of human hematopoietic cells can be tested for their ability to form colonies in soft agar or methylcellulose. One of the earliest progenitor cells in such systems is CFU$_{GEMM}$, which contains granulocytes, monocytes, erythroid cells, and platelet progenitors. From this pluripotent progenitor, more specialized progenitors are formed (*see* Fig. 1.1). Under normal conditions, the majority of stem cells is dormant (G0 phase of the cell cycle). A stem cell divides only to maintain the steady state of hematopoiesis or to meet the body's demand for progenitor cells (stochastic model of hematopoiesis). The daughter cells then either differentiate into determined progenitor cells (e.g., lymphohematopoietic cells) or return to dormancy by reentering the stem cell pool. Stem cells can be enriched and transplanted (stem cell or bone marrow transplantation). The stem cell donor does not experience a detectable loss of stem cells.

There are several hierarchical levels of stem and progenitor cells. In general, the hematopoietic growth factors do not act on true stem cells, but support the survival and the differentiation of committed cells. Although "early-acting" cytokines such as stem cell factor, FLT3-ligand, G-CSF, or IL-6 regulate the earliest progenitor cells, "late-acting" cytokines such as erythropoietin for erythropoiesis or thrombopoietin for megakaryopoiesis support the growth and differentiation of progenitor cells that are already committed to their respective lineage. Many other cytokines play a positive or negative role in the differentiation of hematopoietic cells. A list of the known cytokines is given in Chapter 2.

The gene expression in early stem cells is complex and involves the co-expression of multiple transcription factors. For example, the combination of C/EBP α and Pu 1 directs the expression of the receptor for G-CSF, which is critical for early myelopoiesis. Pu 1 binds to and regulates the promotors of several myeloid growth-factor receptor genes. The Notch family of transmembrane receptors was described in *Drosophila* as a ligand-dependent suppressor of cell differentiation. Similar receptors have recently been found on human stem cells, suggesting that they may also be involved in maintaining an undifferentiated state.

The significance of telomeres present in human stem cells and the activity of telomerase in these cells is currently of interest. Telomeres are specialized structures at the end of chromosomes that change with cell division. Shortening of telomeres is associated with cellular aging. Telomerase is an enzyme capable of extending the length of telomeres. It has now been found that adult stem cells have shorter telomeres than fetal stem cells and that the length of telomeres shortens further after transplantation. The activity of telomerase is generally low in stem cells (which corresponds to their quiescent state), but can be upregulated on entry into the cell cycle. The implications of these findings are not yet clear, but they may indicate that not all stem cells are immortal.

3. ERYTHROPOIESIS

Red blood cells are specialized cells that deliver oxygen to tissues and remove carbon dioxide from the human body. Erythropoiesis, the "making of red cells," involves many different genes and gene products that lead to the production of the mature cell. Erythropoiesis begins at the level of the multipotent stem cell, which then undergoes commitment and differentiation. Listed as follows are the stages of erythroid differentiation:

1. Stem cell.
2. BFU-E (burst-forming unit, erythroid; immature erythroid progenitor).
3. CFU-E (colony-forming unit, erythroid; more mature erythroid progenitor).
4. Proerythroblasts, erythroblasts, normoblasts (morphologically recognizable red cell precursors, they still have a nucleus, multiply by cell division, and progressively decrease in size as hemoglobin content increases).
5. Reticulocytes; mature red blood cells (erythrocyte).

Remnants of ribosomal RNA can be visualized in reticulocytes; no nucleus is present in the mature red cell. The vast majority of nucleated red-cell precursors are confined to the bone marrow.

One proerythroblast gives rise to 12–16 mature red blood cells within 5–10 d. The erythropoietic differentiation is modulated by several cytokines (stem cell factor, IL-3, GM-CSF, and erythropoietin). Erythropoietin is the major cytokine that adapts the production of red cells to the needs of the organism. Both the proliferation and differentiation of CFU-E and late BFU-E are accelerated as a response to erythropoietin. In response to low hemoglobin levels in the blood and tissue hypoxia, the production of erythropoietin by the kidneys is increased. When the serum levels of erythropoietin are increased, both the rate and the speed of erythropoiesis increase. Erythropoietin binds to specific receptors on red cell precursors, consequently activating the Janus 2 kinase (JAK2) by tyrosine phosphorylation. This in turn activates the STAT pathway and Ras signal transduction. A number of transcription factors are involved in the activation of erythroid-specific genes including *GATA1*, *GATA2*, *NFE2*, *SCL*, *EKLF*, and *myb*. During early erythropoiesis, the downregulation of the *SCL* gene precedes the downregulation of the *GATA 2* and *GATA 1* genes. In bone marrow, erythropoiesis occurs in distinct anatomic locations called erythroblastic islands, in which a central macrophage is surrounded by a ring of developing erythroblasts. Important mediators of the cell–cell contact in the erythroid islands include the integrins, the immunoglobulin (Ig) superfamily, and cadherins. In states of chronic tissue hypoxia (e.g., in hemolytic anemias) the proportion of the marrow devoted to erythropoiesis expands and sometimes transforms a large portion of the fatty marrow into active hematopoietic marrow.

3.1. Hemoglobin

Hemoglobin is the molecule responsible for the transport of oxygen. Under physiological conditions, three types of hemoglobins exist:

- Hemoglobin A ($\alpha_2\beta_2$): major adult hemoglobin (96–98%).
- Hemoglobin F ($\alpha_2\gamma_2$): predominant during fetal development, 60–80% at birth, 0.5–0.8% during adult life.
- Hemoglobin A2($\alpha_2\delta_2$): normally 1.5–3%.

The hemoglobin molecule has a molecular weight of 64,500 and consists of four polypeptide chains, each carrying a heme group. The heme synthesis starts with the amino acid glycine. Later, porphobilinogen, uroporphyrinogen, coproporphyrinogen, and protoporphyrin are formed as intermediate steps. Iron (Fe^{2+}) is supplied from serum transferrin and combines with protoporphyrin to form heme. One heme molecule then binds with one globin chain to form the hemoglobin molecule that avidly binds oxygen.

The release of oxygen from red cells into tissue is strictly regulated. Under normal conditions, arterial blood enters tissues with an oxygen tension of 90 mmHg and a hemoglobin saturation close to 97%. Venous blood returning from tissues is deoxygenated. The oxygen tension is about 40 mmHg, the hemoglobin saturation is 70–80%. The oxyhemoglobin dissociation curve describes the relation between the oxygen saturation or content of hemoglobin and the oxygen tension at equilibrium. The oxygen dissociation curve has a sigmoid shape (*see* Fig. 1.2). Under normal conditions, only the upper part of this curve is used. The affinity of hemoglobin for oxygen and the deoxygenation in tissues is influenced by temperature, by CO_2 concentration, and by the level of 2,3-diphosphoglycerate in the red cells. In the case of tissue or systemic acidosis, the oxygen dissociation curve is shifted to the right and more oxygen is released. The same effect results from the uptake of carbon dioxide, which raises the oxygen tension of carbon dioxide. This facilitates the unloading of oxygen. As the body temperature increases, the affinity of hemoglobin for oxygen decreases, thereby facilitating oxygen release.

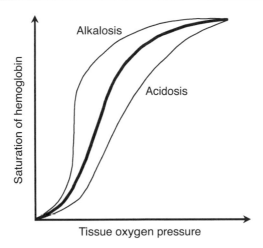

Fig. 1.2. Hemoglobin oxygen dissociation curve.

The oxygen supply to peripheral tissues is influenced by three mechanisms:

1. The blood flow, which is controlled by the heart beat volume and the constriction or dilatation of peripheral vessels.
2. The oxygen transport capacity, which depends on the number of red blood cells and the hemoglobin concentration.
3. The oxygen affinity of hemoglobin.

In anemic patients, the stroke volume of the heart is increased, the heart beats faster (tachycardia), and, in addition, the 2,3-diphosphoglycerate concentration in red blood cells can increase to facilitate the oxygen dissociation in tissues. A compensation mechanism that takes several days or weeks is the increased synthesis of red blood cells.

3.2. Iron Metabolism

With a normal Western diet, 10–15 mg of iron is ingested daily. Under normal circumstances, only 5–10% of this dietary iron is absorbed as Fe^{2+} in the duodenum or, to a lesser degree, in the jejunum. In severe iron deficiency, the proportion of resorbed iron may increase up to 30%. Iron is lost from the body via sweat, urine, and feces. Iron resorption is improved under the normal acidic and reducing conditions of the gastrointestinal mucosa. The mucosal cells of the duodenum are also capable of resorbing dietary heme iron that later dissociates. Iron resorption can increase severalfold according to the body's demand (e.g., during pregnancy, after an acute blood loss, or in menstruating women). Iron absorption proceeds under the influence of the HFE protein (mutated in hereditary hemochromatosis). Under normal conditions, the HFE protein binds to the transferrin receptor at the cell membrane surface. Both proteins (bound to iron and transferrin) are then imported into the cell. Excess iron can be shed from the mucosal villi of the gut, but if the iron supply continues to exceed iron requirements, iron overload will develop. The most common form is the genetic disorder hemochromatosis, but iron overload can also occur in patients with blood disorders who depend on transfusions. In such patients, iron is deposited in the liver, pancreas, heart muscle, and other organs.

Iron is an essential component of hemoglobin. Most of the iron needed for erythropoiesis does not derive from dietary iron, but is liberated from senescent red blood cells phagocytized by macrophages in the reticuloendothelial system. Iron enters the plasma as Fe^{3+}, where it binds to transferrin and can be used again in erythropoiesis. About 30% of the total body iron is stored in the reticuloendothelial system either as transferrin, ferritin, or hemosiderin. The β-globulin transferrin is synthesized in the liver and can bind two atoms of iron reversibly. Normally, transferrin is only one-third saturated. The progenitor cells of erythropoiesis have specific transferrin receptors, thereby enabling the transfer of iron into these developing erythroid cells.

3.3. The Red Blood Cell

The normal erythrocyte has a diameter of about 8 μm and a biconcave disc form that provides the red cell with a maximum surface-for-gas exchange as well as optimal deformability. The bipolar lipid layer of the red cell membrane is stabilized on the inner side by the attachment of the structural proteins actin and spectrin. Defects of these proteins lead to hemolytic anemia. The outer layer is covered with mucopolysaccharides that form part of the structure of blood group antigens. The N-acetylneuraminic acid found in these glycoproteins results in a negative charge of the cell surface.

Because red cells have lost their nuclei, they are no longer capable of synthesizing proteins, including enzymes. Red cells remain viable and functional for an average of 120 d. The necessary energy for red cell metabolism is supplied by the Embden-Meyerhof pathway, which generates adenosine triphosphate by metabolizing glucose to lactate. This anerobic process also results in the formation of nicotinamide-adenine dinucleotide, which is essential for the reduction of methemoglobin to functionnally active hemoglobin.

Hemoglobin is split into globin and heme in the reticuloendothelial system. Both components can be recycled. The globin chains are metabolized into amino acids consequently used for the synthesis of new proteins, and iron is used for further heme synthesis. The remaining protoporphyrin is metabolized to bilirubin. The bilirubin is conjugated in the liver and excreted via bile secretions into the intestine. Intestinal bacteria metabolize bilirubin into stercobilinogen and stercobilin, which are excreted via feces. Part of these hemoglobin degradation products are reabsorbed and excreted via urine as urobilin and urobiliogen.

4. MYELOPOIESIS

Under the influence of cytokines such as G-CSF, a myeloid progenitor cell, CFU-G, is formed. This cell then differentiates into the morphologically recognizable myeloid precursors: myeloblasts, promyelocytes, myelocytes, and metamyelocytes. Normally these cells do not appear in peripheral blood. Myeloblasts are rather large cells (12–20 μm in diameter) and have a large nucleus with fine chromatin and several nucleoli. No cytoplasmic granules are present. The normal marrow contains up to 5% of myeloblasts. Cell division of myeloblasts results in the formation of promyelocytes, slightly larger neutrophilic precursors with granules in their cytoplasm. These cells in turn give rise by cell division to myelocytes, which have smaller granules (secondary or specific granules). At this stage, a differentiation of the myelocytes into the neutrophil, eosinophil, and basophil series can be recognized. Further cell division produces metamyelocytes. These cells can no longer divide and have a somewhat indented nucleus and numerous granules in their cytoplasm.

Between the mature neutrophil and the metamyelocyte, so-called "juvenile," "stab," or "band" forms are observed in which the nucleus is not yet fully segmented. Such cells occur normally in the peripheral blood (less than 8% of circulating neutrophils) and are increased under hematopoietic stress, such as during infections.

The normal number of neutrophilic granulocytes in the peripheral blood is about 2500–7500/μL. Neutrophilic granulocytes have a dense nucleus split into two to five lobes and a pale cytoplasm. The cytoplasm contains numerous pink-blue or gray-blue granules. Two types of granules can be distinguished morphologically: primary or azurophilic granules, which appear at the promyelocyte stage, and secondary granules, which appear later. The primary granules contain myeloperoxidase, acid phosphatase, and acid hydrolases, whereas lysozyme, lactoferrin, and collagenase are found in the secondary granules. All granules are of lysosomal origin.

According to cytokinetic studies, the time required for the division and maturation of a myeloblast to a mature granulocyte is 6–12 d. It has been estimated that 1.5×10^9 granulocytes/kg are produced daily in the healthy organism. Most of these cells stay at various stages of maturation in the bone marrow, from where they can be mobilized in case of hematopoietic stress. Following their release from the bone marrow, granulocytes circulate for no longer than 12 h in the blood. Approximately half of the granulocytes present in the bloodstream are found in the circulating pool, whereas the other half is kept in a marginated pool attached to blood vessel walls. After granulocytes move from the circulation into tissues, they survive for about 5 d before they die while fighting infections or as a result of senescence.

The major function of granulocytes (neutrophils) is the uptake and killing of bacterial pathogens. The first step involves the process of chemotaxis, by which the granulocyte is attracted to the pathogen. Chemotaxis is initiated by chemotactic factors released from damaged tissues or complementary components. The next step is phagocytosis or the actual ingestion of the bacteria, fungi, or other particles by the granulocyte. The recognition and uptake of a foreign particle is made easier if the particle is opsonized, which is done by coating them with an antibody or complement. The coated particles then bind to Fc or C3b receptors on the granulocytes. Opsonization is also involved in the phagocytosis of bacteria or other pathogens by monocytes. During phagocytosis a vesicle is formed in the phagocytic cell into which enzymes are released. These enzymes, including collagenases, aminopeptidase, and lysozyme, derive from the secondary granules of the granulocyte. The final step in the phagocytic process is the killing and digestion of the pathogen. This is achieved by both oxygen-dependent and -independent pathways. In the oxygen-dependent reactions, superoxide, hydrogen peroxide, and OH radicals are generated from oxygen and NADPH. The reactive oxygen species are toxic not only to the bacteria, but also to surrounding tissue, causing the damage observed during infections and inflammation.

4.1. Eosinophils

Eosinophils, which make up 1–4% of the peripheral blood leukocytes, are similar to neutrophils but with somewhat more intensely stained reddish granules. In absolute terms, eosinophils number up to 400/μL. Eosinophilic cells can first be recognized at the myelocyte stage. Eosinophils have a role in allergic reactions, in the response to parasites, and in the defense against certain tumors.

4.2. Basophils

Basophils are seen less frequently than eosinophils; under normal conditions, fewer than 100 cells/μL are found in the peripheral blood. Basophils have receptors for irnmunoglobulin (Ig)E and, in the cytoplasm, characteristic dark granules overlie the nucleus. Degranulation of basophils results from the binding of IgE and allergic or anaphylactic reactions are associated with the release of histamine and heparin.

4.3. Mast Cells

Similarly to basophils, mast cells derive from bone marrow CD34$^+$ progenitors, have receptors for IgE, and store histamine. Mast cells typically migrate into and mature in connective tissues. Mast cells participate in allergic and immunological reactions.

4.4. Monocytes

As already mentioned, monocytes derive from the myeloid progenitor cell (CFU-GM), which replicates and differentiates into monocytes and, later, macrophages under the influence of certain growth factors. After commitment to the monocytic lineage has been made, the cell goes through distinct monoblast and promonocyte stages before developing into a mature monocyte. Circulating monocytes make up 2–6% of all leukocytes (in absolute numbers 200–800/μL). Monocytes are larger than most other cells of the blood (diameter 15–20 pm). The cytoplasm is abundant and stains blue, with many fine vacuoles. Fine granules are often present. The nucleus is large and often indented with clumped chromatin. Monocytes and macrophages (*see* "Macrophages") can phagocytose pathogens, present antigens, and secrete many cytokines.

4.5. Macrophages

After several hours of transit in the blood, the monocytes migrate into different tissues, where they differentiate into macrophages. Macrophages are larger than monocytes, and have an oval nucleus, prominent nucleoli, a blue cytoplasm, and phagocytic vesicles. The different types of macrophages (e.g., Kupfer cells in the liver, alveolar macrophages in the lung, osteoclasts in the bone, macrophages in the bone marrow, peritoneal macrophages) are known as components of the reticulo-endothelial system. Macrophages are long-lived (life span at least 10 d or much longer) and secrete numerous cytokines, enzymes, and enzyme inhibitors. The major cytokines secreted by macrophages are tumor necrosis factor (TNF)-α, IL-1α, and IL-1β (monokines). Macrophages avidly phagocytose and kill bacteria and other pathogens. In addition, macrophages have immunological functions (antigen presentation) and can kill tumor cells. An important function of macrophages is to remove debris (scavenger function) and to regulate the proliferation of stromal cells.

4.6. Dendritic Cells

The existence and function of dendritic cells (D.C. in Fig. 1.1) has only recently been recognized. Dendritic cells are present in many tissues, including in the skin (where they are known as Langerhans cells), in the airways, in lymphoid tissues, in solid organs, and in blood and bone marrow. Morphologically, they appear as large mononuclear cells with stellate processes. The major function of dendritic cells is to present antigens. Most types of dendritic cells derive from hematopoietic progenitor cells. Some, like follicular dendritic cells, derive from lymphoid or stromal cells. Methods for culturing and expanding human dendritic cells have recently been developed. Dendritic cells can be grown from CD34$^+$ bone marrow progenitor cells or from CD14$^+$ blood monocytes. The cytokines GM-CSF and IL-4 are needed at the beginning of the culture and further maturation of the cells is reached under the influence of monocyte-derived factors. Mature dendritic cells have a characteristic marker profile: they strongly express class II human leukocyte antigens (HLAs) as well as co-stimulatory and adhesion molecules. In vivo, dendritic cells capture and process antigens, migrate to lymphoid organs, and secrete numerous cytokines to initiate immune responses. Dendritic cells stimulate quiescent B- and T-lymphocytes. They are very potent stimulators of T-cell responses: small numbers of dendritic cells and low levels of antigen induce a strong T-cell immunity. Under certain circumstances, dendritic cells can also tolerize the organism to self-antigens, thereby preventing autoimmune reactions. A new approach aimed at overcoming the deficient antitumor immunity of cancer patients has recently been described in which dendritic cells are primed with tumor antigens in vitro and then reinfused into the patient.

5. MEGAKARYOPOIESIS

Platelets are small cell fragments (average size 3–4 µm) that are important for hemostasis and coagulation. The normal platelet count is between 150,000 and 450,000/µL. Platelets derive from megakaryocytes, which are very large cells with a large, multilobulated nucleus. The mean DNA content of megakaryocytes is at least eight times that of other somatic cells. One megakaryocyte can produce at least several thousand platelets. The formation and release of platelets is related to a preformed structure in the cytoplasm of megakaryocytes, the so-called "demarcation membrane system." Megakaryocytes derive from megakaryocyte progenitors (CFU-Mega, see Fig. 1.1), which in turn originate in the hematopoietic stem cell. Megakaryocytes are mainly found in the bone marrow but can transit to many organs, including the lung, where part of the platelet release occurs. The maturation of megakaryocytes and the production of platelets occurs under the influence of thrombopoietin (TPO; for details see Chapter 2). TPO acts, together with certain other cytokines like IL-6 and IL-11, on early megakaryocyte progenitors as well as mature megakaryocytes. Under physiological conditions, the serum levels of TPO are low at normal or elevated platelet counts and high in individuals with low platelet counts. Details on the physiology of platelets are described in Chapter 19.

6. LYMPHATIC TISSUES AND IMMUNE RESPONSE

6.1. Development and Organs of the Lymphoid System

The common or pluripotent hematopoietic stem cell differentiates at an early stage into lymphoid and myeloid progenitor cells. From these lymphoid stem cells, the two main classes of lymphocytes, B- and T-cells, develop. The lymphocytes populate the major lymphatic organs, but can also be found circulating in the peripheral blood. Two types of lymphoid organs can be distinguished: the central lymphoid organs (bone marrow, thymus) and the peripheral lymphoid organs (lymph nodes, tonsils, spleen, mucosa-associated lymphoid tissue). The central lymphoid organs are the original site of lymphopoiesis and lymphoid maturation, whereas the peripheral lymphoid organs specialize in trapping antigen and initiating adaptive immune responses. In the peripheral blood, 80–85% of the lymphoid cells belong to the T-cell lineage, whereas in the peripheral lymphoid tissues most lymphoid cells belong to the B-cell lineage.

6.2. B-Lymphocytes

The major task of B-lymphocytes is the production of antibodies (humoral immunity). The first steps of B-cell differentiation take place in the bone marrow, where lymphoid progenitors differentiate into pro-B- and pre-B-cells. A surface marker that is expressed very early in B-cell ontogeny is CD19. The initial stages of B-cell development depend on the interaction between cell surface molecules and secreted products of stromal cells with their receptor–ligand partners on lymphoid progenitors. Numerous cytokines and growth factors (e.g., TNF, IL-1, IL-2, IL-6, IL-7, IL-10, interferon [IFN]-γ) direct the growth and differentiation of B-cells. In the peripheral blood, where they make up 4–6% of all mononuclear cells, B-cells bear additional surface markers (e.g., CD20, CD22). The specificity of B-cell immunity is reached via surface receptors for antigen (in most cases IgD or IgM). After leaving the bone marrow and circulating in the blood, the mature B-cells migrate into the follicles of the secondary lymphoid organs (e.g., spleen, lymph nodes, and other tissues). Following the contact with an antigen, B-cells differentiate into antibody-secreting plasma cells or into B-memory cells. B-memory cells are long-lived and reside for the most part in lymph nodes. Without antigen stimulation, B-cells have a short life span.

The lymphoid follicles provide the necessary environment for B-cells to maintain their existence as mature recirculating antigen-specific cells. The antigen-specific repertoire of B-cells is generated by the sequential rearrangement of Ig gene segments. This developmental program involves changes in the expression of other cellular proteins and is directed by transcription factors. If an intact Ig chain is generated, then this type of rearrangement is terminated, and the next step in the rearrangement cascade can begin. If successive rearrangements fail to generate first a heavy chain (pre-B-cell receptor) and then a light chain, which can be assembled into a complete immunoglobulin molecule, the B-cell ceases to develop further and goes into apoptosis (programmed cell death). The end result of the successive rearrangements of immunoglobulin genes is a B-cell with a surface Ig of a single specificity.

An efficient antibody response and immune defense can only be achieved in cooperation with T-lymphocytes. However, before the T-cells can recognize the antigen and induce the proliferation of B-cells and their differentiation into plasma cells or memory cells, certain criteria must be met. First, antigen-presenting cells must process the antigen (which may be bound to the receptors of B-cells). Next, the processed antigen must be associated with the molecules of the major histocompatibility complex.

6.3. T-Lymphocytes

T-lymphocytes also derive from stem cells located in the bone marrow. However, before becoming functional cells, the precursor cells migrate to the thymus where they proliferate, differentiate into mature cells, and are finally released into the blood. At the same time autoreactive T-cells are eliminated. The earliest stage of T-cell development is the prothymocyte. Immature T-cells co-expressing the surface markers CD4 and CD8 are located primarily in the cortex of the thymus. During maturation, the T-cell precursors lose either CD4 or CD8 and migrate to the medulla. A large majority of thymocytes is eliminated during this process. During differentiation, antigen-specific surface receptors are formed. These antigen-receptors recognize either bacterial antigens on antigen-presenting cells or new antigens on tumor cells, transplanted cells, or virally infected cells. Taken together, T-lymphocytes specialize in cell-mediated immunity. They do not react with intact antigens but with antigen fragments presented in association with molecules of the major histocompatibility complex. There are two main classes of T-lymphocytes circulating in the peripheral blood: CD4-positive cells (helper cells) and CD8-positive cells (suppressor or cytotoxic T-lymphocytes), explained as follows.

- CD4-positive T-lymphocytes recognize foreign antigens in association with HLA class II molecules and have, for the most part, helper or inducer functions. CD4-positive cells secrete lymphokines after the presentation of the antigen by macrophages has taken place. These cytokines activate macrophages but can also stimulate the proliferation of B-cells and induce the production of antibodies by plasma cells. The secretion of IL-2 also contributes to the development of cytotoxic T-lymphocytes.
- CD8-positive T-lymphocytes react with foreign antigens in association with class I molecules and are the specific effector or killer cells of cell-mediated immunity. CD8-positive lymphocytes also have suppressor functions and control the proliferation of other T-cell subsets as well as the function of B-cells.

6.4. Natural Killer Cells

Natural killer (NK) cells belong to the lymphoid lineage, although some have markers of the monocyte/myeloid lineage. Morphologically, NK cells are characterized as large granular lymphocytes. NK cells are defined by their ability to kill some tumor cells by antigen-independent mechanisms (natural immunity). The physiological function of NK cells is still being debated and includes the removal of certain tumor cells or of virally infected cells. NK cells can be expanded and cultured in the presence of IL-2. Such expanded NK cells (lymphokine-activated killer cells) have been used in the experimental treatment of tumors. Recently, a family of inhibitory receptors on natural killer cells was described. These molecules are specific for some members of the major histocompatibility complex and inhibit the activation of NK cells.

7. PLASMA COMPONENTS

The blood plasma contains all proteins and factors necessary for the integrity of the organism. Some of these factors are involved in coagulation, and others function as transport proteins, hormones, or immunoglobulins. Most of the plasma proteins are synthesized and secreted in the liver. By means of electrophoresis, the major proteins of the serum or plasma can be resolved into five bands, designated albumin, α_1, α_2, β, and γ fractions. Specialized proteins can be further analyzed with antisera (immunoelectrophoresis).

The major protein of plasma or serum is albumin. Albumin maintains the colloidal osmotic pressure of human serum and is a transport protein for many hormones, ions, vitamins, and other factors.

Next in the order of electrophoretic mobility are the α-1-globulins. Among them are acid-α-1-glycoprotein, α-1-lipoprotein, and α-1-antitrypsin.

The β-2-globulin fraction contains β-2-macroglobulin, β-2-haptoglobulin (important as a binder of free hemoglobin), ceruloplasmin, β-2-lipoprotein, and transcobalamin as well as many other proteins.

The γ-globulin fraction contains transferrin (an iron-binding protein) and many other proteins.

The γ-globulin fraction contains most, but not all, normal immunoglobulins (e.g., IgG, IgA, IgM, IgD, and IgE). A global deficiency of the normal immunoglobulin fraction can be recognized by a low or absent γ fraction in the serum electrophoresis.

8. DIAGNOSTIC PROCEDURES IN HEMATOLOGY

8.1. Bone Marrow Aspiration

Because the bone marrow is the main site of hematopoiesis as well as of many hematological disorders, a bone marrow aspiration is essential for the evaluation of the clinical situation. Leukemias, autoimmune thrombocytopenias, myelodysplastic syndromes, and most lymphoproliferative disorders especially cannot be diagnosed without a bone marrow aspiration. Other hematological disorders, such as an obvious iron deficiency anemia or a pernicious anemia caused by vitamin B_{12} deficiency, do not need a bone marrow aspiration performed routinely.

A bone marrow aspiration is usually performed at the posterior iliac crest. If special precautions are taken, the bone marrow can also be aspirated at other locations (e.g., the sternum or anterior iliac crest). The skin over the posterior iliac crest is carefully disinfected and the surrounding area is covered with sterile drapes. The skin and the periosteum are infiltrated with a local anesthetic. For anxious patients, a short-acting intravenous narcotic or sedative (e.g., mepridine, benzodiazepine) may be helpful. For the aspiration, a special needle is advanced 5–10 mm through the periosteum before the trocar is removed. A syringe is then connected with the needle and small portions of marrow (0.5–3 mL) are gently aspirated.

A bone marrow aspiration yields samples for cytomorphology, cytogenetics, surface markers, and molecular studies. In some chronic infections, bone marrow cultures are also indicated. For the optimal morphological evaluation, ethylenediamine tetraacetic acid (EDTA) is used as an anticoagulant; for other studies like cytogenetics or surface markers, heparin is used.

A bone marrow aspiration provides information about the state of maturation and the proliferation of the three hematopoietic lineages (erythropoiesis, myelopoiesis, and thrombopoiesis). If bone marrow spicules are present, the overall cellularity and the relative contribution of the three lineages can be evaluated. Special morphological features (e.g., dysplasia or nuclear asynchrony) can be assessed. Atypical cells (leukemic cells and lymphoma or carcinoma cells) can be recognized and further classified by cytochemistry. The iron stores of the bone marrow can be examined with special stains.

8.1.1. FLOW CYTOMETRY

Flow cytometry discriminates leukemic or other cells according to their marker expression. For flow cytometry, the cells are incubated with fluorescent antibodies. The immunophenotyping can be performed with heparinized blood or bone marrow or EDTA-anticoagulated samples. Flow cytometry also gives information about the granularity of cells (forward and sideward scatter) and can be performed with antibodies labeled with different fluorescent compounds (multiparameter analysis). An example for immunophenotyping is given in Chapter 10. A list of the currently described CD markers is found in Appendix 2.

8.1.2. IMMUNOCYTOCHEMISTRY

Immunocytochemistry combines the morphology of blood or bone marrow cells with antibody staining. For this method, antibodies labeled with peroxidase (brown staining) or alkaline phosphatase (blue staining) are used.

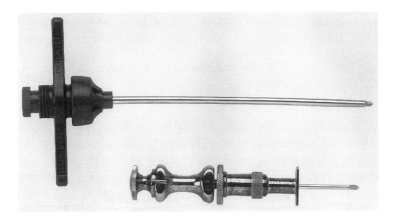

Fig. 1.3. Needles used for bone marrow aspiration and biopsy.

8.2. Bone Marrow Biopsy

In contrast to bone marrow aspiration, a bone marrow biopsy provides information about the histology of the bone marrow. A bone marrow biopsy is performed at the posterior iliac crest with a larger biopsy needle (trephine biopsy, Jamshidi, or similar type of needle). For a bone marrow biopsy, a small cutaneous incision must be made. When the biopsy needle has penetrated the cortical layer and the trocar has been removed, the needle is rotated and advanced with firm movements for about 2 or 3 cm. After this, the needle is rotated without further advancing and then removed. The biopsy core (10–20 mm long and 2–3 mm wide) is then placed in a fixative. If a hypoplastic leukemia is suspected, a touch imprint can be made by gently rolling the biopsy cylinder on a slide. A bone marrow biopsy has a superior diagnostic value in the staging of malignant lymphomas, the assessment of the cellularity in aplastic anemias, and the evaluation of the infiltration by a multiple myeloma. Generally, a bone marrow biopsy provides more information about the architecture and the topographic relationship of normal and malignant cells than does a bone marrow aspiration. A bone marrow biopsy provides less information about cytological details. A bone marrow biopsy is also indicated when an aspiration yields a dry tap. In many cases, a bone marrow fibrosis prevents the aspiration of nucleated cells. In such cases, a biopsy demonstrates the degree of fibrosis and, if present, the infiltration with abnormal cells.

Possible side effects of a bone marrow biopsy or aspiration are bleeding or infection. To prevent bleeding, a local pressure should be applied for several hours. Two commonly used needles for bone marrow aspiration and biopsy are shown in Fig. 1.3.

8.3. Peripheral Blood Film

The differential count of white cells can be done automatically, and this is reliable in most cases. However, the visual inspection of the peripheral blood yields valuable information. The morphology of the red cells can be examined (for details of common red cell abnormalities, *see* Chapter 5.). The presence and morphology of abnormal or uncommon cells, like circulating leukemia and lymphoma cells, myeloma cells, or activated lymphoid cells can be assessed. The number of platelets can be estimated semiquantitatively. Cases of pseudothrombocytopenia (*see* Chapter 20), for example, can be diagnosed by inspecting the blood film.

SUGGESTED READING

Banchereau J, Steinman RM. Dendritic cells and the control of immunity. *Nature* 1998; 392:245–252.
Burrows PD, Cooper MD. B cell development and differentiation. *Curr Opin Immunol* 1997;9: 239–244.
Cross MA. Enver T. The lineage commitment of haemopoietic progenitor cells. *Curr Opin Gen Dev* 1997;7:609–613.
Gewirtz AM. Megakaryocytopoiesis: the state of the art. *Thromb Haemost* 1995; 74:204–209.
Hsia CCW. Respiratory function of hemoglobin. *N Engl J Med* 1998;338:239–247.
Janeway CA, Travers P. Immunobiology. In: *The Immune System in Health and Disease,* 3rd ed. New York and London: Garland, 1997.
Migliaccio AR, Migliaccio G. The making of an erythroid cell. Molecular control of erythropoiesis. *Biotherapy* 1998;10:251–268.
Ogawa M. Differentiation and proliferation of hematopoietic stem cells. *Blood* 1993; 81:2844–2853.

2 Molecular Biology and Cytokines

Reinhold Munker, MD
and Amanda Sun, MD, PhD

CONTENTS

1. INTRODUCTION

The proliferation and differentiation of hematopoietic cells is regulated by the interaction of multiple genes, transcription factors, and proteins.

The genetic information is encrypted in DNA. The cell synthesizes messenger RNA (mRNA) via transcription. The corresponding proteins are synthesized (translation) in the cytoplasm. Molecular biology is of special importance to the clinical hematologist, as leukemias and lymphomas are clonal neoplasms and can be detected by DNA analysis if a genetic marker lesion is known. The discovery of DNA sequences in normal cells that are homologous to RNA viruses led to the description of oncogenes. These genes, also called proto-oncogenes, are responsible for cell growth and differentiation in normal cells. In several neoplasms, a mutation or abnormal expression of oncogenes is present. The loss of antioncogenes also contributes to the initiation and progression of tumors. Other genes that permit the survival of malignant cells are the group of antiapoptotic genes. There is reasonable hope that the elucidation of the molecular pathogenesis of leukemias and lymphomas will lead to new treatment possibilities.

From: *Contemporary Hematology: Modern Hematology, Second Edition*
Edited by: R. Munker, E. Hiller, J. Glass, and R. Paquette © Humana Press Inc., Totowa, NJ

Cytokines are proteins involved in cell-to-cell communication. They are produced and secreted by both normal and malignant cells. Some cytokines have growth-stimulatory properties; others inhibit cell growth or induce cell death. Most cytokines bind to specific receptors on the cell surface. The number of known cytokines and related molecules has expanded enormously in recent years. Some cytokines, like the family of interferons (IFNs), the family of colony-stimulating factors (CSFs), and interleukin (IL)-2 have entered into clinical practice. It can be foreseen that in the next years, even more cytokines and cytokine antagonists will become important in clinical hematology.

2. RECOMBINANT DNA TECHNOLOGY

Recombinant DNA technology has made possible the isolation and characterization of genes from the human genome. This method involves the use of enzymes (restriction endonucleases) that recognize and cleave double-stranded DNA at certain points. In addition, other nucleic acid-modifying enzymes and plasmids (extrachromosomal DNA from bacteria) enable further re-engineering of DNA. This can be done, for example, by inserting the desired DNA sequences into these plasmids, expanding them in vitro, and then retrieving large quantities of recombinant proteins in eukaryotic cells. Any tissue can be examined for the presence of certain genes by Southern blotting. Minute amounts of DNA can be amplified with PCR and then visualized on gels. In Northern blots, RNA is separated on gels and then specific mRNA is detected after hybridization with cloned DNA fragments. In Western blots, the presence and molecular weight of proteins in cell extracts or body fluids is examined by immunological methods.

3. CLONALITY OF TUMORS

The clonality of human tumors is one of the major principles underlying malignant transformation. Clonality means that a tumor is derived from a single transformed cell (and retains some characteristics of this cell). Usually, it takes several years until a tumor has grown from a single cell to the stage where it can be diagnosed clinically. Virtually all hematological neoplasms (leukemias, lymphomas, and myeloproliferative and myelodysplastic syndromes) are clonal. One of the few exceptions is the lymphoproliferative disorder associated with the Epstein-Barr virus (EBV), which is clinically malignant, yet polyclonal in many cases. In some elderly persons, or in the immediate period after bone marrow transplantation, monoclonal or oligoclonal cells can be demonstrated in the absence of a malignancy.

The criteria for malignant growth are abnormal morphology, clinical aggressiveness, genetic changes, and clonality. The general rule is that all or most of these criteria should be present in order to diagnose a malignant tumor. There are several methods to establish clonality in hematological disorders. Some of these methods are used only in research laboratories, whereas other methods have entered clinical routine.

3.1. Cytogenetics

The study of chromosomes, or cytogenetics, aids in the diagnosis of many human tumors and is a common method used to establish the clonality of abnormal cells found in the bone marrow, the peripheral blood, or any other tissue. The normal human somatic cell is diploid, meaning that each of the 22 chromosomes is present in two copies. In addition, the sex chromosomes, XX in females and XY in males, are present in all somatic cells. The cells of sperm or oocytes that have 23 single chromosomes are haploid. The normal human chromosomes are numbered 1–22 in decreasing order of size. Each chromosome has two arms, the shorter "p" arm and the longer "q" arm, which meet at the centromere. Chromosomes are usually visible only during metaphase. In order to study chromosomes, the cells are cultured in media and then arrested in metaphase with colchicine. Special stains are used to identify regions and bands of chromosomes. Common changes in chromosomes are gains and losses of chromosomes, translocations, deletions, and inversions. The genetic changes of pathogenetic or diagnostic relevance are not random, but involve all or most chromosomes studied; this establishes clonality. In a translocation, part of one chromosome is moved to another chromosome. A well-known translocation is t(9;22), where part of chromosome 9 is moved to chromosome 22 and vice versa. This translocation is also known as the Philadelphia chromosome and is diagnostic of chronic myelogenous leukemia (see Fig. 8.1). One refers to a deletion when part of a chromosome is missing. The deletion of part of a chromosome and its reattachment to the breakpoint in the opposite direction is called an inversion (denoted as inv). Sensitive cytogenetic methods can detect chromosomal changes in most leukemias and lymphomas. When even more sensitive molecular methods are used (see "Molecular Cytogenetics"), changes in the DNA of tumor cells can be demonstrated in virtually all hematological neoplasms. Some cytogenetic changes have prognostic relevance. Examples are t(15;17) and inv(16), which are markers for a better-than-average prognosis in acute myelogenous leukemia, and t(9;22), which is associated with an unfavorable prognosis in acute lymphoid leukemia. New cytogenetic aberrations often appear when a leukemia or lymphoma undergoes progression, as in the case of chronic myelogenous leukemias that acquire new cytogenetic abnormalities when entering the accelerated phase and then the blast crisis. The acquisition of new cytogenetic aberrations is called "clonal progression" or "clonal evolution" and is a poor prognostic sign. The analysis of chromosomes ("karyotyping") is usually done only with a limited number of cells (in routine cytogenetic analysis 15–25 metaphases are examined). Minor clones of aberrant cells can therefore be missed. Some cytogenetic aberrations are frequent in hematological neoplasms but not specific for a particular disease. For example, t(3;21) can occur in acute myelogenous leukemia as well as in the blast crisis of chronic myelogenous leukemia.

3.2. Molecular Cytogenetics

A further refinement in the area of cytogenetics has been achieved through the ability to clone the breakpoints for most translocations and other genetic changes in tumor cells. So-called fusion genes encoding novel RNAs and proteins are occasionally created by the genetic changes in tumor cells. An example is the *BCR-ABL* fusion gene resulting from the translocation t(9;22). The analysis of fusion genes can clarify certain mechanisms of transformation, as in the case of lymphoma cells with the translocation t(14;18), which express a protein inhibiting apoptosis. The most sensitive method to assay fusion genes is the PCR. PCR can be used for the study of minimal residual disease after intensive treatment or bone marrow transplantation, but PCR is not quantitative in routine use. With the same methods, point mutations or the expression of oncogenes can be assayed. The analysis of protein (Western blot), RNA (Northern blot), and DNA (Southern blot) is not as sensitive as PCR but permits an approximate quantification. The fraction of malignant cells that can be recognized by Western, Northern, or Southern blot is in the range of 1–5%. PCR can recognize one malignant cell in 10^5 normal cells if a specific molecular marker for the tumor cell is known. A new method known as fluorescence *in situ* hybridization (FISH) can also analyze nondividing interphase cells, allowing determination of the type of cell with a particular mutation or translocation. A disadvantage of FISH is that the currently available probes yield a rather high background. Molecular genetic methods such as PCR and FISH are intended as complements, not substitutes for, the classical cytogenetic methods. In order to perform PCR or FISH, the type of mutation must first be known.

3.3. Rearrangement of Immunoglobulin Genes or of the T-Cell Receptor

During the ontogeny of normal B-cells, the genes for the heavy and light chains of the different immunoglobulin molecules are rearranged sequentially. Similarly, the genes encoding the α, β, γ, and δ chains of the T-cell antigen receptor are rearranged in normal T-cells. In malignant B- or T-cells, the immunoglobulin genes or the T-cell receptor genes have clonal rearrangements. Again, these rearrangements can be studied by Southern blot (which is semiquantitative) or by PCR (which is the most sensitive method). The study of immunoglobulin gene rearrangements also detects cells at an early stage of B-cell development, but is not specific for the B-cell lineage, as acute myeloid leukemias occasionally have rearranged immunoglobulin genes.

3.4. Light-Chain Restriction

The analysis of light chains using flow cytometry or immunocytochemistry is a simple tool to detect clonality in neoplasms that express light chains (κ or λ) on their surface or in their cytoplasm. Mature lymphoid neoplasms (e.g., chronic lymphocytic leukemia or follicular lymphomas) express surface light chains, whereas tumor cells of multiple myeloma or some acute lymphoblastic leukemias express only cytoplasmic light chains. The normal ratio of κ to λ expressing B-cells in humans is about 2:1. If a significant imbalance of light-chain expression is found, clonality is likely.

3.5. Loss of Heterozygosity

Loss of heterozygosity (LOH) refers to the loss of genetic material from one allele at a specific gene locus. LOH is tested with PCR amplification of polymorphic microsatellite markers for a particular gene or locus. LOH is specific for the detection of clonally derived cells, but is not sensitive enough for the study of minimal residual disease. In addition, some normal persons have clonally derived cells that can be detected with LOH; therefore, control tissues should be studied. LOH studies as well as the study of the inactivation of genes on the X chromosome are only performed in specialized research laboratories.

3.6. X-Inactivation Assays

These studies are performed with genes located on the normal X chromosome. An example for such a gene is glucose-6-phosphate dehydrogenase (G6PD), which has two allelic forms, A and B. Normal females have two X chromosomes and may be homozygous for A or B or heterozygous (AB) in all somatic cells. Normal cells in heterozygote females are approx 50% of the A-type and 50% of the B-type. Using a simple enzyme assay for G6PD, it has been shown that myeloproliferative syndromes are clonal disorders involving myeloid, monocytic, and other cell types. These studies can only be performed in heterozygotes. More recently, the inactivation of other genes located on the X chromosome was studied by DNA- or RNA-based methods. An example is the gene encoding the human androgen receptor locus. Again, these studies can only be performed in females. The inactivation of the gene of interest on the X chromosome is studied by the analysis of methylation or transcription. An advantage of X-inactivation assays is that no prior knowledge of mutations or gene rearrangements is necessary. A caveat for these assays is that adequate controls are required because some individuals have a more or less than 50% likelihood of gene silencing on the X chromosome. Clonal cells can also be detected by this method in some older individuals without a malignancy being present.

3.7. Small RNA Molecules in Hematology

Recently, two types of small RNA molecules, microRNA (miRNA) and small interfering RNA (siRNA), have emerged as sequence-specific posttranscriptional regulators of both prokaryotic and eukaryotic gene expression. Below, a brief overview of miRNA and siRNA and their implications in hematological research is given.

3.7.1. miRNA

MiRNAs are a family of about 22 nucleotide small, functional, noncoding RNAs that have been shown to play important roles in various biological processes, including developmental timing, apoptosis, cell proliferation, fat metabolism and hematopoietic differentiation.

Hundreds of miRNA genes have recently been found in both animals and plants. In animals, miRNAs are transcribed by RNA polymerase II through sequential processing in the nucleus and cytoplasm. MiRNAs are initially transcribed as long transcripts (pri-miRNAs), which are cleaved by the nuclear endonuclease Drosha to generate the intermediate short, 60-70 nt hairpin structures (pre-miRNAs). Pre-miRNA is subsequently transported to the cytoplasm by exportin-5 and cleaved by RNase III Dicer to about 22 nt RNA duplex. One strand of the duplex is the mature miRNA, and miRNA regulates gene expression at the transcriptional and/or translational level.

One group reported the identification of more than 100 miRNAs from mouse bone marrow. Among them, three (miR-181, miR-223, and miR-142s) were specifically expressed in hematopoietic tissues. MiR-181 was preferentially expressed in B lineage cells. Overexpression of miR-181 by a retrovirus vector in hematopoietic stem cells led to an increase of cells in the B lymphoid compartment. The results indicate the potential role of miRNA in hematopoietic differentiation.

miRNA profiling in human B cell chronic lymphocytic leukemia (CLL) was performed by another research group. Significant difference in the expression pattern was observed between normal and CLL patient samples. More recently, it was discovered that the expression of miR-155 is increased in human B cell lymphomas. This observation has linked miRNA to the pathogenesis of human lymphatic malignancies.

In an in vivo model, "antagomirs" were created ablating endogenously overexpressed miRNAs. As a secondary phenomenon, multiple other genes were repressed in mice treated with "antagomirs." Ultimately, "antagomirs" or similar molecules might be useful for treating human diseases including leukemia and cancer.

3.7.2. SiRNA

RNA interference is an evolutionarily conserved process of posttranscriptional gene silencing through siRNAs that mediate mRNA degradation. This phenomena was first described in C. elegans, and was found in different organisms such as plants, fungi, flies and mammals. DsRNAs are processed by the highly conserved RNase III Dicer and cleaved into 21-23 nt small interfering RNAs (siRNAs). siRNAs are then packaged into RNA-induced silencing complexes (RISC). The RISC directs the base pairing and cleavage of the target mRNA. In mammalian cells, dsRNA larger than 30 bp can also trigger interferon/antiviral response, leading to nonspecific silencing of cellular genes. The success of the direct introduction of chemically synthesized small duplex RNA into mammalian cells without triggering interferon response has allowed the development of many strategies to introduce siRNA. RNAi has been rapidly growing as an effective tool for study of gene function and for therapeutic applications.

Many hematopoietic genes have been targeted by siRNA, including BCR-ABL, AML1/MTG8, CD4 and CD8. Using a cell line bearing the BCR-ABL rearrangement, RNAi can achieve sequence-specific silencing of the BCR-ABL oncogene. Transfection of a 19 nt dsRNA specific for the BCR/ABL fusion mRNA into K562 leukemic cells depleted the corresponding mRNA and oncoprotein, and induced apoptosis. Reduction of BCR-ABL mRNA levels was also observed in primary CML cells upon introduction of anti BCR-ABL siRNA by electroporation. RNAi shows promise as a technology for future therapeutic development.

4. DIAGNOSTIC APPLICATIONS OF MOLECULAR BIOLOGY AND GENE THERAPY

A number of hematological diseases (e.g., thalassemias, sickle cell anemias, leukemias, and lymphomas) have a genetic basis, and the introduction of molecular methods has allowed for a more refined diagnosis of these disorders. For example, certain cases of chronic myelogenous leukemia were recognized that do not have the classical Philadelphia chromosome yet were shown by molecular analysis to harbor the *BCR-ABL* fusion gene. The classification of non-Hodgkin's lymphomas has been made more reproducible, as molecular and immunological methods have been employed for diagnostic purposes. The defective genes in hematological disorders may be inherited (germ-line defects) or acquired (somatic mutations). Because many of the molecular defects were defined, the replacement of defective genes by gene therapy is a logical treatment. For gene transfer, human DNA sequences are introduced into a packaging system or vector (discussed in the following paragraphs) and transferred into the cell of interest. The vectors also often carry genes for antibiotic resistance, which allows later selection of transduced cells. The transduced cells synthesize proteins according to the DNA sequences transferred. Gene transfer can replace missing or defective genes or introduce genes usually not found in the target cells.

At present, human somatic gene therapy is at a turning point. It was shown for the first time that gene replacement could actually have major clinical benefit (normalizing the immune defect of children with X-linked severe combined immunodeficiency [SCID]). Almost at same time, the first major or serious complications were observed after gene therapy. A patient died from an infection or inflammatory response related to the adenoviral vector used for gene transfer. Out of 11 patients cured by gene therapy of X-linked SCID, two developed acute leukemia by insertional mutagenesis (see Chapter 10). These tragic events have tempered the enthusiasm that surrounded gene therapy and have led to additional safeguards for clinical protocols. However, basic research continues to make progress and new protocols are currently under development. Gene therapy can also promote an effective immunotherapy by making tumor cells immunogenic. The types of vectors used, some of the problems involved, and the first clinical applications of gene therapy are discussed in this chapter.

4.1. Viral Vectors and Gene Delivery Systems

4.1.1. RETROVIRAL VECTORS

This widely used modality of gene transfer has permitted the transfer of genes into cell lines, experimental animals, and patients. Retroviral vectors are based on the Moloney murine leukemia virus and can integrate only into dividing cells. The retroviruses used for gene transfer are made replication incompetent. Unfortunately, the efficiency of gene transfer is generally low and only 8–9 kb of foreign DNA can be transferred using these vectors. Furthermore, retroviruses integrate randomly into the host genome, which can theoretically cause insertional mutagenesis.

4.1.2. ADENOVIRAL VECTORS

Adenoviral vectors can also infect nonproliferating cells. These viruses are generally stable and can be purified. The uptake of adenoviral vectors is episomal; therefore, no long-term expression is achieved. Adenoviruses usually mediate a strong expression of the integrated genes. Up to 15 kb of foreign DNA can be transferred. The induction of antibodies that decrease the efficacy of repeated administration can cause a problem when using adenoviral vectors.

Adeno-associated virus is a defective parvovirus and can also be used in gene transfer experiments. This virus is nontoxic but difficult to prepare on a large scale. Adeno-associated virus integrates into the host genome and potentially infects a wide range of target cells.

Foamy viruses are retroviruses that belong to the spumavirus family of nonpathogenic viruses. Recent studies showed that foamy viruses transduce hematopoietic stem cells more effectively than oncoretroviral vectors.

4.1.3. FOAMY VIRUSES

Foamy viruses are retroviruses that belong to the spumavirus family of nonpathogenic viruses. Recent studies showed that foamy viruses transduce hematopoietic stem cells more effectively than oncoretroviral vectors.

4.2. Nonviral Vector Systems

Liposomes are a simple, nontoxic, and noninfectious modality of gene transfer. The efficiency of gene transfer, however, is rather low, as liposomes compete with serum in vitro and the DNA transferred in liposomes is degraded in the cell.

At present, further vectors based on viruses (e.g., herpesviruses and lentiviruses) are being developed. A common problem of all the currently used gene transfer systems has been that only a minority of cells can be infected and the expression of the transferred gene is lost after some time.

4.3. Clinical Gene Therapy Protocols

Gene therapy is an attractive idea for hematological disorders, in which stem cells can be treated, and for cancer in general, in which patients have limited options after relapse.

The first group of studies aims at the *replacement of missing genes*. A small group of children with adenosine-deaminase (ADA) deficiency has been treated by gene transfer. These patients have severely defective T- and B-cells (SCID). As a consequence of the deficient enzyme, adenosine and desoxy-adenosine triphosphate accumulate in cells, thus interfering with DNA synthesis. T-cells from children with ADA deficiency were infected in vitro with ADA-expressing retroviruses, then re-infused into the children after in vitro culture. The first children in which the ADA gene was transferred obtained about 25% of the normal ADA levels and had fewer infections than before. The administration of transfected lymphocytes has to be repeated every 3–6 mo. More recently, some patients underwent nonmyeloablative conditioning with busulphan prior to transplantation with oncoretrovirally transduced CD34+ cells. As expected, a transient myelosuppression was observed, but otherwise the procedure was well tolerated. The transduction efficiency of clonogenic progenitors was between 21 and 25%. At preliminary analysis, the peripheral blood B-, T-, and natural killer (NK) cells showed levels of gene marking between 70 and 100%. The transfer of other genes is also under investigation. As mentioned, SCID could be successfully corrected by gene therapy. X-linked SCID is due to a defect in the common γc-chain of the IL-2 cytokine receptor family. Without specific treatment, SCID is fatal within the first year of life. Two groups (one in France, one in Great Britain) treated children with SCID by gene therapy.

In Gaucher's disease, several groups have transferred the gene coding for glucocerebrosidase into stem cells from bone marrow or blood. In Hurler syndrome, a storage disease, the first clinical trials with gene transfer into hematopoietic stem cells are being performed. In hemophilia, attempts are being made to replace the gene coding for factor VIII or IX by transducing skin or other tissues. Hemophilias are attractive disorders for gene therapy because a low level of transgene expression (1–5%) might offer major clinical benefit. Currently, the results of 6 phase I/II clinical trials are under evaluation. It appears that the vectors used had little toxicity but did not lead to any lasting transgene expression. More recently, gene therapy trials for hemophilia B were initiated using recombinant adeno-associated virus, which has not been associated with human diseases. Chronic granulomatous disease is another disease in which the genetic defects have been characterized and gene replacement has entered phase I clinical studies. Gene replacement studies also aim at replacing mutated genes in tumor cells, for example, by the replacement of the missing or mutated *p53* gene in solid tumors and the alteration of abnormal growth in leukemic cells that have a leukemia-specific translocation. The goal of reversing malignant growth can theoretically also be accomplished by downregulating the expression of oncogenes and certain growth factor genes with antisense oligonucleotides or small interfering RNAs.

The second group of clinical protocols are *gene-marking studies*. The aim of these studies is not to cure a disease but to follow the fate of transplanted or transduced cells in vivo. Small amounts of blood or other tissues are taken and the presence or absence of the marker gene is demonstrated with PCR. From these marker gene experiments, it was shown that relapse of acute leukemias after autologous bone marrow transplantation derives both from the host (residual leukemic cells surviving the conditioning) and from the graft (autologous stem cells contaminated with leukemic progenitor cells).

The third group of studies aims at stimulating a *local or systemic antitumor immunity* by transducing tumor cells with cytokine genes (e.g., the genes for granulocyte/macrophage colony stimulating factor [GM-CSF], IL-2, or tumor necrosis factor [TNF]). The transduced tumor cells are irradiated and then reinjected into the host.

In some animal models, "bystander effects" are observed whereby only a fraction of the tumor cells is transduced, but the subsequent immune reaction also eliminates or attacks nontransduced tumor cells. A similar approach is also taken with tumor-infiltrating lymphocytes. These cells are genetically modified, irradiated, and then re-injected into the patient. A new development involves transducing tumor cells with peptide transcription units. The proteins synthesized by the transduced cells bind to class I human leukocyte antigen molecules and thereby can stimulate a T-cell-dependent immune response against the tumor. The modification of dendritic cells may also promote a potent cellular immune response directed against tumors. Many groups are focusing on the generation of antitumor vaccines aimed at making the immune system recognize hitherto poorly immunogenic tumor cells. Many tumor cells fail to express the co-stimulatory molecule B-7. If B-7 is transferred, the tumor cells can become immunogenic and can be eliminated by the immune system. In patients with AIDS, several groups are trying to restore cellular immunity either by immunizing asymptomatic patients with transduced cells or enhancing the degradation of HIV-mRNA by ribozymes, small interfering RNAs, or other mechanisms.

Finally, a diverse group of studies aims at modifying the general behavior of normal or malignant cells. An example is the transfer of a multidrug resistance gene to hematopoietic stem cells, thereby making them resistant to chemotherapeutic drugs. This procedure could permit the use of higher doses of drugs for the treatment of a malignant tumor, at least theoretically. The transfer of suicide genes can also be used to eliminate tumor cells. The first clinical application of a suicide gene was in patients with glioblastomas. Vectors coding for thymidine kinase were injected into these brain tumors. After integration, a drug (gancyclovir) then activated the suicide program of the transduced tumor cells. A similar approach has also been used in the adoptive transfer of T-lymphocytes. These cells are transduced with a suicide gene and then transfused into a recipient to induce a graft-vs-leukemia reaction. Once a significant graft-vs-host reaction has developed, the suicide program of the transduced cells is activated, thereby stopping any noxious effects.

5. CYTOKINES

5.1. Colony-Stimulating Factors

CSFs were originally defined as substances that stimulate the colony growth of blood cells in soft agar or methylcellulose. The first hematopoietic growth factors described were granulocyte colony-stimulating factor (G-CSF), GM-CSF, macrophage colony-stimulating factor (M-CSF), and IL-3. Accordingly, G-CSF supports the in vitro growth of granulocyte colonies, GM-CSF supports the growth of mixed colonies with both granulocytes and monocytes/macrophages, and M-CSF stimulates the growth of pure macrophage colonies. IL-3 promotes the growth of mixed colonies that may also contain red cell precursors and megakaryocytes. In the meantime, additional cytokines or ILs have been described that also influence the differentiation of hematopoietic cells in vitro and in vivo.

In this section, we discuss the basic biology of CSFs and their clinical applications in hematological disorders.

5.1.1. BASIC BIOLOGY

G-CSF is a glycoprotein with a molecular weight (MW) of 18 kDa, which can be synthesized by numerous cells, including monocytes, fibroblasts, and epithelial and endothelial cells, but not T-lymphocytes. Substances that induce the secretion of G-CSF are bacterial products or other cytokines.

GM-CSF is a glycoprotein with an MW of about 14–35 kDa, which is synthesized by mast cells, T-lymphocytes, endothelial cells, fibroblasts, and thymic epithelial cells. In vitro, bacterial products, other cytokines, and phorbol esters can induce the synthesis of GM-CSF.

M-CSF is also a glycoprotein, has an MW of about 45–70 kDa, and is synthesized by monocytes, macrophages, fibroblasts, epithelial and endothelial cells, and osteoblasts. M-CSF is also induced by other cytokines.

IL-3 has an MW between 14 and 28 kDa and is produced by T-lymphocytes and mast cells in response to mitogens, phorbol esters, calcium ionophores, and an immunoglobulin (Ig)E receptor activation.

The genes for most human CSFs are located on chromosome 5, with the exception of the G-CSF gene, which is found on chromosome 17.

The action of cytokines is mediated via high- and low-affinity receptors on the cell surface. These receptors are specific for each CSF; however, cross-modulations occur, for example, between IL-3 and GM-CSF. Most factors (G-CSF, M-CSF, and GM-CSF) not only support the proliferation and differentiation of progenitor cells, but also increase the functional capacity of mature cells (granulocytes and monocytes).

5.1.2. CSFs LICENSED FOR CLINICAL USE

GM-CSF is available in the United States as a recombinant cytokine expressed in yeast (sargramostim). In other countries, GM-CSF is also available as a recombinant protein expressed in *Escherichia coli* (molgramostim). The recommended dose of sargramostim is 250 μg/m^2 (given by intravenous or subcutaneous injection). The indications for sargramostim approved by the Food and Drug Administration (FDA) are: promote recovery of myelopoiesis in patients with acute myelogenous leukemia (AML) older than 55 yr who received induction chemotherapy; mobilize autologous stem cells; promote myeloid recovery after autologous or allogeneic stem cell (bone marrow) transplantation; and improve myelopoiesis in patients with delayed engraftment after autologous (allogeneic) engraftment.

G-CSF is available in the United States as a recombinant protein expressed in *E. coli* (filgrastim). In other countries, G-CSF is also available as a recombinant protein expressed in a mammalian cell line (lenograstim). The recommended dose of filgrastim is 5 µg/kg (administered by subcutaneous or intravenous injection). The FDA has approved these indications for filgrastim: support myeloid recovery after chemotherapy for AML; mobilize peripheral blood stem cells; accelerate myeloid recovery after myelosuppressive chemotherapy or bone marrow or stem cell transplantation and severe chronic neutropenia. Because CSFs are expensive and in many instances shorten neutropenia but do not improve the ultimate prognosis of the underlying malignancy, the American Society for Clinical Oncology (ASCO) has developed guidelines for the use of CSFs after myelosuppressive chemotherapy. A primary prophylaxis is only recommended if the risk of febrile neutropenia is ≥40% per cycle of chemotherapy. If a patient has experienced febrile neutropenia during a previous cycle of chemotherapy, the use of myeloid growth factors appears justified to maintain dose-intensity in curable malignancies (testicular cancer, Hodgkin's and non-Hodgkin's lymphoma).

5.1.3. USE OF CSFs IN PATIENTS WITH HEMATOLOGICAL DISORDERS

The cloning of the genes for CSFs and the production of recombinant proteins has made large-scale clinical use of these cytokines possible. In contrast to other cytokines such as TNF and IL-2, the CSFs are generally well tolerated. Some patients treated with G-CSF experience bone pain, and have a slight enlargement of the spleen as side effects. Lethargy, bone pain, and slight fever are symptoms observed in some patients treated with GM-CSF and, especially at higher dosages, cases of phlebitis, generalized edema, and pericarditis were encountered (capillary leakage syndrome).

In vivo, the plasma half-life of the CSFs is in the range of minutes to hours. Subcutaneous administration results in a more sustained plasma level and possibly in a better clinical efficacy than intravenous bolus injections. The doses of CSFs tested in various studies until now have ranged between 1 and 30 µg/kg/d. G-CSF stimulates a dose-dependent leukocytosis (increase of neutrophils) in patients and in normal individuals, whereas GM-CSF also increases the number of eosinophils and monocytes. The action of the hematopoietic growth factors is reversible within days after discontinuing their administration.

The hemopoietic growth factors G-CSF and GM-CSF are widely used in patients with acquired neutropenia. G-CSF is especially well tolerated. According to most studies, the period of neutropenia can be shortened by several days in high-risk patients who have undergone autologous or allogeneic stem cell transplants or other high-dose chemotherapy, thus reducing the likelihood of infection. The general use of these factors in all patients who undergo high-dose therapy is not recommended because of the high cost involved. Only patients who have a high likelihood of serious infections should be treated prophylactically. The increase in the dose of cytostatic drugs is limited not only by neutropenia, but also by other toxicities that cannot be ameliorated by the CSFs. The use of CSFs in patients with a high likelihood of infection also applies to other situations such as severe aplastic anemia. In summary, the use of CSFs in patients with acquired neutropenia is mainly supportive, but may improve the prognosis in high-risk situations.

A clear indication for the use CSFs is idiopathic neutropenia. In congenital neutropenia (Kostmann syndrome), for example, the patients suffer from septicemias, pneumonias, and other infections from early infancy. After treatment with G-CSF, the number of neutrophils normalizes and chronic ulcerations and infections heal. Several patients have now been treated for more than 15 yr with few side effects. GM-CSF is less effective in patients with Kostmann syndrome and increases more eosinophils than neutrophils. In cyclic neutropenia, G-CSF does not eliminate the cyclic variations of neutrophils, but greatly reduces infectious complications. Other acquired neutropenias (autoimmune or idiopathic) also benefit from hematopoietic growth factors.

5.2. Pegfilgrastim

Pegfilgrastim is filgrastim (G-CSF) bound to polyethylene glycol, which significantly increases the in vivo half-life compared with native recombinant G-CSF. Therefore, one injection of pegylated G-CSF per cycle of chemotherapy is sufficient to stimulate neutrophil recovery. The side effect profile is comparable to G-CSF. The indication of pegfilgrastim as approved by the FDA is to reduce the risk of neutropenia following myelosuppressive chemotherapy. The recommended dose of pegfilgrastim is 6 mg given by subcutaneous injection.

5.3. Thrombopoietin

Thrombopoietin (TPO) or megakaryocyte growth and development factor (MGDF) is the major physiological regulator of megakaryocytes and platelet production. The gene for human TPO is located on chromosome 3q27. The mature protein has 332 amino acids. TPO is heavily glycosylated and has an MW of around 70 kDa. TPO is the ligand for the c-MPL receptor, which is present on early hemopoietic progenitor cells, megakaryocytes, and platelets. The m-RNA for TPO is expressed in the liver, kidney, and to a lesser extent in stromal cells of spleen and bone marrow. Signaling via c-MPL involves activation of the JAK[Janus kinase]/STAT and Ras signaling pathways. The serum levels of TPO are high in thrombocytopenic patients and low in normal individuals. TPO stimulates both the proliferation and maturation of cells committed to megakaryocyte production. Recombinant TPO has been given to patients who were thrombocy-topenic following chemotherapy. In these patients, platelets increased with a latency of 8–12 d. The dose of TPO administered was in the range of 0.1–1 µg/kg daily. Platelets produced or stimulated by TPO are functionally normal. The yield of platelets obtained by platelet pheresis from healthy donors treated with TPO is increased two- to threefold, however, in such individuals, the risk of thrombosis with high platelet counts must be considered. According to some studies, TPO is synergistic with other growth factors in mobilizing progenitor cells. Potential clinical applications of recombinant TPO are as prophylaxis for thrombocytopenia following chemotherapy and delayed platelet recovery fol-lowing autologous transplantation. Recombinant TPO continues to be used in clinical trials for the treatment and prophylaxis of thrombocytopenia. The clin-ical trials of a pegylated form of TPO were stopped after a subset of patients developed neutralizing antibodies to TPO (with severe thrombocytopenia in a few patients). Currently, a small-molecule agonist of the TPO receptor is under-going clinical trials for thrombocytopenia.

5.4. Erythropoietin

Erythropoietin (EPO) is produced by kidney cells (in embryonic life also in the liver) and is stimulated by tissue hypoxia. EPO is encoded by a gene on chromosome 7 and has an MW of 1.8 kDa (34–39 kDa in its glycosylated form). It promotes the proliferation and differentiation of erythropoietic cells from progenitor cells. Recombinant EPO is widely used for the treatment of renal anemia (see Chapter 5). Subcutaneously injected EPO is also used for other indications such as aplastic anemias, myelodysplastic syndromes, anemias fol-lowing chemotherapy, and anemias of chronic disease; however, in these indi-cations, the effect of EPO is less predictable. The normal EPO serum levels are between 4 and 26 mU/mL. Recombinant EPO can be expected to improve hematopoiesis if the endogenous EPO level is normal or moderately increased. The recommended dose of recombinant EPO is 100–150 U/kg three times weekly. In patients with renal disease, the recommended dose is lower (50 U/kg three times weekly). Side effects of recombinant EPO include hypertension or hyperviscosity and are mainly observed in patients with renal anemia treated with a high dose of EPO. The improvement in hematocrit may take up to 12 wk after beginning treatment with EPO. EPO is also effective in many cases of HIV-associated anemia (see Chapter 17). A new indication for EPO is the anemia observed in preterm infants. At doses of 200 U/kg, most preterm infants improve their hematocrit and many avoid blood transfusions. Another indication of EPO is the treatment and prophylaxis of anemia in Jehova's witnesses who refuse blood transfusions for religious reasons.

Table 1
Currently Known Interleukins and Interferons and Their Characteristics

Interleukins	
Interleukin (IL)-1	Originally described as endogenous pyrogen or lymphocyte-activating factor, it exists in two forms (IL-lα and IL-1β) and is pleiotropic and a mediator of many inflammatory and immunological reactions. IL-1 is secreted by activated monocytes and endothelial cells, cleaved from a precursor peptide (molecular weight [MW] 33 kDa) to a mature protein (MW 17 kDa) by the enzyme IL-1-converting enzyme. IL-1 receptor antagonist occurs as a natural inhibitor of IL-1.
IL-2	Previously known as T-cell growth factor, it has an MW of about 15 kDa and is encoded by a gene on chromosome 4. IL-2 plays a central role in the expansion and activation of antigen-reactive T-lymphocytes. IL-2 has autocrine and paracrine effects on T-cells, but also activates natural killer (NK) cells and other cell types. IL-2 is used in the experimental tumor therapy with lymphocyte-activated killer (LAK) cells and tumor-infiltrating lymphocyte (TIL) cells. LAK cells can be expanded in the presence of 1L-2 and show some activity in patients with melanomas and other cancers. TIL cells have been isolated from tumors and similarly expanded with IL-2.
IL-3	*See* Subheading 5.1.
IL-4	Secreted by activated T-lymphocytes (especially TH2 cells), MW of about 18 kDa, acts both on B- and T-lymphocytes. IL-4 activates quiescent B-lymphocytes and inhibits the action of proinflammatory cytokines on monocytes and macrophages.

(continued)

5.5. Darbepoietin-α

Darbepoietin is a modified form of EPO (five amino acids were modified to permit the attachment of two additional carbohydrate side chains). This modification leads to a more than threefold longer in vivo half-life. The indications for darbepoietin approved by the FDA are anemia of chronic renal insufficiency and anemia secondary to chemotherapy. The effects and side effects of darbepoietin are comparable to EPO. The advantage for patients is less-frequent dosing. The recommended initial dose in patients with chronic kidney failure is 30–50 µg/kg given intravenously or subcutaneously. The target hemoglobin in kidney failure is 11–12 g/dL. In patients who receive chemotherapy, one injection of darbepoietin per cycle was found effective to prevent anemia.

Table 1 (Continued)

Interleukins	
IL-5	Homodimeric protein with an MW of about 50 kDa, secreted by activated T-cells and mast cells, major biological function is to promote the growth and differentiation of eosinophils. Increased serum levels of IL-5 have been found in hypereosinophilic syndromes.
IL-6	Pleiotropic cytokine (MW 26 kDa), produced by activated monocytes, macrophages, endothelial cells, fibroblasts, and some tumor cells. Major stimulators of IL-6 production are other cytokines like tumor necrosis factor (TNF)-α or IL-1, mediator of acute phase and inflammatory reactions, stimulating the growth of differentiated B-cells and the generation of cytotoxic T-cells. IL-6 acts on hematopoietic progenitor cells together with colony-stimulating factors and promotes the growth of myeloid and megakaryopoietic colonies. IL-6 acts as an autocrine growth factor in multiple myeloma and other malignancies.
IL-7	Glycoprotein, with an MW of 25 kDa, stimulates early B- and T-cells, is expressed in the stromal cells of thymus, spleen, bone marrow, and other tissues, and is recognized as a growth factor for mature T-cell lymphomas such as Sezary syndrome.
IL-8	Small molecule secreted by monocytes and stromal cells (chemokine), recruits granulocytes, is involved in the pathogenesis of adult respiratory distress syndrome, and has pyrogenic activities.
IL-9	Pleiotropic cytokine secreted by activated CD4 cells, has an MW of 30–40 kDa. IL-9 acts on T-cells and mast cells, has a synergistic activity with IL-3 on early erythropoietic cells. m-RNA for IL-9 is found in tumor cells of Hodgkin's disease and anaplastic large-cell lymphomas.
IL-10	Anti-inflammatory properties, MW 18 kDa, produced by activated T-cells, B-cells, and macrophages. IL-10 inhibits the secretion of proinflammatory cytokines like TNF-α, IL-I, IL-6, IL-11, and interferon (IFN)-γ. The apoptosis of B-cells is inhibited in the presence of IL-10.
IL-11	Cloned from stromal cells, is considered as an additional hemopoietic growth factor. IL-11 stimulates the development of megakaryocytes (together with other cytokines), promotes the hematopoietic reconstitution after chemotherapy, and has immunomodulatory effects. IL-11 has an MW of approx 20 kDa. Recombinant IL-11 (oprelvekin) was approved by the Food and Drug Administration for the prevention of severe thrombocyto-

(continued)

Table 1 (Continued)

Interleukins	
	penia and patients with nonmyeloid malignancies after myelosuppressive chemotherapy. The recommended dose of oprelvekin is 50 µg/kg once daily (given subcutaneously).
IL-12	Exists as a heterodimer, has an MW of 75 kDa, is secreted by monocytes or macrophages after stimulation by endotoxin or by activated B-lymphocytes. IL-12 strongly induces the secretion of IFN-γ by T-cells and NK cells and augments the cytotoxicity of NK cells. IL-12 also induces the proliferation of activated T- and NK cells.
IL-13	Structural homology with IL-4 is produced by a subpopulation of activated T-lymphocytes. IL-13 activates B-lymphocytes (e.g., IL-4).
IL-15	Produced by epithelial cells and monocytes, stimulates the proliferation of activated T-lymphocytes. IL-15 has a functional similarity to IL-2 and binds with the β and γ chain of the IL-2 receptor.
IL-16	IL-16 monomer has an MW of 14 kDa, is produced by CD8-positive T-cells, serves as a chemoattractant for CD4-positive lymphocytes, eosinophils, and monocytes. IL-16 binds to the CD4 molecule and is considered to be immunomodulatory and proinflammatory.
IL-17	Produced by activated T-cells, proinflammatory activities. IL-17 induces the production of other cytokines (e.g., IL-6 and IL-8) from stromal cells.
IL-18	Previously described as IFN-γ-inducing factor, related to the IL-1 family. IL-18 is pleiotropic, but generally has proinflammatory activities. Similar to IL-10, IL-18 requires the IL-1β-converting enzyme for cleavage to its active form. Most activities of interleukin-18 are due to a receptor complex that recruits the IL-1 receptor-activating kinase and the consequent translocation of nuclear factor (NF)-κB.
IL-19	Homolog of IL-10, activity at present not well described.
IL-20	Homolog of IL-10, activates keratinocytes.
IL-21	Pleiotropic cytokine, influences proliferation, effector function, and differentiation of B-, T-, NK-, and dendritic cells. Has a private receptor (IL-21 receptor) which activates the JAK/signal transducers and activators of transcription pathway upon ligand binding).
IL-22	Induces inflammatory responses.
IL-23	Induces IFN-γ production and proliferation in T-cells.

(continued)

Table 1 (Continued)

Interleukins

IL-24	Member of IL-10 family, produced by activated monocytes and T-helper cells, can function through receptors or intracellularly as cytotoxic agent.
IL-25	Member of IL-17 family, induces production of IL-4, IL-5, and IL-13.

5.6. Stem Cell Factor

Stem cell factor (SCF) is the ligand for the c-kit proto-oncogene. SCF has an essential role in embryonic development and serves as a growth factor of early hematopoiesis. In vitro, SCF acts synergistically together with G-CSF, EPO, and IL-3 in stimulating hematopoietic colonies. SCF also plays a critical role in mast cell production and function, melanocyte production, germ cell function, and gastrointestinal motility. The gene for human SCF is localized on chromosome 12. When administered to experimental animals, SCF leads to an increase in red blood cells, neutrophils, lymphocytes, eosinophils, and basophils. The receptor for SCF (c-kit) is expressed in acute myelogenous leukemias and certain lymphomas. Human SCF is available in Australia, New Zealand, and Canada as a recombinant protein (ancestim) and was found to increase the mobilization of peripheral blood stem cells in patients who failed a previous mobilization with chemotherapy and/or G-CSF. The recommended dose is 20 μg/kg/d subcutaneously. Because some patients developed anaphylactoid reactions due to mast cell activation, a premedication with inhaled β-mimetics and antihistamines is recommended.

5.7. FLT3 Ligand

FLT3 ligand is a cytokine widely expressed in human tissues. A transmembrane form can be cleaved to generate a soluble form that also has biological activity. The FLT3 receptor is a tyrosine kinase and has a restricted expression (early myeloid and early lymphoid progenitor cells, myeloid leukemias, and certain lymphomas). Based on studies of its expression and function, FLT3-ligand is categorized together with SCF as an early hematopoietic cytokine. Both cytokines require the interaction with other early acting or lineage-specific cytokines. In contrast to SCF, FLT3-ligand does not act on early erythroid cells. A potential clinical application of FLT3-ligand is the expansion of stem cell grafts. FLT3-ligand also stimulates lymphoid progenitors, dendritic cells, and NK cells. Activating mutations of the FLT3 receptor are observed in about 30% of acute myelogenous leukemias (*see* Chapter 9).

5.8. Tumor Necrosis Factor-α

TNF-α is a protein with an MW of 17 kDa, produced mainly by activated monocytes and encoded by a gene on chromosome 6. TNF was originally characterized by its action on certain murine tumors. The physiological relevance of TNF is cell-to-cell interaction and immunoregulation. Lymphotoxin is a related cytokine produced mainly by lymphoid cells. Circulating TNF can be measured in septic shock (endotoxemia) and during acute graft-vs-host reactions. The systemic treatment with TNF in human cancer has showed considerable toxicity and has had only sporadic antitumor effects.

5.9. Fas Ligand

Fas ligand, like TNF, is a type II transmembrane protein with an MW of 38–40 kDa. Fas ligand is produced by activated T- and NK cells, for example, in areas of immune privilege like the testis or the anterior eye chamber. An ectopic expression of fas ligand is found in tumor cells such as colon cancer and melanoma, Fas ligand is cleaved by metalloproteinases and interacts with a receptor present on activated cells and other cell types (Fas, CD95). The physiological function of fas ligand is the transmission of death signals to sensitive cells.

5.10. TNF-Related Apoptosis-Inducing Ligand

TNF-related apoptosis-inducing ligand (TRAIL) is a type II membrane-bound TNF family ligand that is homologous to Fas ligand. TRAIL has the unique property of selectively killing tumor cells and sparing most normal cells. The main function of TRAIL is to induce apoptosis in sensitive cells and activate the transcription factor nuclear factor (NF)-κB. TRAIL has five receptors: DR4 and DR5 transmit death signals, DcR1 and DcR2 act as decoy receptors, and a soluble receptor (osteoprotegerin). The tumor specificity of TRAIL is unclear, but may be related to its intracellular signal transduction.

5.11. Transforming Growth Factor-β

TGF-β is a 14-kDa molecule that is synthesized as a 25–28 kDa homodimeric polypeptide. Three different isoforms of TGF-β are expressed in many tissues, especially in lymphoid cells, monocytes, megakaryocytes, and platelets. The dominant activity of TGF-β is suppression of cell growth, which is illustrated by its ability to inhibit the T-cell response to mitogens. By indirect mechanisms, TGF-β also stimulates some cells, thus promoting angiogenesis and wound healing, for example. TGF-β is expressed in a number of tumor cells including Hodgkin's lymphoma with nodular sclerosis.

5.12. Interleukins

A list of the currently known interleukins (abbreviated as IL-1 through IL-25) and their characteristics are briefly described in Table 1.

5.13. Interferons

IFN-α is widely used for the treatment of hematological diseases (hairy cell leukemia and chronic myelogenous leukemia). IFN-α and IFN-β belong to the group of type I IFNs, whereas IFN-γ is a type II (immune) IFN. Originally, the IFNs were characterized as antiviral substances. However, it was later found that their main activity is immunomodulation. The type I interferons, for example, stimulate the activity of NK cells and modulate the synthesis of immunoglobulins. Moreover, IFN-α has direct effects on tumor cells, such as increasing the expression of cell surface antigens, including class I histocompatibility antigens. This cytokine also has a direct antiproliferative action, possibly through the induction of 2',5'-oligo-adenylate synthetase and inhibits several cell growth-associated proteins. The dose of IFN-α used for the treatment of blood diseases is administered subcutaneously in the range of 3×10^6 U given three times a week to 5×10^6 U given daily. This dose often must be modified, however, as a result of such side effects as fever, chills, myalgias, lethargy, and, less frequently, cardiovascular and metabolic disturbances, interstitial nephritis, confusion, and neuropathies. The pyrogenic side effects subside spontaneously in most cases, and can be controlled with antipyretics. For other side effects, the dose of IFN needs to be altered or the treatment discontinued. About 3–5% of patients develop neutralizing antibodies that render the treatment ineffective. Common hematological side effects of IFN-α are neutropenia and thrombocytopenia.

IFN-β. IFN-β has been found to be less effective than IFN-α against hairy cell leukemia and chronic myelogenous leukemia. A positive response to IFN-β treatment has recently been observed in patients with multiple sclerosis.

IFN-γ. IFN-γ is produced by activated T-lymphocytes. The immunological and antiviral effects of IFN-γ are different from those of the type I IFNs. IFN-γ activates monocytes and macrophages, leads to an increase in the expression of Fc receptors, augments the production of superoxide, and enhances phagocytosis and bactericidal capacity. It increases the cytotoxicity of NK cells and the immunoglobulin synthesis of B-lymphocytes. Like IFN-α, IFN-γ inhibits the growth of some tumor cells in vitro and enhances the cell surface expression of numerous antigens including class I and class II histocompatibility antigens. Clinically, IFN-γ is less active than IFN-α in the treatment of hematological disorders. More recently, it was shown that children with the granulocyte defect chronic granu-lomatous disease have fewer infections when treated with subcutaneous IFN-γ.

SUGGESTED READING

Alexander WS, Begley CG. Thrombopoietin in vitro and in vivo. Cytokines Cell Mol Ther 1998;4:25-34.

Ambros V. The functions of animal microRNAs. Nature. 2004;431:350-355.

Bartel DP. MicroRNAs: genomics, biogenesis, mechanism, and function. Cell 2004;116:281-297.

Czech MP MicroRNAs as therapeutic targets. N Engl J Med 2006;354: 1194-1195

Lyman SD, Jacobsen SEW. c-Kit ligand and flt3 ligand: stem/progenitor cell factors with overlapping yet distinct activities. Blood 1998;91:1101-1134.

Nathwani AC, Davidoff AM, Lynch DC. A review of gene therapy for haematological disorders. Br J Haematol 2005;128:3-17

Scherr M, Battmer K, Winkler T, et al. Specific inhibition of bcr-abl gene expression by small interfering RNA. Blood. 2003;101:1566-1569.

Thomson AW (ed.). The Cytokine Handbook, 3rd ed.. San Diego: Academic, 1998.

3 Supportive Care in Hematology

John Hiemenz, MD
and Reinhold Munker, MD

CONTENTS

1. INTRODUCTION

Patients with hematological malignancies such as leukemias and lymphomas are predisposed to a wide spectrum of infections that need special attention. These patients are immunosuppressed not only as a result of the immune defects associated with the underlying disease, but also because of the treatment regimens that generally further decrease the patient's resistance to infections. An intensive transfusion support with platelets, red cell concentrates, immunoglobulins, cytokines, and other drugs is necessary. Many patients also need antiemetic agents, nutritional support, pain medication, and, very often, venous catheters. All of these measures are considered supportive care and apply in a similar fashion to the high-dose treatment of solid tumors. Supportive care measures, along with the treatment and prophylaxis of infections, are discussed in this chapter. Transfusion support is discussed in Chapter 22.

From: *Contemporary Hematology: Modern Hematology, Second Edition*
Edited by: R. Munker, E. Hiller, J. Glass, and R. Paquette © Humana Press Inc., Totowa, NJ

2. DIAGNOSING SUSPECTED INFECTION
IN NEUTROPENIC PATIENTS

The immune system can be compromised by the underlying disease, the treatment of the disease, or many procedures and devices utilized in support of treatment of the underlying disease (e.g., central venous catheters). Neutropenia has been recognized as the major risk factor for development of opportunistic infection in patients with hematological malignancy or undergoing cancer chemotherapy. Bodey and colleagues studied the relationship between the neutrophil count and the development of severe infection in 52 patients treated for acute leukemia at the National Institutes of Health from 1959 to 1963 *(1)*. In the presence of severe neutropenia, defined as less than 100 cells/mm^3, there were 43 episodes per 1000 d with a marked drop in infection rate as the neutrophil count rose. In addition, the risk of infection increased with increasing duration of neutropenia. This relationship between neutropenia and life-threatening infection has been reported by numerous investigators since the initial publication by Bodey et al. in 1966 *(2,3)*. The Infectious Diseases Society of America (IDSA) defines neutropenia as an absolute neutrophil count of less than 500 cells/mm^3, or <1000 cells/mm^3 with a predicted decrease to less than 500 cells/mm^3 *(4)*. Although the risk of neutropenia has been recognized for more than 40 yr, other qualitative defects in humoral and/or cellular immunity may also increase the risk of infection with a variety of pathogens including bacterial, fungal, and viral pathogens. Examples include infections with encapsulated bacteria in patients with dysgammaglobulinemia due to underlying myeloma or infections due to cellular immune deficiency such as *Pneumocystis carinii* pneumonia or cryptococcal meningitis in the patient with Hodgkin's lymphoma, and invasive aspergillosis or cytomegalovirus (CMV) pneumonia in the leukemic patient with chronic graft-vs-host disease (GVHD) on immunosuppressive therapy *(5)*. All of these patients may have a normal or elevated neutrophil count.

When faced with fever in the neutropenic patient, defined by the IDSA as a single oral temperature of 38.3°C (101.0°F) or 38.0°C (100.4°F) for 1 h or longer, the diagnosis of severe infection must be considered. This situation is consider an emergency and should lead to prompt evaluation and initiation of empirical antimicrobial treatment. Evaluation includes a thorough history and physical examination *(4)*. The history should include the nature and status of the underlying disease, chemotherapy received, other immunosuppressive drugs such as steroids, use of cytokines, and past and recent infections as well as previous procedures. Initial examination should assess all sites of possible infection. The profoundly neutropenic patient may have minimal signs or symptoms of inflammation with 50 to 75% of cases having no definable source of infection when fever develops. The clinician should carefully inspect the eyes, oropharynx, and skin (with particular attention to vascular catheter tunnel and exit sites, bone marrow aspirate sites, nails, and nailbeds) *(2)*. The perineal and perirectal areas are frequently missed but are critical areas to inspect initially and on a regular basis when fever persists. Evidence of perirectal or perianal infection in the neutropenic patient may require modification of initial empirical antimicrobial treatment. Surgical intervention may be warranted for drainage of developing abscess(es) *(6)*. It is also important to carefully inspect the scalp, as hair may hide evidence of infection.

In addition to a thorough physical examination, laboratory evaluation of the febrile neutropenic patient includes a hemogram, electrolytes, renal, and liver function tests. Cultures of blood and urine should be obtained, as these are the most common sites of microbiologically documented infection. A minimum total of two sets (aerobic and anaerobic) of blood cultures should be obtained for the initial evaluation. It has been recommended that, in addition to drawing one set of cultures from a peripheral venipuncture, one set of blood cultures should be obtained from each lumen in patients with central venous catheters. In this group of patients, it is often difficult to obtain peripheral venous access even for simple blood sampling. The need to routinely obtain cultures from the peripheral vein in cancer patients with central venous catheters, therefore, has often been questioned. In a recent retrospective review, DeJardin et al. found a high predictive value of negative blood cultures drawn from central venous catheters of febrile cancer patients *(7)*. These authors have suggested that peripheral venipuncture was thus not routinely required unless blood cultures from the central venous catheter were found to be positive. A routine chest radiograph should be performed to exclude or diagnose pneumonia. Performance of the chest radiograph, however, should not delay initiation of empirical antibacterial therapy immediately after cultures are obtained.

Further diagnostic steps should be taken if clinically indicated. In addition to blood and urine, cultures should be obtained from any other site(s) found on exam to be suspicious for possible focus of infection. If skin lesions are present, biopsy or aspiration should be performed. Biopsy specimens should then be sent for cytology and/or histopathology with special stains for microorganisms as well as culture for bacteria, fungi, and viruses (e.g., *Herpes simplex* and *Varicella zoster*). In the setting of diarrhea, stool culture for bacterial pathogens, screening for the presence of *Clostridium difficile* toxin, as well as evaluation for ova and parasites should be considered. Cerebrospinal fluid (CSF) should be obtained from a lumbar puncture (or Ommaya reservoir when present) in patients who have neurological symptoms or a change in mental status to diagnose meningitis. Bacterial surveillance cultures from the oropharynx, urine, and stool have been performed on a regular basis in neutropenic patients at a number of institutions. Although information obtained from these cultures may be valuable for epidemiological purposes, they are not recommended for the management of the individual patient. In the absence of specific signs or symptoms of infection, bacterial surveillance cultures have little value in predicting infection, rarely change antibiotic therapy, and are costly *(2)*.

High-resolution computed tomography (CT) of the chest should be considered in any patient with abnormalities on routine chest radiograph to better define possible pulmonary infection. CT scan should also be considered despite negative routine radiograph of the chest if symptoms or signs of pulmonary infection exist such as cough, shortness of breath, or hypoxemia, or if there is persistent or recurrent fever after a week of broad spectrum empirical antibacterial therapy *(8)*. Bronchoscopy with bronchoalveolar lavage (BAL) should be performed in patients with abnormal radiograph or CT scan to obtain specimens for cytology, culture, and stains for bacteria, fungal, and viral pathogens. If viral pneumonia is suspected, specimens may be examined for viral DNA by PCR.

Tests for inflammatory cytokines such as C-reactive protein, procalcitonin, interleukin-6, and interleukin-8 may correlate with the presence of an infection in neutropenic patients, but none are specific or reliable and they cannot be used for treatment decisions in the acute situation. The presence of galactomannan in blood has been utilized for a number of years in Europe as a surrogate marker of invasive aspergillosis and was recently approved for use in the United States by the Food and Drug Administration for a similar indication. The sensitivity and specificity of this test may vary in different populations of patients (i.e., children versus adults, neutropenic versus non-neutropenic hosts) and therefore results must be taken in context with the clinical situation. β-glucan is another surrogate marker for invasive fungal infection and may apply to a broad group of pathogens that possess a high concentration of β-glucan in their cell wall *(9–11)*.

3. TREATING INFECTIONS IN NEUTROPENIC PATIENTS

A large array of pathogens is responsible for infections in immunosuppressed and/or neutropenic patients with hematological disorder. The source of infection may be from the normal endogenous flora or may result from nosocomial acquisition from the exogenous environment. Gram-negative rods (*Escherichia coli*, *Klebsiella pneumoniae*, *Pseudomonas aeruginosa*, *Enterobacter* spp., and others) usually arise from the gastrointestinal tract and may cause serious infections in compromised patients. Antimicrobial developments in the 1980s and 1990s led to an increase in the armamentarium of antimicrobial agents available to treat these common Gram-negative pathogens (e.g., extended-spectrum β-lactams, carbapenems, quinolones) *(2,4)*. Unfortunately, increased exposure to these agents empirically and prophylactically has led to the selection of Gram-negative pathogens with broad-spectrum antimicrobial resistance. Organisms with broad antibacterial resistance such as *Acinetobacter anitratis* and *Stenotrophomonas maltophilia* are usually acquired from the hospital environment *(3,12,13)*. The incidence of infection with Gram-positive cocci (Coagulase-negative staphylococci, *Staphyloccocus aeurus*, α-hemolytic such as *Streptococcus mitis,* and *Enterococcus* spp.) has increased over the last decade, and now accounts for the majority of microbiologically documented bacterial infections in the neutropenic host in many institutions *(3,12,13)*. Although the increased use of indwelling central venous silastic catheters has been considered to be the cause of the increase in Gram-positive bacteria infections, the oropharynx and gastrointestinal tract are also considered sources of infection. Severe mucositis after intensive chemotherapy and the use of quinolone prophylaxis have been found to be independent risk factors that can increase the risk of α-hemolytic streptococcal sepsis. Bacteremia with α-streptococcus can lead to septic shock accompanied by adult respiratory distress syndrome (ARDS), more commonly seen with Gram-negative rod bacteremia *(14)*. Approximately 10–20% of neutropenic patients with microbiologically documented bacterial infections are infected with anerobic bacteria (anaerobic streptococci, *Clostridia* spp., *Bacteroides* spp.) or mixed (Gram-positive, Gram-negative, aerobic, and/or anaerobic) infections.

All neutropenic and febrile patients are at risk of fungal infections. Patients with T-cell dysfunction caused by an underlying hematological disorder or its treatment may also be at increased risk for fungal infection. GVHD after allogeneic blood or marrow transplantation is a well-known risk factor for invasive mycosis that may last for months or years *(15–17)*. The use of monoclonal antibodies with anti-T-cell activity for treatment of lymphoproliferative malignancies or GVHD has been recognized as a risk factor for development of invasive fungal infections *(18)*. *Candida albicans* and *Aspergillus* spp. have accounted for the majority of invasive fungal infections in patients with hematological disorders. However, a shift toward the non-albicans *Candida* spp. and an increase of *Aspergillus* spp. as the major cause of fungal-related morbidity and mortality has been seen in many institutions *(19)*. In addition, infection with a wide variety of previously uncommon opportunistic fungal pathogens has been noted over the last two decades. These emerging pathogens include a number of septate filamentous fungi such as *Fusarium* spp. and *Scedosporium* spp. that may mimic *Aspergillus* spp. on microscopic inspection of tissues. Nonseptate filamentous fungal infections with *Zygomycetes*, previously considered a complication of uncontrolled diabetes, has been increasing reported in patients with hematological malignancies or after hematopoietic stem cell transplantation. Invasive infections with the dematiaceous molds, as well as a variety of yeast including the *Trichosporon* spp. have also been reported. It is important to be familiar with these potential pathogens, as they may have variable sensitivities or be frankly resistant to amphotericin B, the newer triazoles, and/or the echinocandins *(20)*.

Viral infections in patients with hematological disorders are most commonly the consequence of reactivation of members of the herpesviruses (*H. simplex, V. zoster,* CMV, HHV-6, etc.) and will be discussed in a later chapter. Community respiratory viruses such as influenza, parainfluenza, adenovirus, respiratory syncytial virus (RSV), and rhinovirus have been reported to cause outbreaks of infection in highly susceptible patients and must be taken into account when considering antiviral therapy and infection control practices for a hematology and/or transplant clinic or ward *(21–23)*. Adenovirus and polyoma type BK virus have been associated with hemorrhagic cystitis, particularly after hematopoietic stem cell transplantation. Less common viral pathogens include echovirus, cocksackie virus, rotavirus, polyoma type JC virus, and parvovirus B19 and should be considered in the appropriate setting.

3.1. Empirical Treatment

In patients with neutropenia (<500 neutrophils/mm^3) and unexplained fever (≥38.3°C), broad-spectrum antibiotic treatment should be started without delay. Although recent studies suggest that patients with fever and neutropenia classified as "low risk" may be treated with ciprofloxacin and amoxicillin-clavulanate through the oral route *(24,25)*, most would consider patients with hematological disorder at "high risk" requiring hospitalization and intravenous antimicrobial therapy. Historically, the classic therapy to begin with was a combination of an aminoglycoside with an extended-spectrum penicillin. Extensive clinical trials and more recent IDSA guidelines, however, suggest the following options:

- Monotherapy with either an extended-spectrum cephalosporin with activity against *P. aeruginosa* such as cefepime or ceftazidime.
- Another option for monotherapy is to use a broad-spectrum carbapenem, with activity against *P. aeruginosa* , such as imipenem/cilistatin or meropenem.
- Combination therapy may still be used as initial therapy for the febrile neutropenic patient. The IDSA recommends the routine addition of an aminoglycoside when treating with an antipseudomonal penicillin, although there have been recent data that support the use of piperacillin/tazobactam as a single agent *(4,27)*. When combination therapy is felt to be indicated, an aminoglycoside plus either an antipseudomonal penicillin, cephalosporin (cefepime or ceftazidime), or carbapenem (imipenem/cilistatin or meropenem) is recommended. In patients with suspected- or proven-resistant Gram-positive bacterial infections, vancomycin should be combined with any one of cefepime, ceftazidime, imipenem/cilistatin, meropenem (with or without an aminoglycoside), or an aminoglycoside plus an antipseudomonal penicillin (Table 1).

Table 1
Empirical Treatment of Fever of Unknown Origin in a Neutropenic Patient

A. Single-agent treatment
    Extended-spectrum cephalosporin (cefepime or ceftazidime)
    Carbapenem (imipenem/cilistatin or meropenem)
B. Combination treatment
    Extended-spectrum penicillin + aminoglycoside
    Extended-spectrum cephalosporin (cefepime or ceftazidime) + aminoglycoside
    Carbapenem (imipenem/cilistatin or meropenem) + aminoglycoside
    Extended-spectrum penicillin + aminoglycoides + vancomycin
    Extended-spectrum cephalosporin (cefepime or ceftazidime) or carbapenem
    (imipenem/cilistatin or meropenem) + vancomycin

Examples of patients at risk of having resistant Gram-positive infection include those suspected of catheter infection based on clinical findings, those colonized with methicillin-resistant *S. aureus* (MRSA) or penicillin- or cephalosporin-resistant pneumococci, and those with documented Gram-positive bacteremia before antimicrobial susceptibility has been defined. Vancomycin should also be considered as part of early empirical antibacterial therapy in patients with hypotension or cardiovascular instability. Fever and neutropenia should be considered a dynamic process with continued and ongoing evaluation of the patient. Antimicrobial therapy should be adjusted based on culture results, the clinical course of the patient, and persistence of fever.

With persistent or recurrent fever in the neutropenic patient after 3 to 5 d of broad-spectrum antibacterial coverage without a documented source of infection, the empirical addition of broad-spectrum antifungal coverage is considered the standard of care to reduce the risk of morbidity and mortality caused by invasive mycosis *(28)*. Although overall survival was not improved in the studies performed at the National Cancer Institute and by the European Organisation for Research and Treatment of Cancer (EORTC) more than two decades ago, the incidence of documented invasive fungal infections was significantly reduced when amphotericin B deoxycholate was empirically added to ongoing antibacterial therapy *(28,29)*. Over the last 10 yr, a number of alternative antifungal agents have been shown to be equally effective yet less toxic as compared with amphotericin B for empirical therapy of the persistently febrile neutropenic patient. These include members of the class of lipid formulations of amphotericin B, extended spectrum triazoles, and the echinocandins *(30–34)* (Table 2). Attempts to make a definitive diagnosis of infection should continue with thorough examination, cultures, and chest radiography including CT of the lungs with

Table 2
Empirical Antifungal Therapy for Patients With Persistent Fever and Neutropenia

A. Polyenes
    Amphotericin B deoxycholate
    Lipid formulations of amphotericin B
        Liposomal amphotericin (AmBisome)[a], amphotericin B complex (Abelcet)
B. Azoles
    Itraconazole (intravenous formulation with cyclodextran)[a]
    Voriconazole (intravenous and oral formulation)
C. Echinocandins
    Caspofungin[a]

[a]Approved for this indication by the Food and Drug Administration.

bronchoscopy and BAL if abnormal *(8)*. Serological tests for evidence of invasive fungal infection using galactomannan and β-glucan may be helpful; however, false-positive and false-negative tests have been noted *(9–11)*.

3.2. Documented Bacterial Infections

Bacterial infections should be treated according to the antibiotic spectrum and the clinical pattern of sensitivity. A marked increase in antibiotic resistance has occurred over the last decade. The most common resistant bacteria encountered in patients with hematological disorders include MRSA, methicillin-resistant *S. epidermidis,* vancomycin-resistant enterococcus (VRE), and β-lactamase producing Gram-negative bacilli *(12,13)*. The National Nosocomial Infections Surveillance System (NNIS) noted a steady increase in MRSA to more than 50% of isolates from 300 hospitals reported to the database in 1999 and over 55% MRSA in 2000 *(35,36)*. Although viridans streptococci are found as part of the normal microbial flora, they have been isolated as pathogens with increasing frequency in patients with hematological disorders. Risk factors include severe neutropenia, mucositis, treatment with high-dose cytosine arabinoside, and antimicrobial prophylaxis with either a fluoroquinolone or trimethoprim-sulfamethoxazole. Although most patients respond to therapy, a toxic shock-like syndrome with hypotension, a maculopapular rash, palmar desquamation, and ARDS has been reported in as many as 25% of cases *(15,37)*.

The increased use of vancomycin for the treatment of proven or probable MRSA, viridans streptococci, or for empirical therapy of febrile neutropenic patients is considered to be one of the major risk factors for the increasing incidence of VRE seen in the 1990s. Other risk factors noted have been the use of oral vancomycin for the treatment of *C. difficile*-related enteritis, use of drugs with anaerobic activity, gastrointestinal procedures, mucositis, acute renal failure, glucose intolerance, or diabetes *(38–40)*. Compared with the mean rate of growth of vancomycin-resistant isolates of enterococci reported to the NNIS database over the prior 5 yr, the rate of growth between 1998 and 2000 appeared to be decreasing *(35,36,41)*. It is hoped that this trend will continue as a result of both better infection control practices and more judicious use of vancomycin. Newer antimicrobials such as linezolid and quinupristin/dalfopristin have been developed for the treatment of VRE *(42,43)*. Although the initial experience had suggested that linezolid might have more hematological side effects (especially thrombocytopenia) compared with the other antimicrobial agents, recent reports in both children and adults suggest that the toxicity profile is not worse than that of vancomycin *(44,45)*. Even with these newer agents, however, resistant organisms have already been reported *(46)*.

Most Gram-negative bacterial isolates from patients with hematological disorders remain sensitive to standard antibacterial agents. Patients will usually respond to appropriate therapy if there is eventual recovery from immune dysfunction. As with the Gram-positive bacteria, however, there has been a gradual increase in isolation of multi-drug resistant Gram-negative organisms like *S. maltophilia (12)*. These infections usually occur in the most complicated patients with uncontrolled malignancy, prolonged hospitalization, prolonged immune suppression, and multiple courses of prior antibiotic therapy.

3.3. Documented Fungal Infections

Oropharyngeal candidiasis is often diagnosed clinically with classical signs of erythema, white plaques, and ulcers. Presumptive diagnosis of infection with *Candida* spp. by inspection only, without examination of wet mount or Gram stain of exudate material, may not be accurate. Infection with *H. simplex,* bacterial infections, and noninfectious causes of mucositis in patients with underlying hematological disorders may mimic oral lesions due to *Candida* spp. Local treatment can be attempted with nonresorbable antifungal agents (nystatin or clotrimazole), but if this fails, or if the patient is severely neutropenic, systemic treatment may be indicated. For patients not already receiving azole prophylaxis, fluconazole is the most commonly used antifungal agent for the systemic treatment of oropharyngeal candidiais. Typically, this infection is due to *C. albicans,* which is usually highly susceptible to treatment with fluconazole. In the unusual setting of oropharyngeal infection refractory to systemic therapy with fluconazole, documentation of persistent or recurrent fungal infection should be attempted. Treatment with a broader-spectrum antifungal agent that covers the non-albicans species of *Candida* would then be recommended. Broader-spectrum antifungal drugs would include amphotericin B, one of its lipid formulations, or an echinocandin. Although alternative triazole such as itraconazole or voriconazole could be considered, cross resistance between azoles has been seen among the non-albicans *Candida* spp.

Most experts would therefore recommend using either an echinocandin or amphotericin B product in this setting. Esophageal candidiasis is common in patients with AIDS and hematological neoplasms undergoing chemotherapy. A typical symptom is a burning pain on swallowing. Esophageal candidiasis can also be treated with local or systemic antifungal therapy. If the patient has already been on fluconazole prophylaxis, or has failed systemic therapy with fluconazole, the same attempts to document persistent fungal infection and switch to alternative therapy with an echinocandin or amphotericin product are recommended.

Deep-seated or invasive candidiasis is a spectrum of infections. It may present as isolated candidemia, infection of a single organ (endocarditis or endophtalmitis), or wide-spread disseminated infection involving the liver and spleen (hepatosplenic candidiasis), kidneys, and/or other organs. Some clinicians will differentiate disseminated candidiasis into acute and chronic forms. Acute disseminated candidiasis is a syndrome of acute, life-threatening infection presenting as persistent fungemia, hypotension, and multi-organ failure in the neutropenic patient. Cutaneous and skeletal muscle involvement frequently occurs in the acute form of invasive candidiasis. In contrast, chronic disseminated candidiasis is established by hematogenous spread of infection during neutropenia. It is not accompanied by hypotension and frequently previous blood cultures failed to document fungemia prior to the patient manifesting signs and symptoms of infection. As marrow function recovers and neutropenia resolves, radiological manifestations of chronic infection are seen in the liver and spleen on ultrasound, CT, or most reliably on magnetic resonance imaging (MRI). The patient may have presented with persistent or new fevers, but may also have had minimal temperature elevations with anorexia, weight loss, or failure to thrive along with an isolated increase in alkaline phosphatase. This clinical presentation warrants further evaluation to rule out chronic disseminated fungal infection. Although frequently referred to as "hepatosplenic candidiasis" because of the radiological manifestations in the liver and spleen, this infection may be widely disseminated involving many other organs. Confirmation of the diagnosis of fungal infection with biopsy and culture of liver and/or other accessible lesions should be attempted in order to direct appropriate therapy. Although most of these infections are caused by *Candida* spp. disseminated infection with other bacterial, fungal, or protozoal pathogens may have similar clinical presentations *(47,48)*.

Disseminated candidiasis requires prompt and aggressive therapy. Sources for *Candida* fungemia include not only indwelling central venous catheters, but also the gastrointestinal tract. The need for routine removal of central venous silastic catheters (Hickman® and Broviac® [C.R. Bard, Inc.], etc.) for successful treatment of candidemia has therefore been controversial. Fungemia with certain species of *Candida* (e.g., *C. parapsilosis*) however is clearly felt to be line-related, necessitating removal of the indwelling catheter. If the catheter is left in place and fungemia does not rapidly clear with appropriate antifungal therapy, the central line will need to be removed promptly. All patients with positive blood cultures for *Candida* spp. should be treated with an appropriate course of antifungal therapy regardless of immune status and whether or not the central line was removed (49,50).

Isolated candidemia can be successfully treated with 10–14 d of antifungal therapy after clearing of fungemia. Historically, however, appropriate treatment for disseminated candidiasis consisted of prolonged treatment with amphotericin B, possibly combined with flucytosine. Fluconazole is much better tolerated for longer courses of therapy. The use of this azole has usually been reserved for the non-neutropenic patient and as follow-up therapy for patients responding to induction treatment with amphotericin B. Lipid formulations of amphotericin have been shown to be useful in patients with disseminated disease refractory to treatment with conventional amphotericin B and fluconazole (47). A recent randomized trial comparing caspofungin with amphotericin B deoxycholate in the treatment of invasive candidiasis has shown the echinocandin to be equally efficacious and less toxic than the polyene in both neutropenic and nonneutropenic hosts (51).

Infection with *Aspergillus* spp., once the second most-common fungal infection in immunocompromised hosts, is now the most common cause of mortality related to invasive fungal infections in the United States (19). More than two decades ago, Gerson et al. showed that a prolonged severe neutropenia (>2 wk) led to an exponential rise in risk of invasive pulmonary aspergillosis in a group of patients with leukemia (52). More recent studies have focused on the risk of invasive fungal infections in the allogeneic transplant recipient on immunosuppressive therapy for GVHD after marrow recovery (15,53). The most common site of invasive *Aspergillus* infection is the lungs. Infections can also involve the sinuses and other organs and expand in a locally destructive fashion. Pulmonary disease has a characteristic radiological appearance (round mass overlaid by a crescent of air) (8) and may result in catastrophic bleeding. On CT, a nodular lesion is typical and has a surrounding "halo" due to bleeding into the tissues. These lesions will frequently evolve as neutropenia resolves with contraction of tissue surrounded by a crescent of air ("air crescent" sign) (see Fig. 3.1A,B). Although amphotericin B deoxycholate had been the drug of choice for invasive *Aspergillus* infections for four decades, overall response to treatment was poor in patients with underlying hematological disorders with most neutropenic patients dying of fungal disease (48,53,54). Over the last decade, lipid formulations of amphotericin B have become available, allowing higher doses of drug to be delivered safely for longer periods of time (55). Caspofungin was also found to be active in a retrospective trial of the treatment of invasive aspergillosis in patients refractory or intolerant to other standard antifungal therapy (mainly amphotericin B or its lipid formulations). A recent large, multinational, multi-

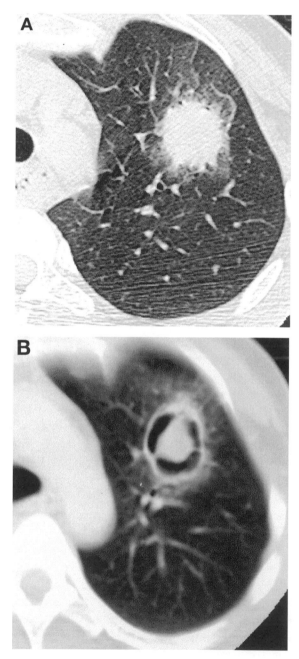

Fig. 3.1. Invasive pulmonary aspergillosis (IPA) in a neutropenic patient with acute myelogenous leukemia. Above, a typical "air halo" can be seen on CT imaging with surrounding ground glass opacity. The patient was starting on antifungal therapy, recovered his blood counts, and developed an "air crescent" sign (*see* lower image) 10 d later. The diagnosis of IPA was confirmed after surgical resection. (Reproduced from ref. *8*, with permission).

institutional randomized clinical trial has led to a major change in the recommended standard therapy for invasive aspergillosis. In this trial, amphotericin B deoxycholate was compared prospectively to the newer triazole voriconazole in patients with proven or probable invasive aspergillosis. This study showed superior response rates and overall outcome in patients who began therapy with voriconazole as compared with those whose treatment was initiated with amphotericin B deoxycholate. This superior outcome was seen even when taking in to account a change to other licensed antifungal therapy, which in the case of amphotericin B deoxycholate, was most commonly a switch to a lipid formulation of amphotericin B because of toxicity. Moreover, the survival benefit with voriconazole was seen even in the neutropenic patient population and those who had received a hematopoietic stem cell transplantation *(56)*. Although one must take into account the increased risk of drug–drug interactions, visual hallucinations, and photosensitivity of the skin not seen with the more narrow-spectrum agent fluconazole, voriconazole now appears to be the drug of choice for the treatment of invasive aspergillosis in the immunocompromised host with a hematological disorder. Unfortunately, a large proportion of these patients were still considered nonresponders and no doubt died from complications of invasive aspergillosis. Although difficult to study in a randomized trial, most experts feel that surgical debridement, when possible, is beneficial in improving overall outcome in patients with invasive filamentous fungal infections like *Aspergillus* *(54,57)*.

The availability of newer agents with activity against *Aspergillus* spp. has led to the consideration of combination therapy for treatment of invasive disease in the immunocompromised host. A number of in vitro studies, in vivo animal models, and retrospective clinical reports have suggested the potential benefit of combination therapy, particularly utilizing a cell wall-active agent such as an echinocandin with a cell membrane-active drug, either voriconazole or a polyene *(58–64)*. Marr et al. suggested an improved outcome with the routine addition of caspofungin to voriconazole in a group of bone marrow transplant recipients treated for invasive aspergillosis at the Fred Hutchinson Cancer Research Center in Seattle. Unfortunately, this was not a randomized trial and long-term follow up of these patients is unknown *(65)*. The continued and increasing importance of infections with *Aspergillus* spp. warrant further prospectively controlled trials of combination therapy.

C. albicans and *Aspergillus* spp. have accounted for the majority of opportunistic invasive fungal infections in patients with hematological disorders. In addition to a shift toward the non-albicans *Candida* spp. and an increase of *Aspergillus* spp. as a major cause of morbidity and mortality in many centers, a wide variety of previously uncommon opportunistic fungal pathogens have been encountered over the last two decades *(19)*. These emerging pathogens include septate filamentous fungi such as *Fusarium* spp. that may be difficult to distinguish from *Aspergillus* spp. on microscopic inspection of tissues, along with an expanding group nonseptate *Zygomycetes*, the dematiaceous molds, as well as a variety of yeasts including the *Trichosporon* spp.. The increasing recognition of these isolates as causes of life-threatening invasive fungal infections in patients with hematological disorders mandates knowledge of the microbiology, epidemiology, and options for the prevention and treatment of these previous uncommon opportunistic pathogens *(20)*.

In neutropenic patients with pulmonary infiltrates, the antibiotic treatment should include other antibiotics in addition to the broad-spectrum coverage outlined in Table 1. If a *Legionella* pneumonia is suspected, erythromycin should be added. The addition of trimethoprim-sulfamethoxazole is indicated if an infection with *P. carinii* (*see* Chapter 18) is suspected. Most patients who develop pulmonary infiltrates should also receive empirical antifungal treatment. Patients with hematological neoplasms are also at risk of infection with *Mycobacterium tuberculosis* and atypical mycobacteriae.

Certain viral pathogens are also responsible for infections in patients with leukemia, lymphoma, and/or neutropenia. Details about herpesvirus infections are given in Chapter 18.

4. PROPHYLAXIS OF INFECTIONS IN NEUTROPENIC PATIENTS

A high standard of personal hygiene is essential for the neutropenic patient. If prolonged neutropenia (longer than 3–5 d) is expected, the patient should be housed in private rooms and strict hand washing should be observed. Potential sources of pathogens (e.g., fresh flowers) should be removed from the patient's room. Contact with infected patients should be avoided under all circumstances. For patients with more prolonged neutropenia, such as recipients of bone marrow grafts, special measures such as isolation in rooms with positive pressure and high-efficiency particulate air (HEPA) filtration may reduce the risk of acquisition of aspergillus spores and the development of subsequent invasive aspergillosis *(66)*. The use of a total protective environment (TPE) with isolation of patients in a "sterile" room with HEPA filters and laminar air flow, a low-bacteria diet, topical antiseptics and washings, and the administration of oral nonresorbable antibiotics (colistin, neomycin, norfloxacin) and antifungal agents (amphotericin B, nystatin) in these high-risk patients led to the reduction in documented infections in some prospective randomized clinical trials. Unfortunately, the lack of a survival advantage has led to the decline in use of TPE in most centers, although many centers continue to use positive pressure and HEPA filtration.

Specific antimicrobial prophylaxis has been found to be beneficial in some settings. Numerous studies have focused on the use of oral absorbable antibiotics (e.g., trimethoprim-sulfamethoxazole, erythromycin, fluoroquinolones, and others). The most commonly used agents utilized for antibacterial prophylaxis are the extended-spectrum fluoroquinolones. Although they may reduce the frequency of Gram-negative infections, they do not have significant enough activity to prevent breakthrough infections with Gram-positive organisms and may also lead to the development of resistant Gram-negative organisms. Oral antibiotics, therefore, should be reserved for certain high-risk situations. Antifungal prophylaxis with fluconazole was shown to be highly effective in prevention of infections with *Candida* (mainly *albicans* species) in bone marrow transplant recipients in several randomized trials in the 1990s. Recent studies are focusing on the utility of newer broader-spectrum agents such as voriconazole and posaconazole in this high-risk group of patients. Unfortunately, like antibacterial therapy, when an effective therapy for one infection is found (e.g., *Aspergillus*), increased or "breakthrough" infection with resistant organisms may be seen (e.g., *Zygomycetes*).

Although previously considered a protozoa, *P. carinii* (also designated as *P. jarvoii*), is now classified as a fungus. Trimethoprim-sulfamethoxazole is active as a prophylaxis of infections with *P. carinii.* (*see* Chapter 18). Although aerosolized treatment with pentamidine and oral dapsone has been used, breakthrough infections have been seen. Trimethoprim-sulfamethoxazole therefore remains the prophylactic agent of choice. Such a prophylaxis is indicated in high-risk situations (e.g., bone marrow transplants, patients with acute lymphoblastic leukemia under high-dose steroids).

Antiviral prophylaxis with acyclovir was shown to be extremely effective in reduction of the morbidity due to mucositis exacerbated by infection with *H. simplex* after bone marrow transplant over two decades ago. Although many centers use acyclovir, valcyclovir, or famciclovir for prophylaxis against infection with *V. zoster* virus, the dose of drug needed is higher and the period of time required for adequate protection is much longer (e.g., 6–12 mo after a hematopoietic stem cell transplant) than that needed for prophylaxis against *H. simplex*. Many clinicians will, therefore, educate their patients, family members, and other caregivers regarding the early signs and symptoms of viral infection. Antiviral treatment for *Varicella* is then withheld until the earliest signs of infection are evident. This approach is only effective if therapy is begun within 48–72 h of the first sign of infection and may serve to reduce the risk of visceral dissemination, reducing the need for prolonged prophylaxis in high-risk patients. For CMV infections (*see* Chapter 18), several drugs are active for prophylaxis (e.g., ganciclovir, foscarnet, cidofovir), but because of their toxicity profile, routine prophylactic use is not indicated. Prospective monitoring of blood for a positive signal for CMV antigen or by quantitative PCR is now standard of care for patients at high risk (i.e., allogeneic blood or marrow transplant recipients, patients receiving therapy with anti-CD52 antibody, etc.) for development of CMV-related disease (e.g., pneumonitis, hepatitis, cerebritis). Pre-emptive therapy with either ganciclovir or foscarnet is given in the presence of a positive signal for CMV to reduce the risk of progression to CMV disease and withheld in patients with a negative signal in attempt to avoid unwarranted drug toxicity. Recent and ongoing prophylactic studies of newer oral formulations of antiviral agents with activity against CMV (e.g., valganciclovir) are promising. The routine use of hyperimmuneglobulins as a means of antiviral prophylaxis, more common in past years, has fallen in to disfavor because of costs, toxicities, and the improvements in the use of pre-emptive antiviral therapy.

Many treatment protocols for hematological malignancies include the use of hematopoietic growth factors. These factors (granulocyte colony-stimulating factor [G-CSF], granulocyte/macrophage colony-stimulating factor [GM-CSF], and others) generally shorten neutropenia by several days. The rationale, dosage, and side effects of hematopoietic growth factors are discussed in Chapter 2.

5. VENOUS ACCESS

Patients who undergo intensive treatment for hematological malignancies need multiple transfusions, often parenteral nutrition, antibiotics, cytostatic drugs, and multiple other drugs. In these patients, a large lumen venous catheter is indicated. For patients who undergo multiple cycles of chemotherapy (e.g., patients with lymphomas) or who will have prolonged cytopenias (e.g., in bone marrow or stem cell transplantation) or who need prolonged parenteral nutrition, an implanted catheter system is useful (portacath systems, Hickman or Broviac multiple lumen systems, and other catheters). These systems are implanted surgically and can stay for several months if necessary. Portacath-type systems need special needles for access and are recommended for patients who experience shorter cytopenias or who need long-term parenteral nutrition. Hickman-type catheters are suited for patients with acute leukemia or who undergo marrow transplantation. The implanted catheter systems are not free from complications (total rate 2–5%) including bleeding or pneumothorax at the time of implantation and thromboses or infections later on.

If a central venous catheter is the source of bacteremia, an attempt can be made to treat the infection by appropriate antibiotics including vancomycin. If the fever or the local signs of infection do not regress within 24 h, the catheter should be replaced. The catheter should be drawn immediately if signs of a tunnel infection are evident.

Table 3

Antiemetic Regimen for Chemotherapy in Leukemias and Lymphomas

Regimen	Dose
A. Ondansetron +	2×8 mg i.v.[a]
Dexamethasone	10 mg i.v.
B. Ondansetron +	2×8 mg i.v.[a]
Dexamethasone +	5 mg i.v.
Aprepitant	125 mg p.o. d 1, 80 mg d 2, 3
C. Ondansetron	2×8 mg i.v.[a]
D. Metoclopramide ±	3×1–2 mg/kg[b]
Dexamethasone	10 mg i.v.

[a]First dose 1 h before chemotherapy, second and third dose after 4 and 8 h, intravenously (i.v.) or orally.

[b]First dose 1 h before chemotherapy, second and third dose after 2 and 4 h i.v.

A local thrombus in a central venous catheter can often be reopened by injecting 1–3 mL of a solution containing 3000–5000 U/mL of streptokinase or urokinase. The extravasation of cytostatic drugs through a central venous catheter that has been correctly positioned is almost impossible. However, if this occurs as a result of leakage of the catheter, the affected tissue should be infiltrated with 5–15 mL of isotonic saline solution and the catheter should he removed. Necrotic tissue should be excised surgically.

6. FURTHER CONSIDERATIONS

All patients with hematological malignancies need an intensive emotional support. Many patients suffer from anxiety, whereas others develop major depressions or other affective disorders requiring treatment.

Many patients need analgesia. The side effects of commonly used analgesic drugs (e.g., respiratory depression with morphine) and drug interactions must be considered.

Nausea and vomiting are common side effects of many cytostatic drugs and can be prevented or ameliorated by modern antiemetic therapy. Examples of effective regimens are given in Table 3; however, they must be modified individually. The choice of antiemetic agent depends on the emetogenic potential of the chemotherapy. Several other emetic drugs have a similar mechanism of action. The side effects of these antiemetic drugs should be considered. Ondansetron belongs to the class of 5-hydroxytryptamine antagonists and has only minor side effects (headaches, slight elevation of transaminases). Palonosetron (recommended dose 0.25 mg i.v.) is a longer acting 5-hydroxytryptamine antagonist and should be considered in cases of delayed nausea and vomiting. Combinations using aprepitant (a neurokinin-1-receptor antagonist) should be considered in high-emetogenic chemotherapy; however, the dose of dexamethasone (if part of the regimen) should be reduced by half (because dexamethasone is eliminated by CYP3A4).

Metoclopramide is an effective antiemetic agent but has troublesome side effects in 5–20% of patients (extrapyramidal reactions, dystonic reactions, sedation, diarrhea). Steroids are effective in combination regimens of antiemetic drugs and have few side effects if used on a short-term basis. Other drugs (benzodiazepines, cannabinoids) are also useful and effective in antiemetic combination treatments.

REFERENCES

1. Bodey GP, Buckley M, Sathe YS, et al. Quantitative relationships between circulating leukocytes and infection in patients with acute leukemia. *Ann Intern Med* 1966; 64:328–340.
2. Pizzo PA. Fever in immunocompromised patients. *N Engl J Med* 1999;341:893–900.
3. Donowitz GR, Maki DG, Crnich CJ, Pappas PG, Roloston KV. Infections in the neutropenic patient—new views of an old problem. *Hematology* 2001;113–139.
4. Hughes WT, Armstrong D, Bodey GP, et al. 2002 guidelines for the use of antimicrobial agents in neutropenic patients with cancer. *Clin Infect Dis* 2002;34:730–751.
5. de Pauw BE, Donnelly JP. Infections in the immunocompromised host: general principles. In: Mandell GL, Bennett JE, Dolin R, eds. *Mandell, Douglas, and Bennett's Principles and Practices of Infectious Diseases*, 5th ed. Philadelphia: Churchill Livingston, 2000:pp. 3079–3090.
6. Bodey GP. Unusual presentations of infection in neutropenic patients. *Int J Antimicrob Agents* 2000;16:93–95.
7. DesJardin JA, Falagas ME, Ruthazer R, et al. Clinical utility of blood cultures drawn from indwelling central venous catheters in hospitalized patients with cancer. *Ann Intern Med* 1999;131:641–647.
8. Caillot D, Couaillier J-F, Bernard A, et al. Increasing volume and changing characteristics of invasive pulmonary aspergillosis on sequential thoracic computed tomography scans in patients with neutropenia. *J Clin Oncol* 2001;19:253–259.
9. Pazos C, Ponton J, Del Palacio A. Contribution of (1-3) beta-D-glucan chromogenic assay to diagnosis and monitoring of invasive aspergillosis in neutropenic adult patients. *J Clin Microbiol* 2005;43:299–305.
10. Pinel C, Fricker-Hidalgo H, Lebeau B, et al. Detection of circulating *Aspergillus fumigatus* galactomannan value and limits of the Platelia test for diagnosing invasive aspergillosis. *J Clin Microbiol* 2003;41:2184–2186.
11. Walsh TJ, Shoham S, Petraitiene R, et al. Detection of galactomannan antigenemia in patients receiving piperacillin-tazobactam and correlations between in vitro, in vivo, and clinical properties of the drug-antigen interaction. *J Clin Microbiol* 2004;42:4744–4748.
12. Rolston KVI. *Stenotrophomonas maltophilia* infection in cancer patients-frequency, spectrum of infection and antimicrobial susceptibility. European Congress of Clinical Microbiology and Infectious Diseases (ECCMID) 2003;Glasgow, Scotland Abs. 678

13. Safdar N, Maki DO. The commonality of risk factors for nosocomial colonization and infection with antimicrobial-resistant *Staphylococcus aerues,* enterococcus, gram-negative bacilli, *Clostridium difficile,* and *Candida. Ann Intern Med* 2002;136:834–844.

14. Razonable RR, Litzow MR, Kaliq Y, et al. Bacteremia due to viridans group streptococci with diminished susceptibility to levofloxacin among neutropenic patients receiving levofloxacin prophylaxis. *Clin Infect Dis* 2002; 34:1469–1474.

15. Jantunen E, Ruutu P, Niskanen L, et al. Incidence and risk factors for invasive fungal infections in allogeneic BMT recipients. *Bone Marrow Transplant* 1997;19:801–808

16. Yuen KY, Woo PCY, Ip MSM, et al. Stage-specific manifestations of mold infections in bone marrow transplant recipients: risk factors and clinical significance of positive concentrated smears. *Clin Infect Dis* 1997;25:37–42.

17. Fukuda T, Boeckh M, Carter RA, et al. Risks and outcomes of invasive fungal infections in recipients of allogeneic hematopoietic stem cell transplants after nonmyeloablative conditioning. *Blood* 2003;102:827–833.

18. Keating MJ, Flinn I, Jain V, et al. Therapeutic role of alemtuzumab (Campath -1H) in patients who have failed fludarabine: results of a large international study. *Blood* 2002;99:3554–3561.

19. McNeil MM, Nash SL, Hajjeh RA, et al. Trends in mortality due to invasive mycotic diseases in the United States. 1980-1997. *Clin Infect Dis* 2001;33:641–647.

20. Walsh TJ, Groll A, Hiemenz J, et al. Infections due to emerging and uncommon fungal pathogens. *Clin Microbiol Infect* 2004;10;48–66.

21. Ison MG, Hayden FG, Kaiser L, et al. Rhinovirus infections in hematopoietic stem cell transplant recipients with pneumonia. *Clin Infect Dis* 2003;36:1139–1143.

22. Martino R, Ramila E, Rabella N, et al. Respiratory virus infections in adults with hematologic malignancies: a prospective study. *Clin Infect Dis* 2003;26:1–8.

23. Marcolini JA, Malik S, Suki D, et al. Respiratory disease due to parainfluenza virus in adult leukemia patients. *Eur J Clin Microbiol Infect Dis* 2003;22:79–84.

24. Freifeld A, Marchigiani D, Walsh T, et al. A double-blind comparison of empirical oral and intravenous antibiotic therapy for low risk febrile patients with neutropenia during cancer chemotherapy. *N Eng J Med* 1999;341:305–311.

25. Rolston KVI. New trends in patient management: risk-based therapy for febrile patients with neutropenia. *Clin Infect Dis* 1999;29:515–521.

26. Del Favero A, Menichetti F, Marino P, et al. A multicenter, double-blind, placebo-controlled trial comparing piperacillin-tazobactam with and without amikacin as empiric therapy for febrile neutropenia. *Clin Infect Dis* 2001;33:1295–1301.

27. Walsh TJ, Hiemenz JW, Anaissie E. Recent progress and current problems in treatment of invasive fungal infections in neutropenic patients. *Infect Dis Clin North Am* 1996;10:365–400.

28. Pizzo PA, Robichaud KJ, Gill FA, et al. Empiric antibiotic and antifungal therapy for cancer patients with prolonged fever and granulocytopenia. *Am J Med* 1982;72:101–111.

29. EORTC International Antimicrobial Therapy Cooperative Group. Empiric antifungal therapy in febrile granulocytopenic patients. *Am J Med* 1989;86:668–672.

30. White MH, Bowden RA, Sandler ES, et al. Randomized, double-blind clinical trial of amphotericin B colloidal dispersion vs. amphotericin B in the empirical treatment of fever and neutropenia. *Clin Infect Dis* 1998;27:296–302.

31. Walsh TJ, Finberg RW, Arndt C, et al. Liposomal amphotericin B for empirical therapy in patients with persistent fever and neutropenia. *N Engl J Med* 1999; 340:764–771.

32. Boogaerts M, Winston DJ, Bow EJ, et al. Intravenous and oral itraconazole versus intravenous amphotericin B deoxycholate as empirical antifungal therapy for persistent fever in neutro-

penic patients with cancer who are receiving broad-spectrum antibacterial therapy; a randomized controlled trial. *Ann Intern Med* 2001;135:412–422.

33. Walsh TJ, Pappas P, Winston DJ, et al. Voriconazole compared with liposomal amphotericin
    B for empirical antifungal therapy in patients with neutropenia and persistent fever. *N Engl
    J Med* 2002;346:225–234.

34. Walsh TJ, Teppler H, Donowitz GR, et al. Caspofungin versus liposomal amphotericin B for
    empirical antifungal therapy in patients with persistent fever and neutropenia. *N Engl J Med*
    2004;351(14):1391–1402.

35. National Nosocomial Infections Surveillance System. National Nosocomial Infections Sur-
    veillance (NNIS) System report. Data summary from January 1990-May 1999. *Am J Infect
    Control* 1999;27:520–532.

36. National Nosocomial Infections Surveillance System. National Nosocomial Infections
    Surveillence (NNIS) System report. Data summary from January 1992-April 2000. *Am J
    Infect Control* 2000;28:429–448.

37. Tunkel AR, Sepkowitz KA. Infections caused by viridans streptococci in patients with neu-
    tropenia. *Clin Infect Dis* 2002;34:1524–1529.

38. Donskey CJ, Chowdhry TK, Hecker MT, et al. Effect of antibiotic therapy on the density of
    vancomycin-resistant enterococci in the stool of colonized patients. *N Engl J Med*
    2000;343:1925–1932.

39. Edmond M, Ober JF, Weinbaum DL, et al. Vancomycin-resistant *Enterococcus faecium*
    bacteremia: risk factors for infection. *Clin Infect Dis* 1995;20:1126–1133.

40. Patterson DL, Rice LB. Empirical antibiotic choice for the seriously ill patient; are minimi-
    zation of selection of resistant organisms and maximization of individual outcome mutually
    exclusive? *Clin Infect Dis* 2003;36:1006–1012.

41. National Nosocomial Infections Surveillance System. National Nosocomial Infections Sur-
    veillance (NNIS) System report. Data summary from January 1992-June 2001. *Am J Infect
    Control* 2001;29:404–421.

42. Stevens DL, Dotter B, Madaras-Kelly K. A review of linezolid: the first oxazolidinone anti-
    biotic. *Expert Rev Anti Infect Ther* 2004;2:51–59.

43. Raad I, Hachem R, Hanna H, et al. Prospective randomized study comparing quinupristin with
    linezolid in the treatment of vancomycin-resistant Enterococcus faecium infections. *J
    Antimicrob Chemother* 2004;53:646–649.

44. Rao N, Ziran BH, Wagener MM, et al. Similar hematologic effects of long-term linezolid and
    vancomycin in a prospective observational study of patients with orthopedic infections. *Clin
    Infect Dis* 2004;38:1058–1064.

45. Meissner HC, Townsend T, Wenman W, et al. Hematologic effects of linezolid in young
    children. *Pediatr Infect Dis J* 2003;22(S19):186–192.

46. Dibo I, Pillai SK, Gold HS, et al. Linezolid-resistant *Enterococcus faecalis* isolated from a
    cord blood transplant recipient. *J Clin Microbiol* 2004;42:1843–1845.

47. Pappas PG, Rex JH, Sobel JD, et al. Guidelines for the treatment of candidiasis. *Clin Infect Dis*
    2004;38:161–189.

48. Walsh TJ, Hiemenz JW, Anaissie E. Recent progress and current problems in treatment of
    invasive fungal infections in neutropenic patients. *Infect Dis Clin North Am* 1996;10:365–400.

49. Nucci M, Anaissie E. Should vascular catheters be removed from all patients with candidemia?
    An evidence-based review. *Clin Infect Dis* 2002;34:591–599.

50. Walsh TJ, Rex JH. All catheter-related candidemia is not the same: assessment of the balance
    between the risks and benefits of removal of vascular catheters. *Clin Infect Dis* 2002;34:600–602.

51. Mora-Duarte J, Betts R, Rotstein C, et al. Comparison of caspofungin and amphotericin B for invasive candidiasis. *N Engl J Med* 2002;347:2020–2029.
52. Gerson SL, Talbot GH, Hurwitz S, et al. Prolonged granulocytopenia: the major risk factor for invasive pulmonary aspergillosis in patients with acute leukemia. *Ann Intern Med* 1984;100:345–351.
53. Patterson TF, Kirkpatrick WR, White M, et al. Invasive aspergillosis. Disease spectrum, treatment practices, and outcomes. *Medicine (Baltimore)* 2000;79:250–60.
54. Stevens DA, Kan VL, Judson MA, et al. Practice guidelines for diseases caused by *Aspergillus*. *Clin Infect Dis* 2000;30:696–709.
55. Hiemenz JW, Walsh TJ. Lipid formulations of amphotericin B: Recent progress and future directions. *Clin Infect Dis* 1996;22(S2):133–144.
56. Herbrecht R, Denning DW, Patterson TF, et al. Voriconazole versus amphotericin B for primary therapy of invasive aspergillosis. *N Engl J Med* 2002;347:408–415.
57. Caillot D, Mannone L, Cuisenier B, et al. Role of early diagnosis and agressive surgery in the management of invasive pulmonary aspergillosis in neutropenic patients. *Clin Microbiol Infect* 2001;7(S2):54–61.
58. Bartizal K, Gill CJ, Abruzzo GK, et al. In vitro preclinical evaluation studies with the echinocandin antifungal MK-0991 (L-743,872). *Antimicrob Agents Chemother* 1997;41:2326–2332.
59. Arikan S, Lozano-Chiu M, Paetznick V, et al. In vitro synergy of caspofungin and amphotericin B against *Aspergillus* and *Fusarium* spp. *Antimicrob Agents Chemother* 2002;46:245–247.
60. Perea S, Gonzalez G, Fothergill AW, et al. In vitro interaction of caspofungin acetate with voriconazole against clinical isolates of *Aspergillus* spp. *Antimicrob Agents Chemother* 2002;46:3039–3041.
61. Kirkpatrick WR, Perea S, Coco BJ, et al. Efficacy of caspofungin alone and in combination with voriconazole in a guinea pig model of invasive aspergillosis. *Antimicrob Agents Chemother* 2002;46:2564–2568.
62. Petraitis V, Petraitiene R, Sarafandi AA, et al. Combination therapy in treatment of experimental pulmonary aspergillosis: synergistic interaction between an antifungal triazole and an echinocandin. *J Infect Dis* 2003;187:1834–1843.
63. Aliff TB, Maslak PG, Jurcic JG, et al. Refractory aspergillus pneumonia in patients with acute leukemia. Successful therapy with combination caspofungin and liposomal amphotericin. *Cancer* 2003;97:1025–1032.
64. Kontoyiannis DP, Hachem R, Lewis RE, et al. Efficacy and toxicity of caspofungin in combination with liposomal amphotericin B as primary or salvage treatment of invasive aspergillosis in patients with hematological malignancies. *Cancer* 2003;98:292–299.
65. Marr KA, Boeckh M, Carter RA, et al. Combination antifungal therapy for invasive aspergillosis. *Clin Infect Dis* 2004;39:797–802.
66. Sherertz RJ, Belani A, Kramer BS, et al. Impact of air filtration on nosocomial aspergillus infections. Unique risk of bone marrow transplant recipients. *Am J Med* 1987;83:7109–7718.

4 Transplantation of Stem Cells From Bone Marrow, Peripheral Blood, and the Umbilical Cord

Ronald Paquette, MD
and Reinhold Munker, MD

CONTENTS

1. DEFINITIONS AND INTRODUCTION

Hematopoietic stem cells have two important functions: they give rise to all blood cell lineages and they also recapitulate themselves. These processes are thought to occur through asymmetric division, in which one daughter cell is

From: *Contemporary Hematology: Modern Hematology, Second Edition*
Edited by: R. Munker, E. Hiller, J. Glass, and R. Paquette © Humana Press Inc., Totowa, NJ

identical to the parent and the other daughter is committed to further differentiation into mature blood cells. True hematopoietic stem cells occur rarely in the bone marrow, they divide infrequently, and the forces that regulate their proliferation and differentiation are incompletely understood. Stem cells are identified in clinical practice by their expression of the CD34 antigen, which functions as an adhesion protein to the bone marrow stroma. Although hematopoietic stem cells express CD34, only a small fraction of CD34+ cells are capable of giving rise to all peripheral blood cell lineages (pluripotent). The majority of CD34+ cells have limited proliferative capacity, and they have been committed to produce a restricted spectrum of cells types.

Stem cell transplantation (SCT) is the infusion of hematopoietic progenitor cells, in numbers adequate to engraft the bone marrow of the recipient, after the administration of conditioning therapy. The stem cells may be obtained from the patient (autologous), an identical twin (syngeneic), or an individual of a different genetic background who has a compatible tissue type (allogeneic). The suitability of an allogeneic donor, whether related or unrelated to the patient, is determined by typing the tissue antigens of the patient and prospective donor. It is desirable that the tissue antigens, or human leukocyte antigens (HLA), of the donor and recipient are identical. Donor stem cells can be procured from the bone marrow, the peripheral blood, or from umbilical cord blood. Currently, stem cells used to transplant patients with malignant diseases are most frequently procured from the peripheral blood, whereas those used in patients with bone marrow failure states and immunodeficiency disorders usually are collected from the bone marrow. The basic principles of SCT are shown in Fig. 4.1.

2. INDICATIONS FOR SCT

SCT is performed for congenital immunodeficiency and metabolic disorders (lysosomal storage diseases); bone marrow failure states (aplastic anemia, myelodysplastic syndrome); sickle cell anemia; hematological malignancies (leukemias, lymphomas, multiple myeloma); and solid tumors (testicular cancer, neuroblastoma), for which dose-intensive chemotherapy has greater effectiveness than standard-dose chemotherapy. Because of the potentially severe toxicity associated with SCT, it is only applied to patients with adequate pulmonary, renal, hepatic, and cardiac function and performance status. Transplantation should be delayed in patients with active uncontrolled infection. Patients with a malignancy are more likely to be cured by SCT if their disease is in remission or has responded to conventional therapy. The potential for SCT to cure a patient is low when chemotherapy-refractory malignant disease is present.

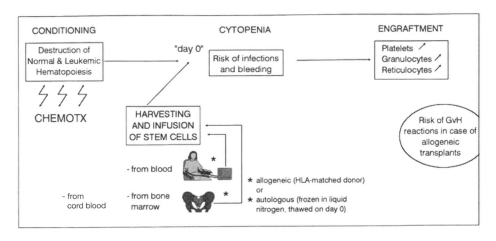

Fig. 4.1. The basic principles of stem cell transplantation.

3. SELECTION OF A TRANSPLANT TYPE

The decision regarding the type of transplant for a specific individual is based on the disease and its remission status, stem cell donor availability, and the age of the recipient. There are benefits and risks that are unique to the use of autologous or allogeneic stem cells. Autologous transplants are typically performed when there is a steep dose–response of the chemotherapy against the malignancy. In this setting, autologous transplantation is simply a way to rescue the patient from treatment-related bone marrow toxicity; the stem cell infusion does not otherwise have therapeutic benefit. The chance of cure following an autologous transplant is more likely when the patient has had a favorable response to preceding chemotherapy. Patients with treatment-resistant disease are unlikely to be cured. Autologous transplants are associated with a low risk of treatment-related mortality (<5%) but a high relapse risk. Because autologous stem cells can be contaminated by malignant cells, the bone marrow must be adequately free of disease prior to stem cell collection in order for this approach to be feasible. In addition, patients who have received extensive prior chemotherapy, especially alkylating agents, may have reduced stem cell numbers that prevent the collection of adequate numbers of cells for transplantation. Allogeneic stem cells are free of disease and have not been adversely affected by prior cytotoxic chemotherapy. However, allogeneic transplantation is associated with the risk of graft-vs-host disease (GVHD), a complication that increases the mortality rate of this approach. Acute GVHD occurs when the T-lymphocytes present in the stem cell graft initiate an immune response against host antigens, causing injury to the skin, liver, and/or gastrointestinal tract. Because the risk of GVHD increases progressively with age, standard allogeneic transplantation is typically limited to patients who are less than 50 yr of age. Although T-lymphocytes can cause GVHD, they also can mediate an immune response against the recipient's malignancy. This phenomenon has been most clearly established as occurring in patients with myeloid leukemias, especially chronic myelogenous leukemia, and therefore it is termed the graft-vs-leukemia (GVL) effect. When allogeneic stem cells are used, the risk of excess early mortality from acute GVHD may exceed or be less than the benefit of the GVL effect depending on the patient's age, disease, and remission status. Therefore, the choice of allogeneic vs autologous stem cells for transplantation in any individual is based partly on the expected risk of acute GVHD vs the potential benefit of a graft-vs-malignancy effect. In addition, allogeneic stem cells must be used for inherited disorders, immunodefiency states, bone marrow failure states, and malignant disorders in which autologous stem cells cannot be harvested or rendered adequately tumor-free.

4. STEM CELL DONOR SELECTION AND EVALUATION

The most important criterion for stem cell donor selection is tissue-type compatibility with the recipient. This is evaluated by performing serological testing of HLA on peripheral blood leukocytes. HLA compatibility between related individuals typically is determined using antisera against the HLA-A, -B, and -DR loci. Because each individual has two alleles at each HLA locus, a total of six antigens are evaluated. Each sibling has a one in four chance of being HLA-identical with the patient. Parents are unlikely to be more than haplo-identical with the child. If there is no related donor available, an unrelated donor search is initiated. The use of unrelated donor stem cells conveys a higher risk of GVHD and is associated with increased early mortality compared to related donor stem cells. This increased risk of mortality is approximately an absolute 10% difference. In evaluating unrelated donors, serological testing is initially used as a screening test. The antibodies used in the serological assays do not discriminate perfectly between different HLA antigens at the molecular level. Amino acid differences can exist between HLA antigens that are found to be the same by serological testing. Therefore, molecular DNA analyses using PCR are used to evaluate potential unrelated stem cell donors who are found to be HLA-compatible with the patient by initial serological screening. Ideally, a 10/10 matched donor is ultimately identified using PCR analysis of HLA-A, -B, -C, -DRB1, and -DQB1 loci. Of these antigens, the DQB1 locus is least important.

Once a compatible donor is identified, a decision must be made regarding the type of stem cells that will be collected. For most transplants, stem cells collected from the peripheral blood are preferred over those collected from the bone marrow. This is because the collection of peripheral blood stem cells (PBSCs) is better tolerated by the donor (*see* "Stem Cell Collection" below) than bone marrow collection. In addition, PBSCs produce survival superior to that of bone marrow in the allogeneic transplant setting. This is because PBSCs engraft 3–5 d sooner than bone marrow (reducing the risk of serious infection), and they decrease the risk of disease relapse. PBSCs contain, on average, 10-fold more T-lymphocytes than bone marrow, which are capable of mediating a GVL effect. Bone marrow collection may be necessary when young children are donors because their blood volume is too small to permit the use of the apheresis machine to collect PBSCs.

All stem cell donors are screened to ensure that they will tolerate the collection procedure and that they are not at risk for transmitting disease to the recipient. Laboratory tests are performed to exclude infection by hepatitis viruses, human T-cell leukemia virus type 1 or 2, or HIV. Bone marrow donors usually donate 1–2 units of blood prior to the procedure, depending on the volume of marrow that will be collected, for reinfusion following the harvest if required for anemia. This is not required prior to PBSC donation.

In the United States, the National Marrow Donor Program (NMDP) maintains a registry of approx 5 million volunteer donors. The NMDP also facilitates international and cord blood bank searches. The NMDP has data on the ethnicity of stem cell donors, and performs outcomes analysis. The success rates of finding a matched donor depend on ethnicity of a patient, being at present highest in Caucasians and Asian-Americans.

5. UMBILICAL CORD BLOOD STEM CELLS

Blood obtained from the umbilical cord at the time of delivery contains a high concentration of hematopoietic stem cells, and it can be used for transplantation. A number of umbilical cord blood (UCB) banks have been established that provide cord blood units for transplantation to unrelated recipients. UCB stem cells are more primitive than those from bone marrow and peripheral blood and the total numbers of cells that can be obtained is low. Therefore, engraftment following transplantation of UCB cells typically is slower than when another source of stem cells is used. The minimum number of UCB stem cells required for engraftment is approx 10% of the number of PBSCs. Nevertheless, the principal limitation of the use of UCB is the low number of stem cells available from a typical collection, and therefore UCB transplants are predominantly performed in children. One potential advantage of UCB is that the T-lymphocytes in the graft are relatively naive. This appears to lessen the risk of GVHD and permits the use of UCB stem cells in patients with a greater degree of HLA disparity than is tolerated using bone marrow or peripheral blood as a source of stem cells. Up to two antigen mismatches are acceptable when selecting an UCB unit for transplantation, although the survival of recipients of 4/6 HLA-matched units is inferior to that of recipients of 5/6 or 6/6 matched units. Additional advantages of this cell source are its ready availability and lack of inconvenience to the donor. Disadvantages include the limited stem cell dose causing delayed hematopoietic recovery, and inability to obtain additional cells from the donor in the event of graft failure or disease relapse. Retrospective studies have demonstrated similar survival results for recipients of unrelated bone marrow and UCB. Therefore, a number of variables including UCB cell dose, degree of HLA disparity between donor and recipient, and the disease to be transplanted, all may play a role in deciding between UCB, peripheral blood, and bone marrow as a stem cell source.

6. STEM CELL COLLECTION

Hematopoietic stem cells normally reside in the bone marrow. As a result, bone marrow harvesting has been a reliable method to obtain stem cells for transplantation. The bone marrow donor receives spinal, epidural, or general anesthesia in the operating room and is positioned in the prone position. The skin over the iliac crests is cleansed with betadine and iodophor, then covered with sterile drapes. The bone marrow is withdrawn by repeatedly inserting a trochar into the marrow space of the iliac crest, aspirating 3–5 mL of bone marrow into a heparinized syringe, removing the trochar and ejecting the marrow into a bag containing heparinized media. The adequacy of the collection is usually checked approximately midway though the procedure by performing a mononuclear cell (MNC) count. An adequate bone marrow collection should contain at least 3×10^8 MNCs/kg of recipient weight. Bone marrow collection continues until the target MNC count is reached. Once the collection is completed, the bone marrow is filtered to remove bone fragments and clots.

Stem cells occur infrequently in the peripheral blood but, following recovery from chemotherapy or after adminstration of several hematopoietic growth factors, they can be induced to enter the circulation. Stem cell mobilization in normal donors is usually performed by administering granulocyte colony-stimulating factor (G-CSF) 10 µg/kg by subcutaneous injection daily until collection is complete. PBSCs also can be mobilized using granulocyte/macrophage colony-stimulating factor (GM-CSF). In patients with malignant conditions chemotherapy is often given, followed by the daily administration of growth factors, to mobilize PBSCs as the neutrophil count recovers. PBSC collection usually begins 5 d after the start of hematopoietic growth factor administration when growth factors alone are used. In patients who have stem cells mobilized with growth factors following chemotherapy, collections may be initiated when the number of CD34+ cells in the peripheral blood reaches the threshold established at each institution. Harvesting of the stem cells is performed using apheresis, a procedure in which a machine continuously withdraws blood from one vein of the donor, removes the MNC fraction by centrifugation, and returns the remainder of the blood through another venous access. The blood is anticoagulated during this procedure with the use of sodium citrate. The cell product obtained in this manner contains predominantly immature granulocytes, lymphocytes, and monocytes; immature hematopoietic progenitor cells including stem cells usually comprise less than 1% of the total cells. The adequacy of stem cell collection can be assessed by analyzing the percentage of cells expressing the CD34 antigen. The number of CD34+ cells administered following myeloablative therapy correlates with the time to engraftment of neutrophils and platelets. The minimum threshold of CD34+ cells required for stable engraftment is approx 10^6 cells/kg. The number of stem cells collected for transplantation usually ranges within $2-5 \times 10^6$ CD34+ cells/kg.

UCB is collected after the baby is delivered and the cord has been clamped. If the placenta has been delivered, it is held up by a clamp with the umbilical cord hanging down. The cord is cleaned with alcohol and the umbilical vein is cannulated with a large needle connected to a bag containing anticoagulant. The blood is collected by gravity drainage. The volume of the cord blood is measured and a MNC count is performed to ensure that a minimum threshold of acceptability is reached. If so, samples are removed for infectious disease and sterility testing, CD34 cell quantitation, HLA typing, and if appropriate, hemoglobinopathy testing. Approximately 1.8×10^8 MNCs/kg or 1.7×10^5 CD34+ cells/kg is considered adequate for transplantation.

7. CONDITIONING THERAPY

The conditioning therapy administered prior to SCT can be used for two potential purposes: in patients with a malignant disorder, it reduces the tumor burden to the minimum possible level, and in patients who are receiving stem cells from a related or unrelated donor, it also suppresses the host immune system and allows engraftment to occur. Conditioning therapy may consist of radiation and chemotherapy or chemotherapy alone. The chemotherapeutic agents employed to condition patients with malignancies may be disease-specific. The drugs are selected to avoid agents used earlier in the course of treatment, to which the malignancy may have developed resistance. In addition, the conditioning therapies are chosen such that their primary toxicities are hematological and their nonhematological toxicities do not overlap, in order to prevent injury to organs other than the bone marrow.

Recently, nonmyeloablative conditioning regimens, using immunosuppressive chemotherapies such as cyclophosphamide and fludarabine, have been investigated as an approach to SCT. Because the GVL effect is critical to the cure of several malignancies following allogeneic BMT, the nonmyeloablative approach uses less-toxic doses of chemotherapy to permit engraftment of the donor immune system. The efficacy of this approach relies on the potential ability of the transplanted immune system to eradicate the recipient's malignancy. The reduced intensity of the conditioning regimen reduces the incidence and severity of acute GVHD. Therefore, nonmyeloablative transplants have been favored in patients with advanced age (>50 yr), those who had undergone a prior autologous transplant with full intensity conditioning, and those with slow-growing tumors for whom dose-intense chemotherapy is not curative (low-grade lymphomas). Although the risk of acute GVHD is diminished, chronic GVHD remains a significant cause of mortality for patients undergoing nonmyeloablative transplantation. Although the results are encouraging in some settings, clinical indications for this approach have not been firmly established.

8. BLOOD PRODUCT ADMINISTRATION

Several unique precautions must be taken when transfusing blood products into SCT recipients (see Table 1). These precautions include prophylactic transfusion of blood products, irradiation of all blood products, administration of cytomegalovirus (CMV)-seronegative blood products to seronegative allogeneic transplant recipients, and avoidance of allosensitization.

Patients with SCT experience pancytopenia following conditioning therapy and before marrow recovery. During this time period, transfusion support is required to prevent symptomatic anemia and life-threatening thrombocytopenia. Packed red blood cells typically are transfused prophylactically when the hemoglobin falls below 9 g/dL. Platelet transfusions are administered when the platelet count is below 10,000/μL in stable patients, or below 20,000/μL in febrile patients. Platelet transfusion is indicated for platelet count <50,000/μL in the setting of active bleeding or head trauma. A single donor platelet unit (one apheresis pack) is preferred over the use of random donor platelets (10 units) for transplant patients to minimize the risk of allosensitization (discussed later).

Because SCT recipients are profoundly immunosuppressed by the conditioning therapy, they are at risk for the development of GVHD (*see* Subheading 11) from lymphocytes present in blood products. Irradiation prevents the lymphocytes from proliferating in response to host antigens and eliminates the risk of transfusion-related GVHD.

Table 1
Guidelines for Blood Product Transfusion in Stem Cell Transplant Patients

Prophylactically transfuse platelets for platelet count less than 10,000/μL in stable patients or less than 20,000/μL in febrile patients.
Use single-donor platelets rather than random donor platelets.
Irradiate all blood products.
Leukocyte reduce all blood products.
Use only cytomegalovirus (CMV)-negative blood products for CMV seronegative allogeneic stem cell transplant patients.
Do not transfuse prospective allogeneic stem cell transplant recipients with blood products from family members prior to transplantation.
Minimize all transfusions in aplastic anemia patients prior to transplantation.

CMV can produce life-threatening pneumonia, hepatitis, or colitis in allogeneic transplant recipients (*see* "Prevention and Treatment of Posttransplant Infections"). Patients who have not been exposed to CMV should receive blood products only from donors who are seronegative for CMV. Leukocyte reduction of blood products using a filter has been shown to reduce the risk of transmitting CMV. Whether or not leukocyte-reduced blood products can substitute for CMV-negative ones is controversial.

Allosensitization, the development of immunity to HLA, must be avoided for two reasons: it can cause patients to become refractory to platelet transfusions and it can increase the risk of graft rejection in patients receiving allogeneic transplants. Because HLA are expressed on platelets, the development of humoral immunity to a wide variety of HLA can lead to rapid clearance of transfused platelets and difficulty in maintaining adequate platelet levels posttransplant. Reduction of leukocytes (which also express HLA) from blood products has been shown to reduce the risk of allosensitization. Therefore, recipients of SCT should all receive leukocyte-reduced blood products. In addition, whenever possible, platelet products should be obtained from a single donor by apheresis, rather than by pooling platelet products from several different donors. Platelet-refractory patients may require transfusions of platelets from HLA-matched donors. Allosensitization that occurs prior to transplant conditioning also can increase the risk of graft rejection, particularly in patients who receive less-aggressive conditioning regimens for nonmalignant diseases. Candidates for allogeneic SCT should never receive blood product transfusions from family members prior to transplantation in order to minimize the risk of graft rejection. In addition, every effort should be made to minimize blood product transfusions prior to transplantation in aplastic anemia patients, who typically receive relatively mild conditioning therapy.

9. PREVENTION AND TREATMENT OF POSTTRANSPLANT INFECTIONS

The profound neutropenia that occurs following the administration of myeloablative therapy subjects transplant recipients to a risk of developing serious bacterial or fungal infections. (Neutropenia is defined here as an absolute neutrophil count of less than 500/μL.) Because many infections that occur during the neutropenic period originate from the gastrointestinal tract, prophylactic "gut sterilizers" have traditionally been used in an attempt to reduce this problem. A poorly absorbed antibiotic such as norfloxacin (400 mg by mouth twice daily), and the oral antifungal agents nystatin (1 million units orally four times daily) and clotrimazole (10 mg troche dissolved in mouth four times daily) are used in many centers to prevent infections. In recipients of allogeneic transplants, itraconazole has been demonstrated to significantly reduce the risk of invasive fungal infections compared with fluconazole. The dose of itraconazole is 200 mg i.v. every 12 h for 2 d followed by 200 mg every 24 h from d 1 to d 100 posttransplant. Itraconazole suspension 200 mg p.o. every 12 h can be substituted for the injection if there is no malabsorption due to GVHD, but the capsule formulation is too poorly absorbed to be effective. Continuation of itraconazole should be considered if steroids are continued beyond 100 d posttransplant. Itraconazole affects cyclophosphamide metabolism, so these drugs should not be given concurrently.

The initial neutropenic fever that occurs in a transplant patient must be treated rapidly and empirically. In the absence of an obvious source, after appropriate cultures are obtained, intravenous antibiotics that have activity against a broad spectrum of Gram-negative bacilli, Gram-positive cocci, and anaerobic organisms should be administered as quickly as possible. Potential regimens are listed in Table 2. Antimicrobial therapy subsequently can be modified if cultures demonstrate the etiology of the infection. If fevers persist in spite of antibiotics and without a source, empiric antifungal therapy may be initiated, especially if a prolonged period of neutropenia is anticipated. In allogeneic transplant patients, an azole antifungal agent with activity against *Aspergillus* is appropriate, including itraconazole or voriconazole (Table 3). Alternatively, amphotericin B may be initiated empirically at a dose of 0.5 mg/kg/d, but full treatment doses (1 mg/kg/d) are required if fungal infection is documented. Patients usually are not at high risk for *Aspergillus* infection and therefore can be treated with empiric

Table 2

Empiric Antibiotic Regimens for Treatment of Febrile Neutropenia
in Adult Transplant Patients

1.	Imipenem 500 mg i.v. every 6 h
2.	Ceftazidime 1 g i.v. every 8 h, alone or with Vancomycin 1 g i.v. every 12 h
3.	Aminoglycoside (with activity against local *Pseudomonas*), and Ceftazidime 1 g i.v. every 8 h, or Piperacillin 3 g i.v. every 4 h
4.*	Ciprofloxacin 400 mg i.v. every 12 h, or Aztreonam 2 g every 6–8 h, and Vancomycin 1 g i.v. every 12 h

*Acceptable for use in most patients with demonstrated penicillin allergy.

Table 3

Empiric Antifungal Agents for Treatment of Febrile Neutropenia
in Adult Transplant Patients

Allogeneic Transplant Patients

1. Voriconazole 6 mg/kg i.v. every 12 h 24 h, then 4 mg/kg every 12 h
2. Itraconazole 200 mg i.v. every 12 h 48 h, then 200 mg every 24 h
3. Amphotericin B
    Empiric therapy: 0.5 mg/kg i.v. qd
    Treatment of documented infection: 1 mg/kg i.v. qd

Autologous Transplant Patients

1. Fluconazole 400 mg i.v. qd

fluconazole. Antimicrobial coverage usually can be discontinued after neutropenia resolves (absolute neutrophil count >500/µL) when it is applied empirically, but a full treatment course is required if a source of infection is identified.

Pneumocystis pneumonia was a major problem following allogeneic bone marrow transplantation (BMT) prior to the routine use of prophylactic measures. Patients now are given trimethoprim/sulfamethoxazole (TMP/SMX; 160 mg/ 800 mg) three times daily for approx 7 d prior to transplantation, stopping 2 d before stem cell infusion. Following marrow recovery, TMP/SMX is administered three times daily with leucovorin 5 mg daily on 2 d per week. *Pneumocystis* prophylaxis is continued until the patient has discontinued all immunosuppressive therapy. Dapsone (100 mg daily) can be substituted for TMP/SMX in sulfa allergic patients.

Patients who are seropositive for CMV are at risk for reactivation of this virus and development of hepatitis, colitis, or a highly fatal interstitial pneumonitis following allogeneic BMT. Prophylactic therapy has markedly reduced the incidence of CMV infection. Patients seropositive for CMV can be treated prophylactically with ganciclovir 5 mg/kg/d for approx 1 wk prior to transplantation, stopping 2 d before stem cell infusion. After the neutrophil count rises above 1000/µL, ganciclovir may be resumed at a dose of 6 mg/kg/d on the 5 d of the week that the TMP/SMX is not given, and it is continued until 100 d posttransplant. Because ganciclovir is myelosuppressive, blood counts must be monitored in order to reduce or temporarily discontinue drug therapy if neutropenia develops. Dose adjustment is also required for renal insufficiency (creatinine clearance <80 mL/min). An alternative strategy is to monitor the blood weekly for CMV reactivation using a quantitative assay, and treat only patients who develop viremia. Patients who are CMV seronegative do not require ganciclovir but should be given blood products only from CMV-seronegative donors. It is controversial whether the use of leukocyte-reduced blood products can replace CMV-negative products for these patients. Seronegative patients who receive stem cells from a seropositive donor rarely develop CMV infection and therefore do not benefit from prophylactic ganciclovir.

Varicella zoster and *Herpes simplex* viruses (HSV) also are commonly reactivated following SCT. Patients with a history of recurrent oral or genital HSV lesions prior to transplantation may benefit from the prophylactic administration of acyclovir (400 mg orally twice daily) during the posttransplant period. Oral mucosal herpetic lesions occur commonly after high-dose chemotherapy and the resultant mucositis can cause substantial morbidity. Direct fluorescent antigen testing for HSV permits rapid identification of this infection. Treatment consists of acyclovir 5 mg/kg i.v. every 8 h. Patients who undergo allogeneic or unrelated SCT and who develop cutaneous zoster lesions are at risk for secondary dissemination. Pulmonary involvement that develops in this setting can be fatal. Therefore, patients with zoster limited to a single dermatome should be treated with intravenous acyclovir 10 mg/kg every 8 h, to prevent secondary spread, until crusting of the lesions has occurred, then the acyclovir can be given orally. More prolonged intravenous treatment is required in the setting of disseminated zoster.

10. GRAFT FAILURE

Graft failure is defined as pancytopenia and a severely hypocellular bone marrow that persists beyond approx 21 d following PBSC transplant or 28 d after a BMT. Risk factors for graft failure in patients receiving autografts include the administration of inadequate numbers of stem cells, poor graft quality due to extensive prior treatment of the patient with alkylating agents, or extensively manipulation of the graft (i.e., if it has been treated with cytotoxic agents for the purpose of purging tumor cells). Patients receiving allografts are at increased risk of graft failure if they have had extensive prior allosensitization from blood products, if the conditioning therapy was inadequate to eliminate the recipient immune system, if they have HLA incompatibility with the donor, if the graft has been depleted of T-lymphocytes, or if the stem cell dose is inadequate. Administration of myelosuppressive medications (e.g., methotrexate) to the patient after stem cell infusion can delay engraftment and increase the risk of graft failure. Persistent or recurrent malignancy in the bone marrow also can cause prolonged pancytopenia posttransplant. The diagnosis of graft failure is made by performing a bone marrow biopsy, and in the setting of allogeneic transplantation, testing the bone marrow for the presence of donor cells by performing restriction fragment length polymorphism (RFLP) analysis. Cytogenetic analysis on the bone marrow is performed if the patient had a malignancy with a known chromosomal abnormality. Treatment with myeloid growth factors such as G-CSF (5–10 µg/kg/d) or GM-CSF (250 µg/m^2/d) may be useful in this setting. In addition, every effort should be made to obtain additional stem cells from the donor for treatment of graft failure in allotransplant patients. Additional immunosuppressive therapy usually is given prior to a second stem cell infusion in these patients to minimize the risk of repeat graft rejection.

11. GRAFT-VS-HOST DISEASE

Patients who receive allogeneic or unrelated stem cells can develop GVHD. Risk factors for this complication include older age of the recipient, HLA mismatch between the donor and recipient, use of an unrelated donor, use of a parous female donor, and increased numbers of T-lymphocytes in the graft.

The syndrome of GVHD is divided into an acute phase that is defined to occur within the first 100 d posttransplant, and the subsequent chronic phase. This acute disease may involve the skin, gastrointestinal tract, and liver. Skin involvement usually develops first and is manifested as palmar, plantar, and auricular erythema. Acute skin GVHD may evolve into a diffuse erythematous maculopapular rash. When skin involvement is severe, bullae and desquamation develop. Acute liver involvement is initially manifested as an asymptomatic rise in the conjugated bilirubin level, with more minor elevations of the serum alkaline phosphatase and transaminase levels. Synthetic function of the liver is initially preserved, but severe disease may progress to liver failure and hepatic encephalopathy. Gastrointestinal GVHD is characterized by diarrhea that may become voluminous. Severe enteric involvement is characterized by shedding of the colonic mucosa, bleeding, ileus with bowel distension, and potential perforation. Involvement of the upper gastrointestinal tract is manifested by oral mucositis, esophagitis, or gastritis. Patients may experience protracted anorexia, nausea, and vomiting. The grading of acute GVHD is shown in Table 4

Table 4
Staging of Acute GVHD

Stage	Skin	Liver (bilirubin)	Gut (diarrhea)
I	Rash <25% BSA	2–3.5 mg/dL	0.5–1.0 L/d
II	Rash 25–50% BSA	3.5–8 mg/dL	1.0–1.5 L/d
III	Erythroderma	8–15 mg/dL	1.5–2.5 L/d
IV	Desquamation	>15 mg/dL	>2.5 L/d

BSA, body surface area

Chronic GVHD is defined to begin at least 100 d after transplantation, but it usually evolves gradually from acute GVHD. Risk factors include previous acute GVHD, older age of the recipient, use of an unrelated or mismatched donor, and infusion of high numbers of T-lymphocytes with the graft. Skin involvement is characterized by a thin epidermis that ulcerates easily, or by lichenified plaques. In contrast, the dermis becomes firm, and joint contractures may develop. Hyperpigmentation usually is present, but vitiligo also may occur. Dermal structures including hair, sweat glands, and nails may be lost. Xerophthalmia causes a gritty sensation in the eyes, and xerostomia may cause dysphagia. Chronic GVHD of the gastrointestinal tract may manifest as oral mucositis, esophageal webs, or malabsorption. White plaques or reticulations may be present on the buccal mucosa. When chronic liver GHVD occurs, the alkaline phosphatase typically is the most elevated laboratory test, the transaminases are affected to an intermediate degree, and bilirubin is the least abnormal. Pulmonary involvement can present as bronchiolitis obliterans. Patients with chronic GVHD have impaired immunological reconstitution and are at increased risk of developing opportunistic infections.

The diagnosis of acute skin GVHD can usually by made clinically, but liver or gut involvement is best established by biopsy because other posttransplant complications, especially infections, can mimic these conditions. Histopathology of the skin reveals vacuolization of the dermal–epidermal junction, and lymphocytic infiltration into the epidermis and perivascular region. Liver involvement is manifested by destruction of epithelial cells lining the interlobular bile ducts and portal lymphocytic infiltration. Colonic or rectal biopsy characteristically reveals vacuolization of single crypt cells ("exploding crypt cells").

Prophylaxis against acute GVHD is tailored to patient risk factors. Patients at high risk for acute GVHD, such as patients older than 40 yr and those receiving mismatched or unrelated grafts may receive methotrexate. Patients with chronic myelogenous leukemia may also receive this drug because of data demonstrating that it improves survival. A common regimen is to administer methotrexate 15 mg/m^2 on day 1, and 10 mg/m^2 on days 3 and 6 following the transplant. Methotrexate acts by killing T-lymphocytes from the graft that are proliferating in response to recipient antigens. Most patients receive cyclosporine or tacrolimus prophylactically. These drugs inhibit T-lymphocyte activation by interfering with interleukin-2 production. Cyclosporine or tacrolimus are typically continued for at least 6 mo posttransplant, during which time blood levels and renal and hepatic function are monitored to avoid drug toxicity. Mycophenolate mofetil may be combined with cyclosporine in high-risk patients. It is converted to mycophenolic acid, which blocks inosine monophosphate dehydrogenase-mediated guanosine nucleoside synthesis, thus inhibiting the proliferation of B- and T-lymphocytes. Intravenous immunoglobulin can be used to prevent CMV infection but it also decreases the risk of GVHD. It usually is infused weekly at doses of 0.5 g/kg until 100 d posttransplant. Glucocorticoids may be used to prevent GVHD in high-risk patients but this treatment does not improve survival. Depletion of T-lymphocytes from the graft effectively diminishes the risk of death due to acute GVHD, but this benefit is offset by an increased risk of death from disease relapse, as a result of a loss of the GVL effect, and from a higher incidence of graft rejection.

Treatment of acute GVHD consists primarily of glucocorticoid administration. Initially, 1–2 mg/kg/d of methylprednisolone, or its equivalent, is given intravenously. If there is no response or the acute GVHD is severe, much higher methylprednisolone doses, up to 1 gm/d for 3 d, may be administered. When gut GVHD is present, cyclosporine should be given intravenously because absorption is unreliable when given by mouth. Other immunosuppressive drugs with complementary mechanisms of action such as mycophenolate mofetil or sirolimus can be added to the immunsuppressive regimen. Antithymocyte globulin can be used (15–20 mg/kg/d for 4–5 d) for severe acute GVHD, but its impact on outcome has not been studied in a randomized, controlled trial. Symptomatic treatment for severe diarrhea should be instituted only after potential infectious etiologies (enteric pathogens, parasites, or *Clostridium difficile*) have been excluded. Thereafter, tincture of opium frequently is useful in reducing the volume of diarrhea. The somatostatin analog, octreotide acetate, beginning at 200 µg/d i.v. in two to four divided doses may be useful in some patients. Limited clinical data suggest that ursodeoxycholic acid 10–15 mg/kg/d may be useful in treating GVHD involving the liver. Isolated severe skin GVHD can be treated with topical steroids.

Chronic GVHD is generally less responsive to immunosuppressive medications than the acute form of the disease. The value of glucocorticoids for the treatment of chronic GVHD is unproven and they increase the risk of infection in this susceptible population. Many treatments have been tried, but none are consistently effective.

12. POSTTRANSPLANT PNEUMONIA

The profound immunosuppression of patients undergoing SCT, especially recipients of allogeneic and unrelated stem cells, places them at risk of developing pneumonia as a result of a wide variety of pathogens. Many of these organisms usually cause self-limited or mild disease in immunocompetent individuals. The large number of potential pathogens makes the choice of empiric therapy difficult, and rapid disease progression can occur when inadequate treatment is rendered. Therefore, establishment of a specific etiological diagnosis often is critical in the management of posttransplant pneumonia.

The approach to a patient with a posttransplant pneumonia depends on the clinical setting. Patients who are noted to have a localized pneumonia prior to receiving antibiotics may be adequately treated with empiric broad-spectrum antibiotics (Table 2) after appropriate sputum and blood cultures have been obtained. However, patients who develop a diffuse or interstitial pneumonia, or those who develop pneumonia while receiving broad-spectrum antibiotics should be evaluated by bronchoscopy. Bronchoalveolar lavage and transbronchial biopsy should be performed. Specimens should be sent for appropriate diagnostic studies, some of which are listed in Table 5. While awaiting the test results, consideration should be given to treating patients empirically for all possible infectious entities. Rapid clinical deterioration often can occur in the absence of appropriate therapy. Once the results of the diagnostic studies are available, the antimicrobial regimen can be simplified. If the bronchoscopic studies are nondiagnostic and the pneumonia is progressing in spite of empiric therapy, thoracoscopic or open lung biopsy should be considered.

Prophylaxis against *P. carinii* should be administered to all recipients of allogeneic or unrelated stem cell transplants, as outlined in "Prevention and Treatment of Posttransplant Infections." This infection rarely occurs in patients who receive appropriate prophylaxis. Treatment of *P. pneumonia* consists of TMP/SMX at 15–20 mg/kg/d i.v. (of TMP) divided into three to four doses. Patients allergic to sulfa drugs can receive pentamidine 4 mg/kg/d i.v.

Aspergillus spp. are the most common fungal cause of invasive pulmonary infections. Voriconazole and amphotericin B are equally effective at treating pulmonary aspergillosis, but voriconazole does not cause renal insufficiency and is better tolerated. Voriconazole is administered intravenously as a loading dose of 6 mg/kg every 12 h for the first 24 h, then 4 mg/kg every 12 h. Amphotericin B is given intravenously at a dose of 1 mg/kg/d i.v. for adults and 2 mg/kg/d for children. Liposomal amphotericin B can be considered for patients who develop renal insufficiency. Caspofungin can effectively treat some cases of refractory

Table 5
Causes of Pneumonia After Stem Cell Transplantation

Etiological agents	Diagnostic tests
Bacterial	
Legionella species	DFA, urine RIA, culture
Mycobacteria species	Acid fast stain, culture
Nocardia species	Acid fast stain, culture
Routine bacterial pathogens	Gram stain, bacterial culture
Fungal	
Pneumocystis carinii	DFA
Aspergillus spp.	Fungal stain, culture
Candida spp.	Fungal stain, culture
Coccidioides immitis	Fungal stain, culture
Histoplasma capsulatum	Fungal stain, culture
Cryptococcus neoformans	Fungal stain, culture
Mucor, Rhizopus, or *Fusarium* spp.	Fungal stain, culture
Viral	
Cytomegalovirus	Q-PCR, culture, histopathology
Herpes simplex virus	DFA, culture
Varicella zoster virus	DFA, culture
Adenovirus	IFA, culture
Respiratory syncytial virus	DFA, culture
Influenza viruses	IFA, culture
Parainfluenza	IFA, culture
Other organisms	
Mycoplasma pneumoniae	PCR, culture, serologies
Chlamydia pneumoniae	DFA, culture
Diffuse alveolar hemorrhage	
Therapy-related toxicity	
Conditioning chemotherapy	Diagnoses of exclusion
Carmustine	
Cyclophosphamide	
Melphalan	
Radiation therapy	
Recurrent malignancy (lymphangitic)	Histopathology

RIA, radioimmunoassay; DFA, direct fluorescent antibody; IFA, indirect fluorescent assay; Q-PCR, quantitative PCR.

aspergillosis infection, but it has not been compared with voriconazole or amphotericin B as initial therapy. It is administered intravenously as a 70 mg dose on the first day, followed by 50 mg daily.

CMV pneumonia can be effectively prevented in seropositive allogeneic and unrelated SCT patients with prophylactic gancyclovir, as described in "Prevention and Treatment of Posttransplant Infections." Seronegative patients should receive only CMV-negative blood products to prevent infection. CMV pneumonia rarely occurs in recipients of autologous SCT. Treatment requires the administration of gancyclovir 2.5 mg/kg every 8 h for 20 d and intravenous immunoglobulin 0.5 g/kg every other day for 10 doses.

HSV or *V. zoster* pneumonia is treated with acyclovir 10–12 mg/kg every 8 h. Dose reduction may be required if renal insufficiency is present.

Pneumonia caused by common viral pathogens including adenovirus, influenza, parainfluenza, and respiratory syncytial virus (RSV) can be fatal in recipients of SCT. Therefore, family members or health care workers who have any viral illness should not be permitted in the rooms of patients undergoing SCT. No therapy appears to be effective against these viruses once pneumonia is diagnosed. The value of surveillance cultures or prophylactic antiviral therapy have not been adequately studied in the transplant population. Recently, RSV infection of the upper respiratory tract detected by surveillance culture was effectively treated with aerosolized ribavirin 20 mg/mL administered 18 h/d with intravenous immunoglobulin 0.5 g/kg every other day. Established RSV pneumonia was not successfully treated with this regimen. Ribavirin is teratogenic, an irritant, and is difficult to administer safely. Therefore, aerosolized ribavirin should only be used in hospitals that have established adequate safety practices to protect health care workers from toxicity of the drug. A new intravenous formulation of ribavirin may improve its safety profile.

Pneumonia due to therapy-related toxicity typically responds to glucocorticoid administration. Diffuse alveolar hemorrhage that occurs following autologous SCT also may be therapy-related and requires prompt treatment with glucocorticoids. An infectious etiology should be carefully excluded prior to initiating treatment for either of these problems.

13. HEPATIC VENO-OCCLUSIVE DISEASE

Hepatic veno-occlusive disease (VOD) is a disorder characterized by hyperbilirubinemia, hepatomegaly, and ascites that results from blockage of hepatic venules. It is caused by vascular endothelial injury from conditioning chemotherapy and/or radiation. The best-established risk factor is antecedent liver disease or hepatitis. Specific conditioning regimens have not been associated with increased risk of VOD but prior treatment with high-dose chemotherapy does predispose to the development of VOD. The clinical criteria used to diagnose this disorder include the presence of two of the following within 30 d of transplant: jaundice (directed bilirubin >2 mg/dL), tender hepatomegaly, and ascites or unexplained weight gain of more than 5%. Unfortunately, these criteria are not specific and there are no clinical characteristics of VOD that readily distinguish it from other causes of posttransplant jaundice. The differential diagnosis of VOD includes congestive heart failure, cholestasis from drugs or biliary tract disease, hepatitis from infection or drugs, and in allogeneic transplant patients, GVHD.

Evaluation of suspected VOD includes a review of the medications that the patient is receiving to identify any that cause cholestasis or hepatitis. Physical examination is performed to exclude congestive heart failure as an etiology. Blood is drawn for hepatitis serologies if clinically indicated. Ultrasonography is used to exclude obstruction of the biliary tree and to evaluate venous flow in the liver. Transjugular liver biopsy may be required to exclude GVHD. The histopathology of VOD may reveal subintimal thickening of the hepatic venules with lumenal occlusion by reticulum or collagen, but not by thrombus. Centrilobular hepatocyte necrosis also may be present in VOD.

Prophylaxis against VOD with heparin has not been demonstrated conclusively to reduce the risk of this complication, and has been associated with significant risk of bleeding. No treatment has been clearly proven to improve the outcome of patients with established VOD. Recombinant human tissue plasminogen activator has been reported to reverse the course of VOD in some patients, but controlled, randomized clinical trials have not been performed. Supportive care measures remain the standard of care including the management of fluid overload, coagulopathy, and encephalopathy. Patients with advanced liver failure occasionally may be candidates for orthotopic liver transplantation.

14. THROMBOTIC MICROANGIOPATHY

Thrombotic microangiopathy (TM; thrombotic thrombocytopenic purpura or hemolytic uremic syndrome) can occur following either autologous or allogeneic SCT. A number of factors may be important in the pathogenesis of the microvascular injury underlying this disorder including the toxicities of the conditioning regimen and the immunosuppressive drugs administered posttransplant. The use of cyclosporine is associated with the development of this disorder, and GVHD prophylaxis with a combination of cyclosporine, methotrexate, and glucocorticoids may convey a higher risk. TM typically presents as a progressive decline in the hemoglobin and platelet count between 1 and 6 mo posttransplant. Renal insufficiency, neurological symptoms, or fever also may be present. The diagnosis is supported by the presence of intrascular hemolysis (elevated reticulocyte count, serum lactate dehydrogenase, and indirect bilirubin levels; decreased haptoglobin; positive urine hemosiderin) and the presence of fragmented erythrocytes on the peripheral smear. In patients who present with diarrhea and TM, stool should be studied for the presence of *Escherichia coli* strain O157:H7

Discontinuing or markedly reducing the cyclosporine dose may lead to improvement in some recipients of allogeneic transplant. Substitution of other immunosuppressive agents for cyclosporine may be useful, but this approach has not been adequately evaluated. Therapeutic plasma exchange or passage of patient serum through a staphylococcal protein A column using an apheresis machine has been reported to benefit some patients, but these measures are infrequently effective. Inexorable progression of renal failure, refractory thrombocytopenia, and multi-organ system failure are common sequelae.

SUGGESTED READING

Barker JN, Wagner JE. Umbilical cord blood transplantation: current practice and future innovations. *Crit Rev Oncol Hematol* 2003;48:35–43.

Devine SM, Adkins DR, Khoury H, et al. Recent advances in allogeneic hematopoietic stem-cell transplantation. *J Lab Clin Med* 2003;141:7–32.

Karanes C, Confer D, Walker T, et al. Unrelated donor stem cell transplantation: the role of the National Marrow Donor Program. *Oncology* 2003;8:1036–1167.

Laughlin MJ, Eapen M, Rubinstein P, et al. Outcomes after transplantation of cord blood or bone marrow from unrelated donors in adults with leukemia. *N Engl J Med* 2004;351:2265–2275.

Rocha V, Labopin M, Sanz G, et al. Acute Leukemia Working Party of European Blood and Marrow Transplant Group; Eurocord-Netcord Registry. Transplants of umbilical-cord blood or bone marrow from unrelated donors in adults with acute leukemia. *N Engl J Med* 2004;351:2276–2285.

Slavin S, Morecki S, Weiss L, Shapira MY, Resnick I, Or R. Nonmyeloablative stem cell transplantation: reduced-intensity conditioning for cancer immunotherapy—from bench to patient bedside. *Semin Oncol* 2004;31:4–21.

5 Anemias

General Considerations and Microcytic
and Megaloblastic Anemias

Reinhold Munker, MD

CONTENTS

INTRODUCTION
ANEMIAS DUE TO ACUTE BLEEDING
ANEMIAS DUE TO CHRONIC BLOOD LOSS
IRON DEFICIENCY ANEMIA
ANEMIAS OF CHRONIC DISEASES AND OTHER TYPES
    OF ANEMIAS
MEGALOBLASTIC ANEMIAS
SUGGESTED READING

1. INTRODUCTION

Anemias can be secondary to a primary blood disorder (e.g., stem cell failure in aplastic anemia, malignant transformation of stem cells in acute leukemias), but more often, anemias are secondary to other diseases or conditions (e.g., acute blood loss after trauma, chronic blood loss in menstruating women, inadequate nutrition, chronic autoimmune conditions, chronic infections, and many other disorders). An anemia is normally defined as a decrease of hemoglobin below 13.5 g/dL in males and 11.5 g/dL in females. Between the age of 6 mo and puberty, the normal hemoglobin concentration is somewhat lower (between 11 and 15 g/dL). A reduction of the hemoglobin value is often accompanied by changes in other red cell parameters (e.g., microcytic and hypochromic in iron deficiency anemia, macrocytic in vitamin B_{12} deficiency and other conditions). The normal red cell values in adults are shown in Table 1.

From: *Contemporary Hematology: Modern Hematology, Second Edition*
Edited by: R. Munker, E. Hiller, J. Glass, and R. Paquette © Humana Press Inc., Totowa, NJ

Table 1
Normal Adult Red Cell Values

	Males	Females
Hemoglobin concentration	13.5–17.5 g/dL	11.5–15.5 g/dL
Hematocrit (%)	40–52	36–48
Red cell number	4.5–6.5 ($\times 10^{12}$/L)	3.9–5.6 ($\times 10^{12}$/L)
Mean cell hemoglobin (pg)	27–34	
Mean cell volume (fL)	80–95	
Mean cell hemoglobin concentration (MCHC)	30–35	

Anemias are frequently associated with an abnormal red cell morphology. A glossary of the commonly encountered changes in red cell morphology is given in Table 2. Some of these changes are shown in Fig. 5.1 . The major categories of anemias and their clinical manifestations are described in Table 3. In this chapter, the major categories of microcytic, megaloblastic, and other common types of anemias are described, whereas in Chapter 6, the inherited and acquired hemolytic anemias are discussed.

2. ANEMIAS DUE TO ACUTE BLEEDING

Any major bleeding, internal or external, leads to an anemia. First, the patient is hypovolemic and develops tachycardia, then, after several hours, the internal plasma pool or the volume substitution leads to a dilution of the red cell concentration. Acute blood loss is seen in many surgical conditions: trauma, bleeding esophageal varices, perforated ulcers, or aneurysmal ruptures. The treatment of these conditions is urgent (e.g., surgical or endoscopic stoppage of the bleeding, volume substitution, treatment, and prevention of shock). The indication for blood transfusion should be individualized. A commonly accepted threshold below which red cell transfusions are given is a hemoglobin concentration of 8 g/dL. Patients who are adapted to low hemoglobin concentrations may need a transfusion only at a lower hemoglobin value; patients who have had an acute blood loss and are in a critical cardiovascular condition may already need transfusions at hemoglobin values of 9 or 10 g/dL.

3. ANEMIAS DUE TO CHRONIC BLOOD LOSS

Minor but chronic blood loss in the gastrointestinal tract often leads to anemia. Reasons for the blood loss may be cancer in the gastrointestinal tract or benign conditions like hiatal hernias, hemorrhoids, angiodysplasia, or peptic ulcer disease. Hereditary conditions like telangiectasia or a coagulation factor deficiency

Table 2
Abnormalities in Red Cell Morphology and Their Associated Clinical Manifestations

Term	Abnormality	Associated conditions
Acanthocytosis	Irregular membrane	A-β-lipoproteinemia, liver cirrhosis, pancreatitis
Anisocytosis	Frequent variations in size	Nonspecific, iron deficiency, and other anemias
Burr cells	Cells with many short, spiked projections	Renal failure, liver disease, hemolytic-uremic syndrome (HUS), or thrombotic thrombocytopenic purpura (TTP)
Dimorphic red	Distinct population of blood cells	Mixed iron and vitamin B_{12} small and larger cell deficiency, following transfusion
Elliptocytosis	Elliptoid form	Hereditary elliptocytosis, other conditions
Heinz bodies	Hemoglobin precipitates due to oxidation (seen with methylene blue stain)	G6PD deficiency hemoglobin-pathies, thalassemias
Hypochromasia	Poorly hemoglobinized	Iron deficiency anemia, thalassemias, other conditions
Macrocytosis	Cells larger than usual	Liver disease, MDS, compensated hemolysis, vitamin B_{12} or folate deficiency, other conditions
Microcytosis	Cells smaller than usual	Iron deficiency, thalassemias, other conditions
Poikilocytosis	Increased variability in cell shape	Severe iron deficiency, other conditions
Schistocytes	Fragmented red cells	Trauma, burns, HUS, or TTP
Target cells	Target-like cells	Iron deficiency, liver disease, thalassemias, and other hemoglobin disorders

MDS, myelodysplastic syndrome.

may also be responsible. At a certain point, chronic blood loss results in iron deficiency and an iron deficiency anemia results (*see* "Iron Deficiency Anemia").

It is imperative to identify the source of blood loss in all patients with iron deficiency. The treatment depends on the cause (e.g., resecting a colon cancer, treating a hemorrhagic gastritis, treating hemorrhoids). An iron substitution may help to compensate the iron deficiency and thereby hasten the recovery of eryth-

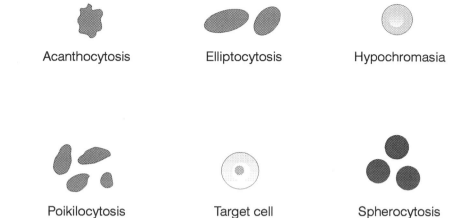

Fig. 5.1. Common changes in red cell morphology.

Table 3
Major Types of Anemias and Their Laboratory Findings[a]

Type of anemia	Laboratory findings
Acute bleeding anemia	Initially, the hemoglobin does not reflect the amount of blood lost
Iron deficiency anemia	Low serum iron with increased total iron-binding capacity, low ferritin.
Anemias of chronic disease	Low serum iron and total iron-binding capacity, ferritin usually not reduced.
Anemias of other diseases: renal insufficiency, hepatic cirrhosis, and hypothyroidism, malnutrition, and others	Serum erythropoietin is inappropriately low in renal insufficiency, TSH is elevated in hypothyroidism.
Megaloblastic anemias	Low serum vitamin B_{12}, increased urinary methylmalonic acid and serum homocysteine levels in vitamin B_{12} deficiency; low serum folic acid level in folate deficiency.
Hemolytic anemias (acute, chronic, congenital, and acquired forms)	Increased reticulocyte count, unconjugated bilirubin, LDH

[a]Anemias associated with other hematological disease entities are not considered here.

Table 4
Etiology of Chronic Blood Loss

Gastrointestinal bleeding	Esophageal varices
	Hiatal hernia
	Erosive gastritis (spontaneous, secondary to aspirin)
	Duodenal ulcer, gastric ulcer
	Colon cancer, gastric cancer
	Ulcerative colitis, Crohn's disease, Coeliac disease, hemorrhoids, angiodysplasia
	Hookworm infestation
	Hereditary hemorrhagic telangiectasia
Urogenital bleeding	Renal cell cancer, bladder cancer
	Gynecological tumors
	Kidney stones
	Increased menstrual blood loss
Other causes	Frequent blood donations

ropoiesis. Blood transfusions are rarely necessary in anemias of chronic blood loss. The major causes of chronic blood loss are described in Table 4. In order to investigate an iron deficiency anemia in an adult, a colonoscopy and, if that is negative, a gastroduodenoscopy should be performed.

4. IRON DEFICIENCY ANEMIA

Iron deficiency is the end result of an iron loss in excess of iron absorption. There are three stages of iron deficiency:

1. The iron stores are reduced but are still sufficient for erythropoiesis.
2. The iron stores are depleted; erythropoiesis is reduced.
3. Manifest iron deficiency anemia has developed (erythropoiesis reduced; hemoglobin has decreased to less than normal).

On a worldwide basis, iron deficiency is among the most frequent causes of anemia. Persons with an increased iron demand, such as pregnant or menstruating women, or children in the stages of growth and development, are the first to develop an iron deficiency anemia. Children fed with cow's milk often develop an iron deficiency because of the low iron content of this milk. In adults, iron deficiency is most often due to blood loss from the gastrointestinal or urogenital tract.

4.1. Pathophysiology

The normal body iron content is 3–5 g. This quantity is contained in hemoglobin, myoglobin, iron stores, and in the reticuloendothelial system (RES); a small amount is contained in serum as ferritin. Iron absorption and iron loss are normally kept constant during adult life. The daily iron demand is 1.3 mg for men and 1.8 mg for women (during the years of menstruation). Adolescents and pregnant women need more iron. Generally, the Western diet contains sufficient iron to compensate for the daily iron losses. Iron resorption takes place mainly in the duodenum and, to some extent, in the jejunum. The mucosal cells regulate intestinal iron absorption. Iron is either directly absorbed and transferred into the circulating blood or stored in the mucosal cells as ferritin. If serum iron is low, iron uptake from the gastrointestinal tract is rapid; if serum iron is elevated or normal, more iron is retained in the mucosal cells. The iron transport from blood to different sites of iron utilization or storage is then performed by transferrin, a specialized transport protein of the β-globulin fraction of human serum. One molecule of transferrin can bind two iron atoms. Normally, about 30% of the total iron-binding capacity is saturated with iron. In the next step, the transferring iron complex is bound to transferrin receptors on the surface of erythroblasts and other cells. Nonutilized iron is then either transported to different storage tissues and accumulated as ferritin or hemosiderin, or excreted via the kidneys. The total iron storage pool is about 800 mg in men and 400 mg in women.

When a negative iron balance occurs, iron resorption first increases from the normal value of 5–10% to a maximum of 20%. If the iron stores are completely exhausted, as can be recognized by a decrease of the serum iron and ferritin and an increase in transferrin, then the erythropoiesis becomes defective. Abnormally small, poorly hemoglobinized (hypochromic) red blood cells are synthesized. After a few weeks, the total hemoglobin concentration decreases (manifest iron deficiency anemia). If the iron deficiency is more severe, the synthesis of other iron-dependent proteins (e.g., cytochromes, myoglobin, flavoproteins) is also impaired.

4.2. Clinical Signs and Diagnosis

The symptoms of iron deficiency anemia depend on its severity. Patients are easily fatigued, may have dyspnea on exertion and have pale skin and pale mucous membranes. An atrophic glossitis, spoon nails (koilonychia), or an angular stomatitis develop. In very severe cases, the patients have dysphagia due to esophageal webs (Plummer-Vinson syndrome). Some patients also develop atrophic gastritis.

An early event in iron deficiency is a decrease in serum ferritin, the major iron storage protein. Normal serum concentration of ferritin is 40–350 ng/mL in men and 20–150 ng/mL in women. The serum values reflect the body iron stores in the reticuloendothelial system. The next laboratory sign of iron deficiency to develop is a decrease in the hemoglobin concentration. At this point, the number of red blood cells can still be normal. If the iron deficiency persists, abnormalities of red cell morphology can be recognized (e.g., poikilocytosis, anisocytosis, hypochromasia). The reticulocytes are generally decreased and the red cell indices (e.g., mean corpuscular volume [MCV], mean corpuscular hemoglobin [MCH], mean corpuscular hemoglobin concentration [MCHC]) are below normal. The bone marrow morphology shows nonspecific changes. The stainable iron, usually seen in bone marrow macrophages after staining with Prussian blue, is decreased or absent. In iron deficiency, the transport protein transferrin is usually increased. The serum iron concentration is generally low, but is not a reliable indicator of the degree of iron deficiency. The transferrin saturation (serum/total iron-binding capacity) is typically less than 10%.

A new parameter for estimating iron deficiency is the measurement of the serum transferrin receptors. In contrast to ferritin, the levels of serum transferrin receptors are usually not influenced by acute or chronic infections. The normal values (as measured by ELISA) are 4–9 µg/L. In iron deficiency, the levels of serum transferrin receptors increase proportionally to the degree of iron deficiency. Increased values, however, are also seen in some myeloproliferative syndromes and anemias with proliferation of the erythroid series.

Early iron deficiency can also be diagnosed by measuring the red blood cell protoporphyrin. The normal value is approx 30 µg/dL of red cells. In iron deficiency, the value increases to greater than 100 µg/dL. Increased levels are also found in lead poisoning and some sideroblastic anemias and porphyrias.

4.3. Treatment

The first step is to identify and treat the underlying cause of the iron deficiency. It is especially important that an underlying malignancy is not overlooked. The standard treatment of iron deficiency is oral ferrous sulfate. One tablet (100 mg, containing 67 mg as ferrous iron) is given before meals and should be continued until the iron deficiency is corrected and the iron stores are replenished (3–4 mo in severe iron deficiency). In severe cases, two or three tablets daily can be given. Ferrous fumarate and ferrous gluconate is equivalent to ferrous sulfate. Most iron preparations are also available as elixir. An increase in reticulocytes should be seen 7–10 d after the iron substitution is begun if the iron is being adequately absorbed. If gastrointestinal side effects occur (e.g., vomiting, abdominal cramps, nausea), iron can be given together with meals or a different formulation can he used, but this decreases the resorption and slows the effect of treatment. A prophylactic iron treatment should he given during pregnancy or for premature newborns. Parenteral iron should only be given when oral iron is not effective or cannot be tolerated. Parenteral iron can be given as bolus injections, as an intravenous infusion, or as an intramuscular injection. For the parenteral substitution, ferric iron (iron-dextran or iron-sorbitol citrate) is used. The amount of iron dextran required can be calculated as follows: iron needed (mg) = [(15–hematocrit [HCT]) × wt lbs)] + 100. The dose range for one injection or infusion is 500–1500 mg. When given by intravenous infusion, the iron preparation should be diluted in 250 mL of 0.9% sodium chloride. A test dose of 0.5 mL should be infused over 1 min; then, if no reaction occurs, the remainder should be given over 30–60 min. Parenteral iron is preferable when gastritis or a duodenal ulcer leads to pronounced side effects or if a severe malabsorption precludes the resorption. Parenteral iron always carries the risk of a hypersensitivity reaction and therefore should be given under close medical supervision. Most cases can and should be managed with oral iron.

5. ANEMIAS OF CHRONIC DISEASES AND OTHER TYPES OF ANEMIAS

5.1. Anemias of Chronic Diseases

A slight anemia (hemoglobin around 9–11 g/dL) is found associated with many chronic infections, rheumatoid disorders, disseminated tumors, lymphomas, hepatitis C, malaria, and other disorders. For the most part, anemias of chronic diseases are not due to iron deficiency, but to iron sequestered in the RES. Inflammatory cytokines like interferon-β and tumor necrosis factor (TNF)-α upregulate the expression of DMT1 with an increased uptake of iron into activated macrophages. The iron sequestration was explained in the past by the increased production of lactoferrin by neutrophils, which then competes with transferrin for iron binding. Iron bound to lactoferrin cannot be utilized by red cell precursors and is instead taken up by the RES. More recently, it was discovered that hepcidin is the mediator of the anemia of chronic diseases. Hepcidin is an acute phase protein induced in liver cells by lipopolysaccharide and interleukin-6 but downregulated by TNF-α. Hepcidin diverts iron traffic through decreased duodenal absorption of iron and the blocking of iron release from macrophages. Further pathomechanisms of the anemias of chronic disease (which are also termed anemias of inflammation) are the impaired proliferation of erythroid progenitor cells and a blunted response to erythropoietin. The anemia of chronic disorders is in general only slowly progressive. The red cell indices are normochromic or slightly hypochromic. If the degree of anemia is severe, a search for other causes should be made. The anemia of chronic disorders has a low serum iron and a normal or elevated (in active inflammation) ferritin. The serum transferrin receptors are normal. Erythropoietin levels tend to be low (if the baseline of the patient's hemoglobin is less than 10 g/dL). The anemia of chronic diseases is best treated by treating the underlying disease. In severe or symptomatic anemia, a blood transfusion is indicated. If the serum ferritin is less than 30 ng/mL, a search for the possible causes of iron deficiency, including screening for blood loss, should be made. More recent studies showed that a cautious treatment of the anemia of chronic diseases with erythropoietin improves the patient's performance status similarly to the anemia of kidney diseases. An overcorrection (hemoglobin >11–12 g/dL) should be avoided. An iron supplementation should be given if a true iron deficiency is documented or if an insufficient response to erythropoietin is observed. In the future, hepcidin antagonists will be developed to overcome the retention of iron within the RES.

5.2. Anemias Due to Malnutrition

Malnourished children or adults in different parts of the world are often anemic. Severe protein malnourishment (kwashiorkor) is always associated with anemia. This anemia is multifactorial (iron, folic acid, protein, dilutional anemia). Treatment of severe malnutrition should be started parenterally with the substitution of protein, electrolytes, iron, and vitamins.

5.3. Anemias Due to Liver Diseases

Chronic liver disease often causes a macrocytic anemia. Biological factors are folate deficiency, chronic blood loss, alcohol-induced changes, hemolysis, and hypersplenism. The red cells sometimes have the morphology of target cells (because of increased cholesterol in the cell membrane). A rare complication of alcoholic liver disease is Zieve's syndrome, in which acute hemolysis is associated with hyperlipidemia and alcoholic hepatitis. Morphologically, acanthocytes are found in the blood smear.

5.4. Anemia of Pregnancy

Starting with the sixth week of pregnancy, a woman's plasma volume increases and reaches a maximum around the 24th week. The red cell mass does not increase proportionally. The end result in many pregnant women is a dilutional anemia. The hemoglobin stabilizes at around 11 g/dL, the hematocrit between 32 and 34%, and the red cells are normochromic. If the hemoglobin is lower, further causes of anemia are most likely present (e.g., a manifest iron deficiency).

5.5. Anemia of Renal Failure

Virtually all patients with chronic renal failure develop an anemia. The anemia is particularly severe in some renal disorders (e.g., analgesic kidney disease). The anemia of renal failure is normochromic and normocytic with low reticulocytes. The major cause of renal anemias is an inadequate production of erythropoietin by the kidneys (see Chapter 2). Additional factors that also contribute to the anemia are a reduced red cell survival, direct toxic effects on erythropoiesis, blood losses during dialysis, infections, and increased aluminum levels in some patients. Patients with chronic renal failure who are not treated with erythropoi-etin have hematocrit values between 20 and 35%.

Severe or symptomatic cases of renal anemia should be treated with recom-binant erythropoietin. Erythropoietin can be given intravenously (after dialysis, three times weekly) or by subcutaneous injection. The recommended doses are between 50 and 150 U/kg. The aim of the erythropoietin treatment is to keep the hemoglobin level above 8 g/dL and to avoid transfusions. The optimum hemo-globin concentration is between 10 and 12 g/dL. Erythropoietin is contraindi-cated if the patient has uncontrolled hypertension, seizures, and problems of vascular access. Potential side effects of erythropoietin are an increase in blood pressure, a thrombotic tendency, and flu-like symptoms. An alternative to recom-binant erythropoietin is pegylated erythropoietin, which needs less frequent dosing (*see* Chapter 2).

5.6. Anemia of Endocrine Disorders

Many endocrine disorders are associated with a certain degree of anemia. Examples are hypopituitarism, Addison's syndrome, and thyroid disease. The anemias of endocrine disorders are, in general, normochromic and normocytic.

5.7. Thalassemia Minor

Individuals with thalassemia minor are asymptomatic and their anemia usu-ally is detected by a routine blood count. The red cells are microcytic, often leading to a misdiagnosis of iron deficiency. However, iron studies typically are normal. Thalassemias result from either a mutation of one β-globin gene or deletion of two α-globin genes. The diagnosis of the thalassemias is discussed in Chapter 6.

5.8. Sideroblastic Anemia

Idiopathic sideroblastic anemia can present with a microcytic, hypochromic anemia. The bone marrow biopsy is diagnostic: it reveals erythroid dysplasia and hyperplasia. Ringed sideroblasts comprise more than 20% of the erythroid series. It was recently recognized that a common pathogenetic mechanism in sideroblastic anemias is the abnormal iron deposition in mitochondria. Two major types of sideroblastic anemias can be distinguished: the rare hereditary sideroblastic anemias and the more common acquired forms, which may be secondary to drugs and toxins (ethanol, zinc, isoniazid, cycloserine) and can also be observed as part of some myelodysplastic syndromes (*see* Chapter 11). As causes of X-linked hereditary sideroblastic anemias, mutations of the ALAS-2 and hABC7 gene were identified. In other forms of hereditary sideroblastic anemias, deletions of mitochondrial DNA and mutations of the WFS1/wolframin gene were found. In some cases of acquired sideroblastic anemias (as part of myelodysplastic syndromes), point mutations of mitochondrial DNA could be identified. As for treatment, any potential toxin should be withdrawn. Some cases of congenital (and acquired) sideroblastic anemia respond to pyridoxine, which should be given (in responsive patients) at a dose of 50–200 mg daily.

5.9. Lead Poisoning

This disorder is usually seen in children who have eaten paint chips tainted with lead, but it also can be seen in adults who have occupational exposure. The clinical manifestations of lead poisoning may include abdominal pain, encephalopathy, peripheral neuropathy, gout, or a proximal renal tubular acidosis. The anemia or lead poisoning is more hypochromic than microcytic, with basophilic stippling of the red cells. There is frequently an element of hemolysis with reticulocytosis. Diagnosis is best made by finding increased free-erythrocyte-protoporphyrin levels, and elevated urinary coproporphyrin III and δ-amino-levulinic acid levels. Serum lead levels are a less sensitive indicator of tissue lead stores.

5.10. Pure Red Cell Aplasia

Pure red cell aplasia is characterized by an absence of erythroid precursors in the bone marrow. This condition can be congenital (Diamond-Blackfan anemia) or acquired. As pathogenesis, defects of progenitor cells and/or an autoimmune or toxic injury to erythroid progenitors have been proposed. In congenital cases of pure red anemia, some patients have mutations in hematopoietic stem cells. In other patients, abnormalities of apoptosis in the red cell precursors were described. Patients with Diamond-Blackfan anemia are treated symptomatically with blood transfusion. Some patients with Diamond-Blackfan anemia respond to steroids or other immunosuppressive agents and enter remission. In refractory patients, a bone marrow or stem cell transplantation may be indicated. An acquired form of pure red cell aplasia is caused by an infection with parvovirus B19 and is seen in advanced HIV infection or chronic hemolytic anemias (*see* Chapter 18). The chronic autoimmune form of pure red cell aplasia is often associated with auto-immune disorders or a T-cell lymphoma or thymoma. It is postulated that these cases are initiated by a T-cell response or antibodies against erythroid progenitor cells. A fraction of such patients respond to immunosuppression, chemotherapy, plasmapheresis, or thymectomy (in cases of thymoma). Pure red cell aplasia is a rare disease. More recently, in Europe an increased number of cases were observed in patients treated with a certain formulation of erythropoietin-α (serum-free, injected subcutaneously). This formulation of erythropoietin was subsequently withdrawn from the market. In most instances, neutralizing anti-bodies against erythropoietin could be demonstrated. It is thought the formulation used made erythropoietin more immunogenic.

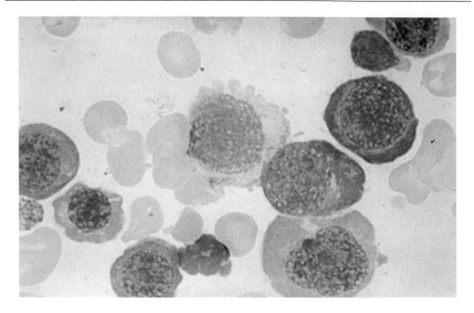

Fig. 5.2. Pernicious anemia (bone marrow aspirate with megaloblastic erythropoiesis, large erythroblasts with immature nuclei).

6. MEGALOBLASTIC ANEMIAS

The megaloblastic anemias are caused by a deficiency of vitamin B_{12} or folates, or by related conditions that lead to impaired DNA synthesis. Characteristically, the maturation of the nucleus in erythroblasts in the bone marrow is delayed as a result of defective DNA synthesis. This discordant maturation is generally termed "megaloblastic." The chromatin of megaloblasts is basophilic and appears lacy and irregular. Sometimes the chromatin is clumped and takes on a bizarre appearance. The proportion of erythropoiesis in the bone marrow is increased. Figure 5.2 demonstrates megaloblastic erythroblasts (*see also* Color Plate 1). The maturation defect in megaloblastic anemias can also be observed in myelopoiesis and megakaryocytes. The megakaryoctes and granulocytes are hypersegmented and the metamyelocytes and band forms are abnormally large. In addition to the anemia, defective maturation of hematopoietic precursor cells leads to leuko- and thrombocytopenia.

6.1. Physiology of Vitamin B_{12}

This vitamin consists of a corrin ring with a cobalt atom in its center attached to a nucleotide portion. Such compounds are termed cobalamins. The pharmacological preparations of vitamin B_{12} (cyanocobalamin and hydroxocobalamin) are biologically inactive. The active forms that are generated by enzymatic synthesis are adenosylcobalamin and methylcobalamin. Adenosyl-cobalamin is the tissue form of vitamin B_{12}, whereas methylcobalamin circulates in blood. The daily requirement for vitamin B_{12}, is about 1–2 μg in adults. A normal diet provides a large excess of vitamin B_{12}. The molecule is liberated in the stomach where it binds to the glycoprotein "intrinsic factor" which is derived from the gastric mucosa. The complex intrinsic factor-vitamin B_{12} is then resorbed in the distal ileum. After resorption, the vitamin dissociates again and then binds to the transport protein transcobalamin (TC) II before entering the enterohepatic circulation. Another transport protein, TCI, is produced by granulocytes. The main storage site of vitamin B_{12} is the liver (2–3 mg, a 1000-fold excess of the daily requirement). Vitamin B_{12} is essential for several enzyme systems:

1. Adenosylcobalamin is a coenzyme involved in the conversion of methyl-malonyl-coenzyme A (CoA) to succinyl CoA,
2. The synthesis of methionine from homocysteine, and
3. The synthesis of S-adenosyl methionine

6.2. Physiology of Folate (Pteroyl Glutamic Acid)

Folic acid is the parent compound of folates that consists of pteridine, p-amino benzoic acid, and glutamic acid. Biologically, tetrahydrofolic acid is the most important compound. The major intracellular compounds are folate polyglutamates, which have additional glutamate moieties attached. Folates are needed in many biochemical reactions (e.g., synthesis of DNA, purines, and thymine) and are essential for all proliferating cells, including hematopoietic cells. Folates are present as polyglutamates in many foods, especially greens, yeast, and liver, but are easily destroyed by cooking. The daily requirement of folates is about 150 μg. Folates are resorbed in the upper jejunum as monoglutamates. The body stores of folates are sufficient for several months.

6.3. Pernicious Anemia

Pernicious anemia is an autoimmune disorder in which antibodies against parietal cells and/or intrinsic factors can be demonstrated. Pernicious anemia is more common in males than in females and has an age peak around 60 yr. Pernicious anemia is often associated with other autoimmune disorders. The gastric mucosa is atrophic and the secretion of intrinsic factor is defective. The earliest gastric lesion in patients with pernicious anemia is an inflammatory infiltrate in the submucosa. Typically, patients with autoimmune pernicious anemia have a type A gastritis, which involves the fundus but spares the antrum.

Autoantibodies to parietal cells and to intrinsic factor are present in the serum and in gastric secretions. The molecular target of the parietal cell antibodies is

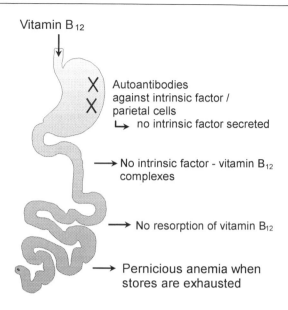

Vitamin B$_{12}$

Autoantibodies
against intrinsic factor /
parietal cells
↳ no intrinsic factor secreted

→ No intrinsic factor - vitamin B$_{12}$
complexes

→ No resorption of vitamin B$_{12}$

→ Pernicious anemia when
stores are exhausted

Fig. 5.3. Pernicious anemia due to vitamin B$_{12}$ deficiency; pathophysiology.

the H$^+$/K$^+$- ATPase in parietal cells that causes gastric atrophy and achlorhydria. Parietal cell antibodies can he found in the serum of approx 90% of patients with pernicious anemia. About 30% of first-degree relatives (who do not have pernicious anemia) also have parietal cell antibodies, whereas low titers of these antibodies are found in only 2–8% of the normal population. Antibodies to intrinsic factor are found in 50–60% of patients with pernicious anemia. Type I autoantibodies block the binding of vitamin B$_{12}$ to intrinsic factor, whereas type II autoantibodies (present in 35–40% of the patients) bind to a different epitope of intrinsic factor.

The pathogenesis of autoimmune pernicious anemia is a selective malabsorption of vitamin B$_{12}$. Development of pernicious anemia is described in schematic form in Fig. 5.3. The vitamin deficiency leads to an ineffective erythropoiesis with megaloblastic features. Lack of vitamin B$_{12}$ is also the cause of disturbances in myelopoiesis, megakaryocyte maturation, and further neurological and mucocutaneous symptoms. It is generally easy to diagnose pernicious anemia. The anemia is macrocytic and the reticulocyte count is low in relation to the degree of anemia. The bone marrow is usually hypercellular, with a decrease of the myeloid/erythroid cell ratio due to a marked increase in cells of the erythroid series. The erythropoiesis shows prominent megaloblastic features. Because of the defective erythropoiesis, laboratory findings of hemolysis are observed (e.g., raised LDH, raised unconjugated bilirubin). Serum levels of vitamin B$_{12}$ are low or very low. Because vitamin B_{12} is required for the conversion of methylmalonyl CoA to succinyl CoA, deficiency of this coenzyme results in increased urinary excretion of methylmalonic acid. Similarly, the conversion of homocysteine to methionine requires vitamin B_{12}; serum homocysteine levels are elevated in vitamin B_{12} deficiency. Both of these tests may be more sensitive indicators of vitamin B_{12} deficiency than measurement of serum vitamin B_{12} levels. An absorption test (Schilling test) is performed with radioactively labeled vitamin B_{12}. An unlabeled dose is given first by intramuscular injection to saturate the vitamin B_{12}-binding sites, and then a radioactively labeled dose is given by mouth. The urine is collected for 24 h to determine if the oral vitamin B_{12} was absorbed. If the absorption is normal, 10–20% of the ingested vitamin B_{12} can be found in the urine. A pathological Schilling test (<3% of tracer found) can be normalized when intrinsic factor is given orally together with vitamin B_{12}. A pathological Schilling test should normalize when it is repeated with the simultaneous oral administration of a purified intrinsic factor.

The onset of pernicious anemia is insidious in most cases. Patients experience fatigue and shortness of breath on exertion and are pale and mildly icteric. The tongue is often beefy red and painful (Hunter's glossitis). Many patients have angular stomatitis, some have an esophagitis with dysphagia. Today, in many cases, an early diagnosis of vitamin B_{12} deficiency is made when asymptomatic patients have a blood count and their vitamin B_{12} levels are determined for unrelated reasons.

Severe vitamin B_{12} deficiency may cause a progressive neuropathy with damage to the peripheral sensory nerves and the posterior and lateral columns (subacute combined degeneration of the cord). If the disease is not treated, the lesions will progress from demyelination to axonal degeneration and eventually neuronal death. Common symptoms are an impaired sense of vibration, paresthesias, and numbness. The patients experience difficulty in walking (positive Romberg's sign). Neuropathologically, the lesions involve both the posterior column and the lateral column. The lesion of the lateral column manifests as limb weakness, spasticity, and extensor plantar responses. Many patients develop mild personality defects or memory loss, and some patients develop frank psychosis. Occasionally the neurological symptoms of vitamin B_{12} deficiency occur with only minor hematological abnormalities.

Blood transfusions are necessary only in rare cases for the treatment of pernicious anemia. The causal treatment is the substitution of vitamin B_{12}, which is given by the intramuscular route (hydroxocobalamin, 1000 µg). After 5–6 d, a strong increase in reticulocytes can be found in the blood and the signs of hemolysis regress. During the first 2–3 wk, six injections should be given. Because erythropoiesis shows a maximum increase, the iron stores may become exhausted and many patients need iron supplements. During the initial treatment of pernicious anemia, the serum K^+ levels may decrease steeply and should be monitored. If a patient with vitamin B_{12}-deficiency anemia is inadvertently treated with folate, the anemia may improve, but irreversible neurological damage may occur (due to a subacute combined degeneration of the cord). Therefore, all megaloblastic anemias need a thorough investigation. Patients with autoimmune pernicious anemia need a lifelong substitution. Maintenance injections (1000 μg) should be given every 3 mo. Prophylactically, vitamin B_{12} should also be given to patients who had a total gastrectomy or ileal resection. For patients with neuropathy, a higher-dose substitution is recommended in the initial treatment phase.

In the older population, a subclinical vitamin B_{12} deficiency is common. Clinically, these patients often have a subtle neurological dysfunction. The secretion of intrinsic factor and the Schilling test is normal in this population. It is thought that this deficiency of vitamin B_{12} is due to reduced gastric secretions, leading to a delayed release of the vitamin from binding substances in food. Further causes are bacterial infections and drugs that suppress gastric acid. A subclinical vitamin B_{12} deficiency may rapidly become symptomatic when anesthesia with nitric oxide (which oxidizes cobalamin) is performed or when folates are given.

6.4. Other Causes of Vitamin B_{12} Deficiencies

Several other conditions besides pernicious anemia may lead to a symptomatic vitamin B_{12} deficiency, including malabsorption of tropical sprue, blind loops syndrome (bacterial overgrowth), fish tapeworms, gastric or ileal resections, and a strict vegetarian diet. Rare causes of megaloblastic anemia are the congenital deficiency of the binding protein TCII and congenital defects in the secretion of intrinsic factor.

6.5. Megaloblastic Anemias Due to Folate Deficiency

Folates may be deficient in malnourished persons and alcoholics. In patients with intestinal disorders, folates may not be resorbed in the small intestine. The causes of folate deficiency are outlined in Table 5. The symptoms of severe folate deficiency are similar to those in severe vitamin B_{12} deficiency. However, there are no neurological signs and symptoms. Serum folate levels are decreased (normal values 3–15 μg/L), and vitamin B_{12} levels are normal. Serum folates rapidly normalize after substitution; therefore, the measurement of red cell folates may be necessary to recognize folate deficiency as cause of a megaloblastic anemia. Folate deficiency during pregnancy is a risk factor for neural tube defects. In recent years, folate deficiency and subsequent elevations of homocysteine were recognized as cause of premature cardiovascular disease. To treat folate defi-

Table 5
Causes of Folate Deficiency

Reduced alimentary intake	Malnutrition, alcoholism, synthetic diets
Malabsorption	Tropical sprue, gluten-induced enteropathy, smoking
Increased demand	Pregnancy, chronic hemolytic anemias, malignancies
Genetic causes	Mutations of genes responsible for folate absorption or metabolism (*MTHFR* and other genes)
Drugs	Inhibitors of dihydrofolate reductase (methotrexate), sulfasalazine, oral contraceptives, phenytoin

ciency, 5 mg daily are given orally for several months. If possible, the underlying disorder, like ileitis, should be treated. For example, many patients with chronic hemolytic anemias need a lifelong maintenance treatment. During pregnancy, a substitution of at least 400 µg daily is recommended.

SUGGESTED READING

Alcindor T, Bridges KR. Review: sideroblastic anemias. *Br J Haematol* 2002;116:733–743.

Baynes RD, Cook JD. Current issues in iron deficiency. *Curr Opin Hematol* 1996;3:145–149.

Durand P, Prost M, Blanche D. Folate deficiencies and cardiovascular pathologies. *Clin Chem Lab Med* 1998;36:419–429.

Hoffbrand V, Provan D. ABC of clinical haematology: macrocytic anaemias. *Br Med J* 1997;314:430–433.

Toh BH, van Driel IR, Gleeson PA. Pernicious anemia. *N Engl J Med* 1997;337:1441–1448.

Weiss G, Goodnough LW. Anemia of chronic disease. *N Engl J Med* 2005;352:1011–1023.

6 Hemolytic Anemias

Reinhold Munker, MD, Ali Mansouri, MD, Snehalata C. Gupte, PhD, and Vishwas Sakhalkar, MD

CONTENTS

1. INTRODUCTION

The different forms of hemolytic anemias are a severe, worldwide health problem. The hemolytic anemias can be classified into acquired and inherited types. The acquired forms are usually caused by the development of autoantibodies against red cells, whereas the latter forms are possibly due to red cell membrane defects, red cell enzyme defects, or abnormalities of the hemoglobin (Hb) molecule. The normal composition of Hb is described in Chapter 1.

All hemolytic anemias have several common clinical features as a result of both increased destruction and an increased compensatory production of red cells. The increased destruction of red cells leads to symptoms of anemia, enlargement of the spleen, the formation of gallstones, and laboratory findings showing hemolysis (raised unconjugated bilirubin and other features). The increased production of red cells is reflected by an elevated reticulocyte count in the blood as well as an increase of erythropoiesis in the bone marrow and leads to bone abnormalities, especially in children with chronic hemolytic anemias. The major features of inherited hemolytic anemias are described in Table 1.

From: *Contemporary Hematology: Modern Hematology, Second Edition*
Edited by: R. Munker, E. Hiller, J. Glass, and R. Paquette © Humana Press Inc., Totowa, NJ

Table 1
Major Characteristics of Inherited Hemolytic Anemias

Hereditary spherocytosis	Dominant inheritance (in most cases), defect of red cell membrane, splenectomy if symptomatic.
G6PD deficiency	Defect of red cell enzyme, hemolytic episodes triggered by certain drugs and other conditions.
Sickle cell anemia	Single-gene disease (HbS), symptoms in homozygotes, severe hemolysis with painful crises, reduced life expectancy, intensive supportive treatment needed.
Thalassemias	α-Thalassemia: α-chain of globin molecule reduced or absent (deletion of three genes: moderately severe hemolytic anemia).
	β-Thalassemia: β-chain reduced or absent (homozygous form: severe hemolytic anemia with reduced life expectancy, chronic transfusions required, iron overload).

2. INHERITED MEMBRANE DEFECTS

2.1. Hereditary Spherocytosis

Hereditary spherocytosis (HS) is the most common hereditary hemolytic anemia in persons of northern European descent (incidence 0.02%). The inheritance is autosomal dominant in most cases. A defect in a major structural protein of the red cell membrane (spectrin, ankyrin, band 3, and/ or protein 4.2) leads to a loss of membrane lipids with decreased osmotic resistance. The defective genes causing spherocytosis were cloned (*ANK1, EPB3, ELB42, SPTA1,* and *SPTB*). The cells of abnormal morphology (e.g., decreased surface area, microspherocytes) can no longer pass through the splenic microvasculature and are phagocytosed.

The severity of the disease is variable. Patients may have a chronic anemia or may be hematologically normal. Some patients show symptoms only during infections or other stressful conditions. Anemic patients have chronic fatigue and many have icteric episodes. Others have colics in the right upper abdomen if they have gallstones. The spleen is always enlarged in HS. Some patients have aplastic crises (due to an infection with parvovirus B19). During such a crisis, the production of red cells is abruptly stopped and a severe anemia follows. Some individuals with HS have a neonatal icterus that later normalizes.

The diagnosis of HS can be made when typical spherocytes are detected on the blood film (diameter <7 μm) and the osmotic resistance is decreased. As an alternative to the osmotic fragility test, the acidified glycerol lysis test can be used. In most patients, the family history is positive. The direct antiglobulin test

(Coombs' test) is always negative. As in other hemolytic anemias, the lactate dehydrogenase (LDH) and unconjugated bilirubin are increased and the serum haptoglobin is decreased. The proportion of reticulocytes is normal or increased. Most patients have an enlarged spleen.

Splenectomy normalizes or improves the hemolytic anemia and is indicated in all symptomatic cases. An exception exists, however, in the case of children less than 5-yr-old, because of the considerable risk of postsplenectomy infections (mainly pneumococcal septicemias). Patients undergoing splenectomy for HS should be vaccinated against pneumococci and *Hemophilus influenzae* and should be advised to take 250 mg penicillin twice daily for an indefinite period. A revaccination against pneumococci is recommended every 6 yr. Recently, a partial splenectomy was proposed to reduce the risk of postsplenectomy infections.

Patients who have a partial splenectomy or who have an accessory spleen that enlarges may need a second operation if a symptomatic anemia recurs. In aplastic crisis, patients with HS may need blood transfusions and other supportive measures. Intravenous immunoglobulin (IVIg) has been used to prevent aplastic crisis in patients with HS by administering it early in the course of the disease. The substitution of folic acid may improve the anemia to some extent.

Cholecystectomy is required in some patients, especially those with intact spleen due to hemolysis leading to unconjugated hyperbilirubinemia, increased pigment stone formation, and cholecystitis. The major features of HS and its management are summarized in Table 2.

2.2. Hereditary Elliptocytosis

Hereditary elliptocytosis (HE), a familial hemolytic anemia, can be recognized by the presence of a sizable proportion of oval or elliptical red cells on peripheral blood films. As with spherocytosis, the inheritance of HE is autosomal dominant. The molecular defects involved are heterogeneous, including mutations of spectrin, protein 4.1, or glycophorin C. Most cases have a mild clinical presentation without evidence of anemia. HE is symptomatic in rare cases of homozygosity, in which infections have been associated with exacerbations of the disease. Patients who are heterozygous for two different mutations (double heterozygosity, hereditary pyropoikilocytosis) may have a severe hemolytic anemia. Symptomatic patients with HE benefit from splenectomy, similarly to patients with spherocytosis.

2.3. Hereditary Pyropoikilocytosis

Hereditary pyropoikilocytosis is a rare form of elliptocytosis with recessive inheritance. The red cells are characterized as micropoikilospherocytes and are thermally unstable. Most patients have a severe hemolytic anemia.

Table 2

Clinical Features and Management of Hereditary Spherocytosis

Features	Spherocytosis trait	Mild spherocytosis	Moderate spherocytosis	Severe spherocytosis
Baseline hemoglobin (g/dL)	Normal	Borderline/normal (11–15)	Slightly/moderately low (8–12)	Moderate/very low (≤7)
Reticulocytes (%)	Normal	Slightly elevated (3–7)	High (≥8)	≥10
Peripheral smear	Normal	Few spherocytes	Spherocytosis	Spherocytes and poikilocytes
Indirect bilirubin (mg/dL)	Normal (0–1)	Slightly high (1–2)	Moderately high (≥3)	Very high (>10)
RBC spectrin (% of normal)	100	80–100	40–80	20–50
Osmotic fragility (unincubated)	Normal	Normal or Slightly increased	Distinctly increased	Markedly increased
Osmotic fragility (24 h incubated)	Slightly increased	Distinctly increased	Markedly increased	Severely increased
Spleen	Normal	Normal, episodically enlarged	Enlarged	Very enlarged
Usual course	Normal	Occasional complications	Multiple complications	Severe complications
Interventions	Genetic Counseling	Counsel + close observation	Observe +? splenectomy ?cholecystectomy	+ splenectomy ?cholecystectomy

Table 3
Factors Causing Hemolysis in Patients With G6PD Deficiency

1. Infections (pneumonias, hepatitis, sepsis), severe illnesses, diabetic ketoacidosis
2. Drugs (acetanilide, nalidixic acid, naphthalene, nitrofurantoin, pamaquine, phenazopyridine, phenylhydrazine, primaquine, sulfacetamide, sulfamethoxazole, sulfanilamide, sulfapyridine, toluidine blue, dapsone, and other compounds)
3. Fava beans (most common in Mediterranean variant)

3. INHERITED ENZYME DEFECTS

The glucose metabolism of red blood cells is regulated by a large number of enzymes. In clinical practice, only two types of enzyme defects are important: the deficiency of glucose-6-phosphate dehydrogenase (G6PD) and the deficiency of pyruvate kinase (PK).

3.1. G6PD Deficiency

Deficiencies of the red cell enzyme G6PD comprise the most common human enzymopathy. It has been estimated that in some Mediterranean countries, as well as in Asia and Africa, 5–20% of the population (in some countries even 60%) have a deficiency of G6PD. The degree of G6PD deficiency is variable, often being found to be more severe in Mediterranean patients than in patients from Africa. In Asia, the incidence varies between 0.1 and 14%. At least 200 million people suffer from G6PD deficiency on a worldwide basis.

G6PD catalyzes the first step of the pentose phosphate pathway (Embden-Meyerhof reaction, conversion of glucose-6-phosphate to 6-phosphogluconate). The G6PD-deficient red cells have a limited capacity to generate nicotinamide adenine dinucleotide phosphate (NADP) and NADPH (reduced form). The lack of reducing potential makes them vulnerable to oxidative stress. Certain drugs, vegetables, and stress conditions (*see* Table 3) induce an acute intravascular hemolysis. It has been speculated that these drugs or conditions induce the formation of free radicals.

G6PD deficiency is a hereditary recessive disorder linked to the X chromosome. The disease is therefore manifested most severely in males, whereas female heterozygotes generally only act as carriers. Females may be affected in cases of extreme lyonization, Turner's syndrome (XO), and 50% of females are affected when both parents are carriers. Because female carriers have the advantage of being protected against malaria, the disease is often prevalent in areas where malaria is endemic. At least 400 different mutations of G6PD are known. Based on the degree of enzyme deficiency, five classes of G6PD deficiency can be distinguished.

- Class I variants: severe enzyme deficiency (rare, chronic active hemolysis)
- Class II variants: severe enzyme deficiency (only intermittent severe hemolysis, frequent in Mediterranean patients)
- Class III variants: moderate enzyme deficiency (10–60% of normal, only intermittent hemolysis, frequent in African-American patients, hemolysis usually associated with infections or drugs)
- Class IV variants: no enzyme deficiency or hemolysis (of limited clinical relevance)
- Class V variants: increased enzyme activity (of limited clinical relevance)

Between hemolytic episodes, patients are hematologically normal. After ingesting fava beans or certain drugs, they rapidly develop severe intravascular hemolysis. Patients develop hemoglobinuria, fever, back pain, and icterus.

The diagnosis of G6PD deficiency can be made by measuring the enzyme activity in red cells. The enzyme measurement should not be made during a hemolytic episode or after transfusion because this will give a falsely elevated enzyme activity. For male patients, a screening test with a fluorescent substrate can give rapid information. During the hemolytic episode the blood film shows numerous fragmented cells and Heinz bodies. Heinz bodies consist of oxidized and denatured Hb and can be visualized as an intracellular inclusion with supravital staining.

The treatment of a hemolytic episode consists of supportive measures. Removal of potential stress factors is obviously necessary and blood transfusions should be given if needed. As a prophylactic measure, all potentially dangerous agents should be avoided in patients with G6PD deficiency. Babies with G6PD deficiency may develop neonatal jaundice and may need an exchange transfusion and/or phototherapy.

3.2. Pyruvate Kinase Deficiency

The inheritance of the red cell enzyme PK deficiency is autosomal recessive. In this deficiency, an impaired nicotinamide adenine dinucleotide (NAD) synthesis and the depletion of adenosine triphosphate (ATP) enhance the hemolysis of erythrocytes. Heterozygotes are usually asymptomatic, whereas homozygotes have a hemolytic anemia of variable severity. By mutation analysis, it was shown that most homozygote patients are actually compound heterozygotes for the two most common mutant forms of the enzyme. In the peripheral blood smear, acanthocytes, echinocytes (sea urchin-like cells), and spherocytes are prominent. Splenomegaly, gallstones, and icterus are commonly observed in symptomatic patients. The diagnosis of PK deficiency can be made by screening tests or by measuring the enzyme activity in the red cells. As in other chronic hemolytic anemias, infections may lead to an exacerbation of the hemolysis. Splenectomy may be beneficial for symptomatic patients who need frequent transfusions. At birth, PK-deficient infants may be severely anemic and often require an exchange transfusion.

3.3. Other Red Cell Enzyme Deficiencies Associated With Hemolytic Anemia

Less common than G6PD and PK deficiency is the deficiency of glucose phosphate isomerase, which may manifest itself by hemolytic crises.

4. HEMOGLOBINOPATHIES

The genetic abnormalities of the Hb molecule are mainly divided into two categories: the structural abnormalities and abnormalities due to the reduced synthesis of normal α- or β-chains of the globin molecule. Sickle cell anemia is the prototype of a structural abnormality, whereas in the thalassemias, a reduced synthesis of the globin chains is encountered. Other structural abnormalities of the Hb molecule cause HbC, HbE disease, and other disorders. Each hemoglobinopathy occurs in homozygous and heterozygous forms. Clinical manifestations are usually only present in the homozygous state. Heterozygotes are referred to as having a trait of the hemoglobinopathy.

4.1. Sickle Cell Anemia

Sickle cell anemia or sickle cell disease (SCD) is an inherited hemolytic disorder that is the result of a mutation in the β-globin gene. The mutated Hb is called HbS. In heterozygotes (sickle cell trait), HbS does not cause major clinical problems. In fact, it gives the carriers a certain advantage vis-à-vis plasmodium falciparum malaria. In contrast, most homozygotes for HbS go through life with major health problems affecting every organ system. Patients with sickle cell anemia have until now a shorter life span than the average. Fortunately, however, advances in the care of these patients, such as early diagnosis, better antibiotics treatment, and better pain control, have contributed to a significant improvement in their life expectancy. In 1973, Diggs reported a mean survival of about 14 yr for homozygous patients whereas in 1994, Platt et al. reported a markedly improved life expectancy of 42 yr for males and 48 yr for females, which was mainly related to prophylactic penicillin, vaccination, and parental education about splenic sequestration. The cure of SCD is still elusive despite major advances in the understanding of its pathophysiology.

4.1.1. PATHOPHYSIOLOGY

A single substitution in the β-globin gene results in the substitution of the sixth amino acid in the β-globin subunit from glutamic acid to valine with hydrophobic properties. This substitution results in a fundamental change in the properties of HbS in the deoxygenated state. In the absence of oxygen and at a critical concentration of HbS there are many intramolecular interactions that form molecular rods, which continue to grow and deform the cell. The sickling phenomenon in turn damages the cell membrane and shortens red cell survival (hemolysis). In addition, there are other factors, such as white cells, endothelial cells, coagulation, and cytokine/inflammation pathways, that affect the sickling phenomenon. Chronic and intermittent tissue hypoxia, and possibly inflammation, eventually leads to tissue damage and organ malfunction. Intravascular hemolysis results in Hb release, which leads to an intense local and systemic inflammatory and cytokine response causing endothelial damage and sludging resulting in ischemia. The systemic component is probably responsible for multifocal cascade of events leading to generalized and/or multifocal symptoms seen in acute attacks. Repeated episodes lead to subintimal proliferation of fibroblasts and smooth muscle, and narrowing and eventual obliteration of endarterioles. These findings first manifest in those organs of body that have maximum acidosis and hypoxia, such as splenic sinusoids and the hyperosmolar environment of renal medulla. Hence, homozygous patients with SCD have usually autoinfarcted their spleen by 5 yr of age and have polyuria, a telltale symptom of poor concentration of urine due to infarction of renal medulla, by 10 yr of age. In milder phenotypes of SCD, splenic function (as inferred from presence of red cell "pits" and absence of Howell-Jolly bodies on peripheral smear or by a radionuclide uptake spleen scan) can remain near normal even beyond the teenage years.

The narrowing and eventual obliteration of endarterioles and even major arteries is classically seen in the internal jugular and middle cerebral arterial distribution in the brain. Poor collateral circulation (from inadequate vessel proliferation leading to "moyamoya"-[Japanese for "puff of smoke"]-type vascular appearance on angiogram) in response to vascular narrowing and ischemia, anemia (hence lower total cerebral oxygen "reserve" capacity and supply), and damage due to inflammation are all responsible for intellectual deficits seen in almost half of older patients with SCD. Acute ischemia or microemboli are the final stress for the already precarious vascular supply that manifests itself as stroke in about 10% of patients with SCD (and as silent infarcts as an incidental finding on computed tomography [CT] or magnetic resonance imaging [MRI] in approx 30%). Ischemic cerebral events manifest mainly between 5 and 10 yr of age. Rupture of the friable overburdened collateral vessels possibly lead to catastrophic and sometimes fatal intracranial hemorrhage that is usually seen in adults with SCD.

The various pathological processes that take place during multiple episodes of intravascular sickling lead to the clinical symptoms. The symptoms are either acute as a result of an ongoing sickling process or chronic as a result of organ dysfunction or failure. The clinical symptoms vary significantly in severity in various sickle genotypes. Many other genes interact with the sickle cell gene and alter the severity of SCD. These genes are referred to as epistatic genes. HbS in a critical concentration can also interact in a heterozygote state with other Hb such as HbC, D, E, as well as with the α- and β-thalassemias. However, all these phenotypes except hemoglobin sickle disease and HbS with β°-thalassemia (when the only β-gene present is nonfunctional and does not produce any β-chains) and HbSD phenotype generally manifest a clinical course that is somewhat milder than homozygous (HbSS) disease. HbS with β-+ thalassemia (when the only β-gene present produces variable amounts of β-chains) and HbS heterozygous with hereditary persistence of fetal Hb (also called HPFH), are the mildest phenotypes of SCD. Various phenotypes of SCD have milder disease when present with a concomitant α-thalassemia trait as a result of a decrease in the mean corpuscular hemoglobin concentration (MCHC). A decrease in MCHC by 3 g/dL lowers the HbS polymer formation threefold.

4.1.2. DIAGNOSIS

The clinical presentation and family history show a number of common features in most cases. Because of the chronic nature of the disease, the Hb is generally low compared to the symptoms of anemia. The blood smear shows sickle cells and target cells. Screening tests for sickling are positive (incubation of red cells under low oxygen conditions, e.g., with dithionate). The definitive diagnosis of SCD is made by means of a hemoglobin electrophoresis or by PCR. In homozygous SCD, the hemoglobin electrophoresis shows the typical band of HbS, whereas the band of normal HbA is absent. Figure 6.1 shows the hemoglobin electrophoresis of a normal individual and of a person with sickle cell anemia. For patients with sickle cell trait, the proportion of HbA and HbS is almost equal however HbA is *always* greater than HbS. Homozygotes for HbS may have a variable proportion of HbF. Cases of SCD with a larger proportion of HbF (20–30%), especially those with pancellular distribution, are associated with an extremely mild clinical course because it delays and decreases the HbS polymer formation significantly.

4.1.3. CLINICAL PROBLEMS

Table 4 shows various clinical problems associated with sickle cell anemia. We will describe some of the most common problems seen in the sickle cell clinic.

4.1.4. ACUTE SICKLE CELL PAIN CRISIS AND CHRONIC PAIN

Some patients with sickle cell anemia often have chronic aches and pains and use multiple analgesics continuously or intermittently. The chronic pain is often interspersed by episodes of acute pain "crises." Although many factors are

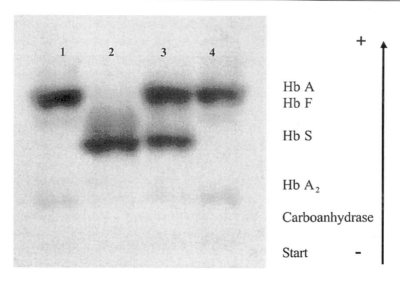

Fig. 6.1. Hemoglobin electrophoresis (normal [1,4], sickle cell anemia [2], and sickle cell trait [3]).

Table 4
Problems Related to Sickle Cell Disease

- Anemia due to ineffective hematopoiesis and chronic hemolysis
- Pain crises due to tissue hypoxia and infarction (caused by red cell sludging) and inflammatory reactions
- Chronic joint disease caused by bone necrosis and inflammation (seen classically in hip joint due to avascular necrosis of femoral neck)
- Acute chest syndrome with gradual development of pulmonary hypertension after multiple such episodes
- Severe infections such as pneumonias and osteomyelitis due to a defective immune system coupled with ischemia
- Chronic vascular disease (stroke, etc.)
- Acute hemolytic crises
- Acute and subacute splenic sequestration
- Aplastic crises
- Priapism
- Chronic organ failure

responsible for these pain episodes, the major problem is tissue hypoxia with or without infarction or inflammation. The painful crises are the most common manifestations of SCD and they often worsen with age. The pain crises appear in an unpredictable fashion or are initiated by stressful factors such as infection, physical or psychological trauma, menstruation, cold weather, and others. The severity and the frequency of the painful episodes also have prognostic significance, which should be factored into the long-term therapeutic management. Although pain control is a challenge for the physician, in most instances, pain can be managed in an outpatient setting with reassurance, hydration, and short- and long-acting narcotics. It is important nevertheless to eliminate all possible precipitating factors if any are identified.

Patient education about healthy living (i.e., good hydration, nutrition, non-competitive exercise, adequate rest, avoiding exposure to cold [wearing gloves and stockings], and periodic follow-ups) is important. Warm soaks may cause symptom relief, but cold compresses or ice *must* be avoided. More recently, inflammation has been identified as a cause of sickling and pain. Therefore, the use of anti-inflammatory drugs should be kept in mind. It is always important to treat pain adequately because chronic pain can affect the patient's outlook on life and lower the quality of life. In addition, it is especially important to treat acute severe pain promptly, adequately, empathically, and with frequent monitoring (for prompt control and to avoid oversedation) in the emergency and inpatient setting. This approach promptly breaks the pain cycle, improves patient self-confidence and compliance, and ensures quicker resolution.

4.1.5. ACUTE CHEST SYNDROME AND PULMONARY HYPERTENSION

Second to pain crises, pulmonary complications are the most common and most feared, being the leading cause of death in the acute and chronic setting. The two main acute problems are infectious pneumonia and acute chest syndrome. Both these problems have similar clinical manifestations: fever, chest pain, and shortness of breath, leukocytosis and pulmonary infiltrate on chest X-ray. However, it is important to make the correct diagnosis because the treatment is different. If the two problems cannot be differentiated from one another, which commonly occurs, the patient should be treated for both. All patients with acute pulmonary problems should be cared for as inpatients with hydration, pain control, oxygen, and antibiotics as well as red cell transfusion or red cell exchange if necessary. Transfusions should be leukocyte-depleted to avoid alloimmunization. One-third of the patients eventually develop pulmonary hypertension.

4.1.6. ACUTE AND CHRONIC BONE AND JOINT PAIN

Patients with sickle cell anemia are predisposed to develop bone infarction. These infarctions result, over a long period of time, in bone and joint dysfunction at the large joints, especially the hip. These lesions cause significant pain and joint malfunction. The bone and joint problems, if severe and repetitive, should be treated with anti-inflammatory and analgesic drugs and physiotherapy. If the joint function cannot be restored the patients should be referred to an orthopedist for further evaluation and treatment. Joint replacement is an option if the less invasive treatments are not helpful.

4.1.7. VASCULAR DISEASE AND STROKE

Vascular disease, especially in the brain, is more common in patients with SCD and manifests far earlier than the population at large. Central nervous vascular accident is the most catastrophic complication of SCD. In more recent years stroke prevention has become possible by using transcranial ultrasonography for early diagnosis and preventive treatment of selected patients as shown by the Stroke Prevention Trial in Sickle Cell Anemia (STOP).

In a series of studies, children at high risk of stroke could be identified with certainty (relative risk = 44, 95% confidence interval 5.5–346) and the impending stroke prevented with chronic blood transfusion or red cell exchange transfusion. Recent data suggests that these patients at "high risk" of stroke need indefinite chronic transfusion after reports of stroke on its discontinuation after years of being on a chronic transfusion program. Stroke in the adult population is not as common as it is in children but it is higher than in the general population in patients with multiple risk factors. The specific risk factors in SCD for stroke are "a previous stroke and silent cerebral infarcts." Familial predisposition has also been mentioned as a risk factor. It should also be noted that now that many patients reach middle age, all other usual risk factors for stroke such as hypertension, hypercholesterolemia, and smoking should be identified and treated. Patients with sickle cell anemia are in particular sensitive to the deleterious effects of high blood pressure. The treatment of strokes is chronic partial exchange red cell transfusion to emergently lower the HbS concentration below 30%. Other treatments (*see* "New Treatments") should be offered as an adjunctive treatment or when transfusion program is not practical because of poor compliance, religious beliefs, multiple alloantibodies, severe iron overload, or other reasons. The exchange red cell transfusion has been used to slow and even prevent iron overload, but at the cost of increased donor exposure, and if started, should be continued probably beyond childhood.

4.1.8. IRON OVERLOAD

Iron accumulates at a different rate in different individuals, and in different organs. Every organ also has a different susceptibility toward the toxic effects of elemental iron.

If they receive repeated blood transfusions, patients with sickle cell anemia are especially prone to iron overload, at an approximate rate of 200 mg of iron per red cell unit. We start treating iron overload when the serum ferritin exceeds 1000 ng/mL. Serum ferritin, however, is not an accurate assessment of iron deposits. The hepatic iron concentration obtained by liver biopsy is more reliable but also more invasive. An alternative noninvasive technique would be to estimate the hepatic iron by a superconducting quantum interface density measurement. However, this is rarely available. MRI is an easier alternative with acceptable results.

The use of iron chelators in β-thalassemia major has shown that it brings significant health improvement and prolongs survival. Iron chelation should also be offered to patients with SCD who have iron overload and has a beneficial effect. However, parenteral iron chelation (Desferroxamine, Desferal®) is costly and cumbersome. In addition, the patient compliance is poor because of its side effects and its complex and restrictive nature related to daily and prolonged slow subcutaneous infusions. Extremely small, lighter infusion pumps may improve compliance. Yet, it is clear that the availability of oral chelators is a great advantage and welcomed by the patients. Although deferiprone (an oral iron chelator, also called L1) has been approved and is used in Europe, it is not approved for use in the United States. In the United States, deferasirox was recently licensed for the treatment of transfusion-associated iron overload (*see* Chapter 23 for details).

4.1.9. ALLOANTIBODY AND AUTOANTIBODY FORMATION

In the United States, 10 to 30% of patients with transfused SCD develop allosensitization leading to alloantibody (mainly C, E, K, and S) and autoantibody formation. The main reason is the discrepancy in minor blood groups in the donor population (predominantly white), and the recipients (most likely African-American). Allosensitization possibly activates the immune system into a hyperactive state leading to further, earlier, multiple, and simultaneous alloantibody and autoantibody formation making it extremely difficult to find compatible blood for transfusion. The formation of auto- and alloantibodies can be decreased by consistently using C, E, and K antigen-matched blood.

4.1.10. SPLENIC AND LIVER SEQUESTRATION

About 25% of patients with SCD develop a sudden massive pooling of blood in spleen that may rarely be asymptomatic. Of these cases, 80% occur before the second birthday. The patients commonly present with pallor, prostration, decreased activity, abdominal pain, massive splenic enlargement frequently associated with an upper respiratory infection or acute chest syndrome, and positive blood culture in 16% of patients. If untreated, 20% die and 50% of survivors will experience a repeat attack. Parental education directed to teaching splenic palpation and seeking immediate help on above symptoms can increase the incidence threefold and decrease mortality 10-fold. Resuscitation, hydration, cautious small transfusion (as the pooled blood is released after transfusion, causing hyperviscosity and stroke), should be followed in some cases by chronic transfusion program until child is more than 2-yr-old. At this time a splenectomy is performed and the patient urged to take penicillin daily for an indefinite period. Liver sequestrations are mild and less sudden because liver is not as distensible as the spleen.

4.1.11. PRIAPISM

Priapism is described as unwanted, often excruciatingly painful, sustained or intermittent (stuttering) erection that is not the result of sexual stimulation and is detrimental to the sexual organ structure and function. Priapism is not uncommon in SCD.

The mechanism of priapism is probably a gradual hypoxemia during the stasis of the blood in the corpora cavernosa and red cell sickling. When priapism takes place in sleep, it also results from sickling of the red cells in the corpora. The glans and corpus spongiosa are often not involved because the latter tumescence is often caused by erection associated with sexual desire. The treatment of priapism is aimed at rapid pain relief and the detumescence of the penis in order to preserve function and prevent complications. The treatment is generally hydration, pain control, and exchange red cell transfusions, if necessary. Partial exchange transfusion must be instituted if the priapism lasts longer than 12 h. If these measures are not effective, irrigation of the corpora can be effective. Surgical creation of shunts is reserved for patients who are resistant to all treatments. On a case report basis, a response was observed to β-agonists. Other drugs such as hydroxyurea or bicalutamide and α-adrenergic agonists have been used with inconsistent results.

Finally, patient education to maintain good hydration, exercise, avoidance of constipation, and sexual counseling are important elements in the treatment plan.

4.1.12. OTHER COMPLICATIONS

There are many other complications associated with SCD, such as dermatopathy, retinopathy, nephropathy, endocrinopathy, and neuropsychiatric problems. It is preferable that the patients are directly referred to experts for these issues.

4.1.13. NEW TREATMENTS

Hydroxyurea was shown to reduce the frequency of pain crises, acute chest syndrome, and the need for blood transfusions. The mechanisms of action of hydroxyurea include increased production of HbF and an alteration of the adhesive properties of leukocytes. Not all patients respond to hydroxyurea; most need regular blood counts and may have side effects. Contraception is necessary for patients who can conceive or become pregnant. Other agents that induce HbF are under investigation. Further future treatments include agents that block endothelia–leukocyte interaction, ion-channel blockers to improve red cell hydration, inhalation of nitric oxide, and gene therapy. Hematopoietic stem cell transplantation (SCT) is the only treatment at present that can cure SCD. In children with severe SCD who had a matched-related donor, a transplant-related mortality of 5% or less and a long-term survival of 90% were reported. At present, few children with SCD have undergone an allogeneic transplantation. Transplants for adults using reduced intensity conditioning, using cord blood or matched-unrelated donors are currently under development.

4.2. Thalassemias

In adults, the predominant Hb molecule has four chains: two α- and two β-chains (HbA). In thalassemias, the synthesis of either the α- or the β-chains is reduced or absent, thus preventing the formation of a normal Hb molecule. In α-thalassemias the α-chain is reduced or absent, whereas in β-thalassemias the β-chain is reduced or absent. The excess globin chains denature in the red cell precursors and cause premature cell death. The two forms of thalassemias (α or β) differ in their clinical presentation and severity. The α-thalassemias are more frequent in persons of African, Mediterranean, or Asian descent, whereas the β-thalassemias are more frequent in persons from Southeast Asia.

4.2.1. β-THALASSEMIAS

Two main variants of β-thalassemias exist: in the β^0-form, no β-chains are produced, and in the β^+-form, a reduced amount of β-chains is produced (10–20%). The molecular pathogenesis of β-thalassemias is heterogeneous. More than 150 different mutations in the β-globin gene have been described. Most lesions are point mutations, and some involve small deletions.

In the β^0-type, the levels of HbF are raised, HbA is absent, and HbA$_2$ has a variable concentration. The β^+-type is associated with raised HbF, a variable amount of HbA, and normal HbA$_2$. The most severe disease develops in homozygous patients (thalassemia major, Cooley's disease). The clinical symptoms begin about 4–6 mo after birth when HbF is normally replaced by HbA. In patients with β-thalassemia, HbF persists. In addition, the free α-chains have toxic effects and lead to an ineffective erythropoiesis. Clinically, homozygous patients with β-thalassemia have a severe hemolytic anemia and are icteric. A hepatosplenomegaly develops. Bone changes develop, as a result of the erythroid hyperplasia in the hematopoietic marrow. These changes are obvious in children with frontal bossing. The bones are prone to fractures as a result of a thinning of the cortex. As a pathogenic cofactor, increased endogenous erythropoietin levels are observed. Furthermore, the iron reabsorption is increased because of anemia. As a result, and also because of repeated transfusions, children with β-thalassemia develop iron overload. They have a pigmented skin and may develop the symptoms of heart failure (hemosiderosis). Bacterial, viral, and fungal infections are common, especially after splenectomy.

4.2.1.1. Laboratory Diagnosis. Patients with β-thalassemia have a hypochromic microcytic anemia, increased reticulocytes with normoblasts, and target cells in the peripheral blood. An iron overload is indicated by elevated iron and ferritin levels in the serum and an increased saturation of the serum iron-binding capacity. Hb electrophoresis reveals the absence or only a faint band of HbA, whereas HbF is increased. HbA_2 ($2\alpha2\gamma$-chains) may also be increased. The molecular defect can be identified by Southern blotting or PCR.

4.2.1.2. Treatment. Patients with homozygous β-thalassemia need regular transfusions to maintain the hemoglobin concentration above 9.5 or 10 g/dL. Chronic transfusions lead to an iron overload; therefore, an iron chelation therapy with desferoxamine should be given to these patients. Details of the chelation treatment with desferoxamine and oral iron chelaters are given in Chapter 23. The substitution of folic acid is beneficial for many patients with β-thalassemia. Patients requiring very frequent transfusions (>220 mL/kg/yr) may benefit from splenectomy. Splenectomy should be deferred until a child has reached the age of 6 yr. All infections should be treated promptly. Splenectomized patients should receive a lifelong penicillin prophylaxis. Patients with β-thalassemia have successfully undergone bone marrow or SCT from human leukocyte antigen (HLA)-identical siblings.

4.2.2. α-THALASSEMIAS

The most severe form (deletion of all four α-genes) is not compatible with life beyond the fetal stage and leads to hydrops fetalis. When only three chains are deleted, a moderately severe hypochromic microcytic anemia results (HbH disease). This hereditary condition is usually caused by deletions removing all but one single α-globin gene (deletional HbH disease). A small number of patients have deletions removing two α-globin genes plus a nondeletional mutation affecting a third α-globin gene (nondeletional HbH disease, generally with a more severe clinical course). HbH disease has a wide phenotypic variability from asymptomatic to severe anemia with hepatosplenomegaly. In a proportion of patients, growth retardation is observed during childhood and iron overload in adults regardless of the number of blood transfusions. This can lead to heart, liver, and endocrine dysfunction. In contrast to α-chains, the free β-chains do not form precipitates but aggregate to tetramers, which are relatively unstable. Red cells with such aggregates have a shortened life span and are sequestered and hemolyzed in the spleen. If only one or two α-chain genes are deleted, the hemolysis is generally well compensated. The hemoglobin concentration is normal in most cases, yet the red cells are hypochromic and microcytic (α-thalassemia trait).

4.2.3. THALASSEMIA INTERMEDIA AND OTHER HEMOGLOBINOPATHIES

Milder forms of thalassemia that do not need transfusions are termed thalassemia intermedia. Patients with this form sometimes have skeletal abnormalities, delayed development, or leg ulcers. The cause of thalassemia intermedia is heterogeneous: some patients have a homozygous β-thalassemia with high levels of HbF and others have heterozygous β-thalassemia with other globin defects.

Genetic screening for hemoglobinopathies is recommended for all women belonging to a high-risk population. The first step is to determine if the mother is heterozygous for the major hemoglobinopathies (e.g., by hemoglobin electrophoresis). If this is the case, the father should also be screened. If he has the same abnormality, there is a 25% chance that the fetus is homozygous and has significant disease. These cases should be referred to a center specializing in the treatment of hemoglobinopathies and offering prenatal counseling. In most cases of hemoglobinopathy, a prenatal diagnosis by DNA analysis and PCR amplification is possible. If the diagnosis of thalassemia major is made early, the option of abortion can be offered to the parents.

4.3. HbC Disease

HbC alleles are common in patients from West Africa. Worldwide, homozygosity for HbC (HbC disease) is the third most common hemoglobinopathy involving a mutated gene (after SCD and HbE). Clinically, HbC disease is generally benign, associated with a mild hemolytic anemia and slight splenomegaly. On blood smears, target cells, microspherocytes, anisocytosis, poikilocytosis, and rod-shaped cells (containing HbC crystals) are found. HbC disease generally requires no treatment, although in severe cases folic acid should be supplemented. Symptomatic disease is observed when HbC alleles are co-inherited with other hemoglobinopathies (e.g., a sickle cell gene).

4.4. HbE Syndromes

HbE alleles are common in patients from Southeast Asia. In the homozygous state, a mild anemia, microcytosis, and target cells are observed.

4.5. Methemoglobinemia

Methemoglobinemia is a condition in which excess methemoglobin (oxidized Hb, unable to carry oxygen) is found in the blood. Normally, the level of methemoglobin is maintained at less than 1% in red cells by NADH diaphorase. Methemoglobinemia may be congenital, resulting from enzyme defects or abnormal Hb, or acquired as a result of toxins or drugs (among others, local anesthetics, sulfonamides, nitrates, and nitroprusside). Clinically, patients with acquired methemoglobinemia are cyanotic and have an altered mental status, especially if the methemoglobin concentration is greater than 20–30%. The cyanosis does not respond to oxygen inhalation. In severe cases (methemoglobin >30–40%), a treatment with the reducing agent methylene blue should be considered. Methylene blue should be avoided in patients who are G6PD-deficient, as it is ineffective and may precipitate hemolysis. For such patients, an exchange transfusion is indicated.

5. ACQUIRED HEMOLYTIC ANEMIAS

5.1. Autoimmune Hemolytic Anemias

These anemias are caused by the development of autoantibodies against red cells and the subsequent destruction of the antibody-coated red cells. There are two types: the autoimmune hemolytic anemias (AIHA) of the warm type with the antibody reacting best at 37°C and AIHA of the cold type with the antibody reacting best at 4°C. Both forms have a positive direct antiglobulin test (Direct Antiglobulin Test [DAT], Coombs' test) demonstrating the presence of antibodies (IgG, IgA, or IgM immunoglobins) or complement (C3, C3d) on the surface of red cells. A negative DAT does not exclude the diagnosis of AIHA, as the antibody may be of weak affinity. Inversely, a positive DAT is not in all cases associated with an overt hemolytic anemia. The principle of the antiglobulin or Coombs' test is outlined in Fig. 22.2. Both forms of AIHA can present as an acute or chronic disorder and can be idiopathic or secondary to other disorders. The hemolysis in AIHA is of the delayed type: the antibody-coated red cells undergo hemolysis in the spleen's reticuloendothelial system. Drug-induced autoimmune hemolytic anemia often is induced by a drug or a metabolite binding tightly to red cells or exposing a neoantigen on red blood cells after drug. In many instances, AIHA is a sign of an acquired immune imbalance.

5.1.1. AIHA OF THE WARM TYPE

The disease is often idiopathic but may also be associated with autoimmune disorders such as systemic lupus erythematosus, certain lymphomas, chronic lymphocytic leukemia; certain drugs such as methyldopa, procainamide, diclofenac, some antibiotics; and cytostatic drugs, as well as with other diseases.

5.1.1.1. Clinical Presentation. AIHA can occur at any age. The hemolytic anemia is of variable severity. Patients experience fatigue, dyspnea, and jaundice, and the spleen may be enlarged. During an acute hemolytic crisis, patients may be febrile. In rare cases, AIHA is associated with an autoimmune thrombopenic purpura (Evan's syndrome).

5.1.1.2. Laboratory Features. The laboratory findings are typical of a hemolytic anemia. Microspherocytes can be seen in the blood film. The DAT is positive, most often as a result of IgG ± complement on the red cells. In rare cases, hemolysis is due to IgA antibodies, which are not detected with commercial IgG/C3 antisera. If the autoantibody is produced at high concentrations, free antibody can also be found with the indirect antiglobulin test. The autoantibodies often have blood group specificity (e.g., recognizing rhesus [Rh], Kidd, or Landsteiner-Wiener [LW] antigens on red cells).

5.1.1.3. Treatment.

1. Blood transfusions may be necessary for severe, symptomatic anemia and should be given according to the same standards used for other anemic patients. If the specificity of the autoantibody is known, red cell concentrates negative for this antigen should be transfused if possible. The presence of alloantibodies resulting from previous transfusions or pregnancy has to be excluded. Because of the presence of autoantibodies, it is often difficult to find compatible red cell concentrates. Hence, the least incompatible blood is transfused with informed consent and adequate monitoring (to recognize an acute hemolytic transfusion reaction).
2. Any underlying cause of AIHA should be treated and any offending drug (e.g., methyldopa) should be withdrawn.
3. Corticosteroids are the standard treatment for AIHA. The starting dose is 1–2 mg/kg prednisone per day, which should be reduced according to the clinical response. Some patients need a maintenance dose for many months. Some critically ill patients may need a higher dose of steroids initially (intravenous methyl prednisone).
4. Splenectomy is indicated for patients who are refractory to corticosteroids, or who need a high-maintenance dose. A preoperative study with radioactively labeled red cells may be helpful to predict the efficacy of splenectomy.
5. An immunosuppressive treatment (e.g., with cyclophosphamide, cyclosporine, or azathioprine) may improve the hemolysis in patients who do not respond well to corticosteroids.
6. High-dose immunoglobulins (similar to the treatment of idiopathic thrombocytopenic purpura, *see* Chapter 20) may be effective in some cases of AIHA.
7. Rituximab (a humanized monoclonal antibody against CD20) has shown efficacy in some cases of refractory AIHA.
8. Plasmapheresis can be used as the last resort; however, the IgG antibody can be present in very high concentration in tissues, so is not cleared by plasmapheresis.

5.1.2. AIHA OF THE COLD TYPE

This disorder may also be idiopathic or associated with infections (e.g., mycoplasma pneumonias, infectious mononucleosis), with lymphomas or as part of the cold agglutinin syndrome. The antibody is almost always IgM and has a binding optimum at lower temperatures. After an exposure to cold temperatures, the antibody binds to the red cells, activates the complement, and initiates hemolysis. As in warm-type AIHA, the red cells are phagocytosed by the reticuloendothelial system, most often in the liver. In contrast to the warm type, intravascular hemolysis is also seen.

5.1.2.1. Clinical Features.
Hemolytic crises and other clinical signs are aggravated in the cold. Many patients develop acrocyanosis when exposed to cold temperatures. Jaundice and splenomegaly may also be present.

5.1.2.2. Laboratory Features. The laboratory features are similar to those for warm-type AIHA, except that the red cells tend to agglutinate in the cold. The DAT is usually positive and shows the presence of complement on red cells. Serum antibodies, if present, are IgM. The specificity of the antibody is often anti-I (anti-i in newborns). In some cases, the antibody has specificity within the ABO, MNS, or LW systems. The cold autoantibodies may be polyclonal (in cases associated with infections or low-grade lymphomas) or monoclonal (in the case of the cold agglutinin syndrome). In the cold agglutinin syndrome, very high titers of the autoantibody may be observed.

5.1.2.3. Treatment. The principal mode of treatment is to avoid exposure to the cold. If an underlying cause of the AIHA can be identified, this cause should be treated. Corticosteroids and splenectomy are rarely effective, because of the intravascular nature of hemolysis. In very severe acute cases, plasmapheresis may be helpful in stopping the hemolysis especially because IgM, being a large molecule, remains in vascular space and can be easily removed. In chronic cases, immunosuppressive agents (e.g., chlorambucil or cyclophosphamide) may be effective. In severe symptomatic anemia, washed red cell concentrates must be transfused to avoid the infusion of additional complement. The transfusion should be made with a blood warmer. In refractory cases, rituximab was found to be effective.

Paroxysmal cold hemoglobinuria is due to a biphasic IgG antibody (reacting both at warm and cold temperatures, Donath Landsteiner antibody). This syndrome is observed in tertiary syphilis and in children after a viral illness. Paroxysmal cold hemoglobinuria is usually self-limited, but may cause significant intravascular hemolysis

5.2. Paroxysmal Nocturnal Hemoglobinuria

Paroxysmal nocturnal hemoglobinuria (PNH) is an acquired clonal stem cell disorder. In PNH, the phosphatidyl-inositol-glycan (PIG) anchor molecules are defective. As the molecular basis of PNH, the mutation of the PIG-A gene on the short arm of the X chromosome has been found. Until now, more than 100 different mutations of the PIG-A gene have been described, including missense and frameshift mutations, splice defects, and other mutations. The defect of the anchor molecules can be present in all or only some hematopoietic lineages. This glycolipid anchor attaches several proteins to the cell membrane that are important for the regulation of complement molecules (among them CD59 [membrane inhibitor of reactive lysis], CD55 [decay accelerating factor], and C8 binding protein). A defect in these molecules leads to a higher sensitivity to complement-mediated lysis and a tendency for thrombosis. Other surface molecules, CD14, CD24, and CD66, are also missing on PNH cells. PNH is a rare disorder that manifests as a chronic hemolytic anemia or as pancytopenia. Some patients have hemolytic crises during the night and become aware of red urine (hemoglobin-uria) in the morning. The major complications include recurring thromboses, such as portal vein thromboses and thromboses of the cerebral vessels or of the cutaneous veins. Sudden severe headaches or abdominal pain should always alert the clinician to the possibility of a thrombosis in any patient with PNH. A chronic iron loss often leads to an iron deficiency anemia.

A common finding is a normochromic, normocytic anemia. Some patients are granulocytopenic and thrombocytopenic. The laboratory signs are consistent with a chronic hemolytic anemia. Increased hemolysis is observed during infections. The diagnosis of PNH was classically made with the acid hemolysis or the sucrose test (the addition of sucrose or acidified serum leads to enhanced in vitro hemolysis). However, it is more convenient and reproducible to measure the expression of anchor molecules in different cell compartments by flow cytometry. A screening test for PNH is to measure different blood cells for the expression of CD55 or CD59. In most patients, three types of PNH cells can be distin-guished: type III cells, which totally lack GPI-anchored molecules; type II cells with a severely reduced expression; and type I cells, which have retained an approximately normal surface expression.

PNH can evolve into other entities (e.g., aplastic anemia, myelodysplasia, and, rarely, acute leukemia) and, vice versa, PNH clones can be recognized in a proportion of patients with aplastic anemia.

The treatment of PNH is mainly supportive. If frequent thromboses occur, the patients should be anticoagulated. A major thrombosis should be treated with thrombolysis and heparin. Iron and folic acid should be substituted. A pulse of corticosteroids may be indicated during a hemolytic crisis. Danazol (an androgen derivative) can also be considered in the treatment of PNH. Blood transfusions should be given if a symptomatic anemia develops. The prognosis of PNH depends on disease severity. Uncomplicated cases may survive with the disease for more than 10 or 15 yr. If PNH leads to progressive complications, a bone marrow or SCT from an HLA-identical sibling may be worth considering and may offer a chance for cure.

5.3. Hemolytic Disease of the Newborn

Among the conditions causing hemolytic disease of the newborn (HDN), the maternal alloimmunization due to blood group incompatibility between the mother and the fetus is the most common. HDN due to ABO antibodies is the most frequent type, whereas Rh antibodies may cause the most severe type of disease.

5.3.1. HDN DUE TO ABO ANTIBODIES

About two-thirds of HDN are due to ABO incompatibility. The HDN pre-dominantly occurs in an infant with the blood group A or B of an O mother. The disease shows a broad spectrum of severity, with mild to moderate symptoms in Caucasians and severe disease in African and Chinese neonates; about one-third of the cases occur in India. The diagnosis of ABO HDN is difficult, as the indirect antiglobulin test is usually negative or only weakly positive and the estimation of IgG anti-A or anti-B is complicated by the presence of a large amount of naturally occurring IgM ABO antibodies. It is necessary to neutralize maternal serum with secretor saliva or to treat it with 2-mercaptoethanol or dithiothreitol prior to the estimation of anti-A or anti-B IgG. Some cases of ABO HDN are associated with microspherocytosis and increased osmotic fragility. The hemoglobin of the infant is generally normal, and reticulocytosis or normoblastosis is present only in severe cases. Mild to moderate ABO HDN can be treated by phototherapy, whereas severely affected infants need an exchange transfusion.

5.3.2. HDN DUE TO Rh ANTIBODIES

Because anti-D immunoglobulins have become available for prophylaxis, the Rh HDN has almost been completely eradicated. Because the Rh antigen exists only on human red cells, the entry of Rh (D)-positive erythrocytes into the maternal circulation is a prerequisite for Rh immunization. In some cases, a fetomaternal hemorrhage before delivery is the cause of sensitization. However, even before the anti-D-prophylaxis was available, not all Rh-negative women who were exposed to Rh-positive erythrocytes became sensitized.

The diagnosis of Rh HDN is easily established when Rh (D) antibodies are detected in the human serum and the antiglobulin test is positive on the fetal erythrocytes. Maternal IgG antibody can cross the placental barrier and coat Rh (D) positive red cells, thus reducing their life span. The disease occurs in intrauterine life and hydrops fetalis is the most severe clinical manifestation. Antenatal assessment is therefore essential to identify a severely affected fetus and rescue it by intrauterine transfusion (IUT). The noninvasive parameters that can predict severity include periodic measurements of Rh antibody levels and periodic ultrasound examinations. A spectroscopic analysis of the amniotic fluid is helpful although it involves amniocentesis (relatively safe under ultrasound guidance). It is also possible to obtain fetal blood to confirm the diagnosis of Rh HDN and to assess the degree of anemia by determining hemoglobin and hematocrit. However, considering the risk involved with this procedure, it should be carried out only when the fetus is suspected to be critically ill and requiring an IUT.

The IUT is usually planned when the mother has high titers of anti-D antibodies, the amniotic fluid shows increasing bilirubin (Liley's zone II or III), and/or ultrasound reveals ascites. If the hemoglobin concentration is more than 2 g/dL lower than the normal value at the same age of gestation, then an IUT is performed. An IUT can be given as early as 18 wk gestation and must be repeated at 1- to 3-wk intervals. Fetuses who had multiple IUTs generally do not need exchange transfusion but may need a simple transfusion at birth. In alloimmunization due to Rh HDN, the delivery is induced after 32 or 34 wk depending on the facilities available in the intensive care unit. Infants who did not require an IUT may require a preventive exchange transfusion immediately after birth. All cases of Rh HDN usually receive phototherapy to convert bilirubin into a nontoxic form. If hyperbilirubinemia is present at birth, an exchange transfusion should always be performed to prevent the possible risk of permanent neurological damage (kernicterus). Other antibodies, such as anti-Kell antibodies, may also cause HDN, although usually of a less severe form than Rh HDN. The management of these cases depends on the degree of severity.

5.4. Special Forms of Acquired Hemolytic Anemias

Vascular changes and a toxic alteration of the endothelium can also cause a shortened survival and premature hemolysis of red cells. In many of these conditions, an abnormal red cell morphology is found (e.g., fragmentocytes, schistocytes in blood smear). Several infections, for example, malaria and babesiosis, may cause a massive hemolytic anemia. In meningococcal sepsis, toxins damage the endothelium and lead to a microangiopathic hemolytic anemia.

5.4.1. HEMOLYSIS DUE TO PARASITIC INFECTIONS

Although **malaria** is rarely seen in the West, it remains a major health problem elsewhere in much of the world. Individuals visiting or inhabiting sub-Saharan Africa, Central or South America, the Middle East, Southern Asia, or Polynesia are at risk for this infectious cause of hemolytic anemia. Malaria is caused by four protozoan species of the genus *Plasmodium*: *P. vivax, P. falciparum, P. malariae,* and *P. ovale*. These protozoans are transmitted into the blood of the host by the saliva of the Anopheles mosquito. The parasites enter the blood as sporozoites and initially infect hepatocytes, where they proliferate and develop into merozoites. The merozoites reenter the blood, where they infect red blood cells, reproduce asexually, and emerge to infect additional erythrocytes. It is important to note that *P. vivax* and *P. ovale* can persist as dormant forms in the liver, which can be reactivated at a later time. The symptoms of malaria include fevers, chills, fatigue, and headache. In addition to these symptoms, patients infected with *P. falciparum* may present with altered mental status, acute renal failure, respiratory distress, or gastroenteritis. These clinical manifestations are due to the tendency of red cells infected with *P. falciparum* to adhere to endothelial cells of the vasculature and cause diffuse microvascular occlusions. Physical examination may reveal splenomegaly, particularly in patients who are chronically infected or in those with *P. falciparum*. Laboratory tests are remarkable for evidence of an extravascular hemolytic anemia. Diagnosis is made by examining a thick peripheral blood smear for the presence of the parasites. Identification of the *Plasmodium* species is determined by examining the morphology of the organisms on the slide. Treatment of malaria depends on the species of the infecting parasite, the severity of the illness, and the likelihood that the organism is chloroquine resistant. Chloroquine-sensitive malaria may persist in Central America, the Middle East, and the Caribbean. Guidelines for the treatment of malaria and prophylactic measures for travelers are given in Table 5.

Babesiosis is a hemolytic anemia due to infection of erythrocytes by piriform (pear-shaped) protozoans. In Europe, the disease is caused by *Babesia divergens* and *B. bovis*, which usually are bovine parasites. On the east coast of the United States, *B. microti*, a rodent parasite, is the etiological organism. On the west coast, a recently identified piroplasm called WA1 has been found in several cases. All of these organisms are transmitted by ticks of the genus *Ixodes*. Babesiosis can also be transmitted by blood transfusions. Babesiosis is usually a mild, self-limited disease, but immunosuppressed patients, and especially individuals who have undergone splenectomy, may have severe and life-threatening disease manifestations. These patients can experience fevers, chills, headache, fatigue, myalgias, and arthralgias at presentation, but respiratory and renal failure may subsequently ensue. Physical examination may reveal icterus and mild splenomegaly. Laboratory results demonstrate an extravascular hemolytic anemia, and frequently thrombocytopenia. A thick smear of the peripheral blood reveals intraerythrocytic parasites, and an intracellular tetrad of merozoites is pathognomonic for babesiosis. Babesia may be overlooked, because parasitemia is often sparse, infecting less than 1% of erythrocytes early in the course of illness. Serological testing can confirm the diagnosis. Treatment consists of quinine sulfate 650 mg po TID and clindamycin 600 mg po three times daily (1200 mg i.v. twice daily) for 7–10 d. As an alternative, the combination of azithromycin and atovaquone was found effective. A chronic carrier state may be established if the treatment is not completed. In severe cases, an exchange transfusion may be life-saving.

Bartonellosis (Carrion's disease or Oroya fever) is endemic in parts of South America and is caused by *Bartonella bacilliformis*. Bartonellosis causes an acute hemolytic anemia and a chronic granulomatous reaction. The infectious agent is transmitted by the bite of sand flies. Untreated, bartonellosis has a high mortality. On peripheral blood smears, the intraerythrocytic bacilli can easily be recognized. Several antibiotics (ciprofloxacin, penicillin, streptomycin) have been found effective for bartonellosis.

5.4.2. MICROANGIOPATHIC ANEMIAS

In these conditions (hemolytic-uremic syndrome, thrombotic thrombocytopenic purpura, *see* Chapter 20) toxins damage the endothelium and the red cells or platelets that come into contact with the endothelium are destroyed. Fragmentocytes may be present in the peripheral blood smear. Similar condi-

Table 5
Treatment and Prophylaxis of Malaria

Treatment of malaria due to *Plasmodium vivax*, *P. malariae*, or *P. ovale*	Inpatient therapy of chloroquine-sensitive disease: chloroquine phosphate 10 mg base/kg i.v. over 8 h, then 15 mg base/kg i.v. over 24 h. Outpatient therapy of chloroquine-sensitive disease: chloroquine phosphate 10 mg base/kg orally (p.o.), then 5 mg base/kg p.o. after 12, 24, and 36 h. Concurrent therapy for patients with *P. vivax* or *P. ovale*: primaquine 0.25 mg base/kg p.o. daily ×14 d (avoid in pregnant women and newborns) Therapy of chloroquine-resistant disease: halofantrine 8 mg/kg p.o., then 8 mg/kg p.o. after 6 h, 12 h, and 7 d with primaquine 0.5 mg base/ kg p.o. daily ×28 d (avoid primaquine in pregnant women and newborns).
Treatment of malaria due to *P. falciparum*	Quinidine gluconate 10 mg/kg IV over 1 h, then 0.02 mg/kg/min with electrocardiogram monitoring until patient is able to take oral medications, then quinine sulfate 10 mg salt/kg p.o. every 8 h with doxycycline 100 mg p.o. twice daily for 7 d. Substitute pyrimethamine-sulfadoxine (pyrimethamine 20 mg/kg and sulfadoxine 1 mg/ kg) for doxycycline in children and pregnant women.
Prophylaxis in areas free of chloroquine resistance	Chloroquine 8.3 mg salt/kg, up to 500 mg, p.o. weekly beginning 1–2 wk before travel and continuing until 4 wk after travel.
Prophylaxis in areas with chloroquine resistance	Mefloquine 250 mg salt p.o. weekly in adults beginning 1 wk before travel and continuing until 4 wk after travel, or doxycycline 100 mg p.o. daily beginning on the first day of exposure and continuing until 4 wk after travel. Both are contraindicated in pregnancy and doxycycline is contraindicated in children.

tions occur after bone marrow transplantation or after the administration of certain drugs (e.g., cyclosporine, cisplatin, mitomycin C).

5.4.3. Disseminated Intravascular Coagulation

Disseminated intravascular coagulation (DIC) results from a number of conditions in which the systemic activation of the coagulation cascades occurs, resulting in the deposition of fibrin thrombi within the microvasculature. The causes of DIC and treatment strategies are described in Chapter 20.

5.4.4. Other Causes of Red Blood Cell Hemolysis

Various forms of trauma can induce red cell fragmentation and intravascular hemolysis. Intravascular red cell injury can be caused by mechanical heart valves or prosthetic vascular devices. External trauma from prolonged marching or running, or playing bongo drums, also can induce red cell fragmentation with hemolysis. Severe burns can directly damage red blood cells. Lead poisoning causes chronic hemolysis in addition to sideroblastic anemia. Copper toxicity due to industrial exposure or Wilson's disease also is associated with red cell hemolysis. Hypophosphatemia, for example, during parenteral nutrition, can shorten red cell survival. Exposure to hypotonic fluid, as in near-drowning, can induce hemolysis. Enzymes produced by clostridial organisms can cause massive intravascular hemolysis. Envenomation by some spiders and snakes also can disrupt red blood cell membranes.

SUGGESTED READING

Abboud MR, Cure J, Granger, S et al. Magnetic resonance angiography in children with sickle cell disease and abnormal transcranial Doppler ultrasonography findings enrolled in the STOP study. *Blood* 2004;103:2822–2825.

Bolton-Maggs PHB, Stevens RF, Dodd NJ, et al. Guidelines for the diagnosis and management of hereditary spherocytosis. *Br J Haematol* 2004;126:455–474.

Charache S, Terrin ML, Moore RD, et al. Effect of hydroxyurea on the frequency of painful crises in sickle cell anemia. *N Engl J Med* 1995;332:1317–1322.

Chui DH, Fucharoen S, Chan V. Hemoglobin H disease: not necessarily a benign disorder. *Blood* 2003;101:791–800.

Claster S, Vichinsky EP. Managing Sickle Cell Disease. *Br Med J* 2003;327:1151–1155.

Gladwin MT, Sachdev V, Jison ML, et al. Pulmonary hypertension as a risk factor for death in patients with sickle cell disease, *N Eng J Med* 2004;350:886–895.

Iolascon A, Miraglia del Giudice E, Perrotta S, et al. Hereditary spherocytosis: from clinical to molecular defects. *Haematologica* 1998;83:240–257.

Platt OS. Sickle cell anemia as an inflammatory disease. *J Clin Invest* 2000;106:337–338.

Rosse WF. Paroxysmal nocturnal hemoglobinuria as a molecular disease. *Medicine* 1997;76:63–93.

Stuart MJ, Nagel RL. Sickle-cell disease. *Lancet* 2004; 364:1343-1360.

Weatherall DJ. The hereditary anemias. *Br Med J* 1997;314:492–496.

7 Leukocytosis, Leukopenia, and Other Reactive Changes of Myelopoiesis

Reinhold Munker, MD

CONTENTS

1. DEFINITIONS AND PATHOPHYSIOLOGY

Most changes in the white blood cell count are reactive and due to an increase or decrease of cells of the myeloid series. By definition, a leukocytosis is present if leukocytes are increased to more than 10,000/μL; in leukopenia leukocytes are below 4000/μL. Infants and small children have slightly different normal values (for the normal values of blood counts, *see* Appendix 3). A neutropenia is present if granulocytes are below 2000/μL, agranulocytosis if granulocytes are below 500/μL. By definition, granulocytes are increased if they are greater than 8000/μL. In leukemoid reactions, leukocytes are increased to more than 30,000/μL. A left shift in the differential count means that the number of band forms (and other

From: *Contemporary Hematology: Modern Hematology, Second Edition*
Edited by: R. Munker, E. Hiller, J. Glass, and R. Paquette © Humana Press Inc., Totowa, NJ

precursors such as metamyelocytes) is increased to more than 5%. In a pathological left shift, more immature precursors such as promyelocytes can be seen in the peripheral blood; this is almost always a sign of a hematological disorder.

The granulocytes of the peripheral blood derive from the bone marrow. The earliest cell is the pluripotent stem cell, which is capable of self-renewal (*see* Chapter 1). Several steps of division and differentiation lead to mature cells (granulocytes), which are capable of fighting infections. The intermediate cells, which can be recognized morphologically, are myeloblasts, promyelocytes, myelocytes, and metamyelocytes. Cells of the myeloid series are produced under the control of interacting cytokines according to the needs of the organism. Approximately 40% of the cells in the peripheral blood are in a reserve pool on the endothelium (marginated pool) and can be mobilized rapidly in case of infection or other stress conditions.

2. DIFFERENTIAL DIAGNOSIS OF LEUKOCYTOSIS (NEUTROPHILIC LEUKOCYTOSIS)

A leukocytosis is a sign of any number of bacterial or other infections. Most cases of infectious leukocytosis are associated with a left shift and neutrophils often show a toxic granulation. The bilobed granulocytes seen in Pelger-Huët anomaly resemble band forms, but this rare condition with autosomal dominant inheritance does not have pathological value (Fig. 7.1, *see also* Color Plate 2). Similar granulocytes are occasionally seen in patients with acute myelogenous leukemia (pseudo-Pelger cells). In severe infections, the granulocytes may develop cytoplasmic inclusions or Döhle bodies (Fig. 7.2; *see also* Color Plate 3).

A massive leukocytosis (leukemoid reaction) most often indicates a severe complication (gall bladder empyema, perforated appendicitis, or bacterial sepsis). Stress reactions with a leukocytosis of 10,000–15,000/µL are common after epileptic seizures, renal colics, or myocardial infarctions. Nicotine and a treatment with steroids or lithium often lead to a leukocytosis. Severe hemolytic anemias and the regeneration from aplasia stimulate hemopoiesis in general and are followed by a leukocytosis. Rare cases of lung cancer and bladder cancer have a paraneoplastic leukocytosis. In these cases, it was shown that the tumor cells produce cytokines such as granulocyte colony-stimulating factor (G-CSF) or granulocyte/macrophage colony-stimulating factor (GM-CSF). Some persons also have an idiopathic or familiar increase in leukocytes.

The major differential diagnosis of a neutrophil leukocytosis discovered in a person without symptoms is an early stage of a chronic myelogenous leukemia (CML) or other myeloproliferative syndrome (*see* Chapter 8). In CML, generally the Philadelphia chromosome or the *BCR-ABL* oncogene can be found, whereas a reactive leukocytosis harbors no cytogenetic aberrations.

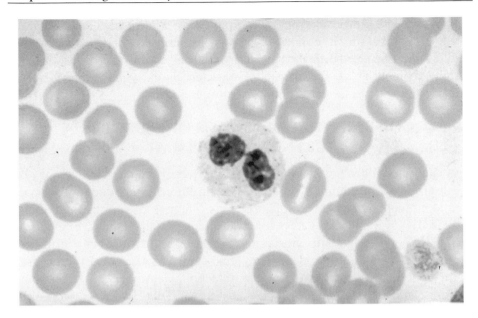

Fig. 7.1. Granulocyte of a patient with Pelger-Hu't abnormality (two round nuclear lobes are connected by a very thin strand and have the appearance of spectacles).

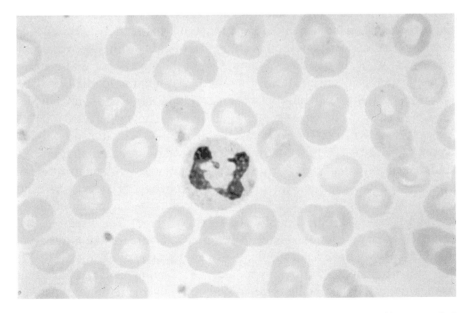

Fig. 7.2. Döhle bodies. Cytoplasmic inclusion in granulocytes, observed in severe infections.

Children with Down syndrome sometimes have a leukemoid reaction in the first few months of life which later subsides spontaneously. A leukoerythroblastic reaction is defined by the appearance of myeloid and erythroid progenitors in the peripheral blood. This is seen in osteomyelosclerosis and when the bone marrow is infiltrated with tumor cells (bone marrow carcinosis).

3. DIFFERENTIAL DIAGNOSIS OF LEUKOPENIA (GRANULOCYTOPENIA)

A slight neutropenia with granulocytes between 1000 and 2000/μL of idiopathic origin or that commonly found in certain ethnic groups does not normally lead to an increased incidence of infections. The risk of serious infectious is increased if the granulocytes are below 1000 and especially if they are below 500/μL. Neutropenia or agranulocytosis can be a side effect of a number of drugs (*see* "Agranulocytosis"). A dose-dependent leukopenia can also occur if large areas of the bone marrow are irradiated. Postinfectious neutropenias are seen after hepatitis, infectious mononucleosis, measles, varicella, and other viral infections. A moderate leukopenia is classic in typhoid fever, but can also be seen with other infections such as tuberculosis or brucellosis. Congenital neutropenias occur in several syndromes such as reticular dysgenesis. Kostmann syndrome is defined as a congenital agranulocytosis. The pancreatic insufficiency and growth retardation associated with Schwachmann-Diamond syndrome often presents with neutropenia and frequent infections. Mutations in the *ELA-2* gene encoding neutrophil elastase were identified in about half of cases with severe congenital neutropenia (SCN). In rare cases, a mutation of the zinc finger transcriptional repressor Gfi1 was identified. It was proposed that mutations of the *ELA-2* gene lead to a mistrafficking of neutrophil elastase. A long-term follow-up of patients with SCN and Schwachmann-Diamond syndrome has shown that 5–10% develop myelodysplastic syndrome or acute myeloid leukemias. The transition to acute leukemias is associated with monosomy 7, ras mutations, and mutations of the G-CSF receptor. Further rare genetic diseases associated with neutropenia are: Hermansky-Pudlak syndrome (mutation of the *AP3B1* gene), Chediak-Higashi syndrome (mutation of the *LYST* gene), Barth syndrome (mutation of the *TAZ* gene), and Cohen syndrome (mutation of the *COH1* gene). The disease entity of cyclic neutropenia is discussed later. Autoimmune disorders like lupus erythematosus frequently have neutropenia due to granulocyte antibodies. The Felty syndrome (rheumatoid arthritis, leukopenia, and splenomegaly) also has an autoimmune etiology. Leukopenia is often found in glycogen storage disorders. Myelokathexis, a rare disorder with morphological aberrations of neutrophils, also manifests as neutropenia. Finally, T-γδ-lymphocytosis, which was recently classified as T-cell large granular lymphocyte leukemia (T-LGL), is often associated with a chronic neutropenia. The lymphocytes in T-LGL are clonal as can be shown with T-cell receptor rearrangement. The characteristic immunophenotype is CD3$^+$, CD16$^+$, and CD57$^+$. Clinically, the patients with T-LGL have frequent infections, occasional splenomegaly, and, rarely, hepatomegaly. Enlarged lymph nodes are uncommon in T-LGL. Sometimes, an isolated neutropenia is of auto-immune origin or is idiopathic. For patients with congenital, idiopathic, and cyclic neutropenias, the clinical course and the treatment are documented in an international registry.

Alloimmune neonatal neutropenia is observed in less than 0.3% of pregnancies and caused by the transplacental transfer of immunoglobulin (Ig)G antibodies to neutrophils. This type of neutropenia is often severe, causing neonatal infections. However, with supportive care including antibiotics, the prognosis is good. The neutropenia resolves by 6–8 wk after delivery.

The differential diagnosis of a newly diagnosed neutropenia includes a wide spectrum of other hematological disorders, including aplastic anemias, leukemias, myelodysplastic syndromes, pernicious anemias, malignancies with bone marrow infiltration, and hypersplenism. These cases almost always have a bicyto- or pancytopenia and other signs and symptoms (e.g., lymph node swelling, dysplastic changes). Further diagnostic work-up includes bone marrow studies with cytology, histology, and immunological and molecular studies.

Treatment depends on the severity of the neutropenia. For a patient on a medication known to be associated with neutropenia, discontinuation of the medication should be the first measure. For a slight neutropenia, it is sufficient to control the white cell count at regular intervals. The etiology of severe neutropenia should be investigated thoroughly. If the patients have frequent infections and if no other etiology of the neutropenia can be found, a treatment with G-CSF (filgrastim, *see* Chapter 2) should be started. Almost all patients with chronic neutropenias or Kostmann syndrome respond to G-CSF and normalize their white cell count. The rare cases of Kostmann syndrome that fail to normalize their white cell counts are candidates for a bone marrow transplant. Leukopenias during the course of autoimmune disorders often respond favorably to an immunosuppressive treatment.

4. DRUG-INDUCED NEUTROPENIA (AGRANULOCYTOSIS)

Agranulocytosis has been described as a potentially severe side effect of a number of drugs, including antithyroid drugs, phenothiazines, and antiarrythmic drugs (incidence 0.01–2% per treatment course). A list of certain drugs associated with a risk of agranulocytosis is given in Table 1

As pathomechanisms, toxic and/or allergic reactions against myeloid progenitors and granulocytes have been recognized. In a proportion of patients,

Table 1
Some Drugs Reported to Cause Neutropenia and/or Agranulocytosis

Antiarrhythmic and other cardiovascular drugs:
 Procainamide, chinidin, aprindin, captopril
Antibiotics and antiviral drugs:
 Penicillins, cephalosporins, sulfonamides, vancomycin, chloroquin, co-trimoxazole,
 sulphasalazine, ganciclovir, zidovudin, dapsone
Anti-inflammatory and antirheumatic drugs:
 Gold compounds, penicillamin, aminopyrine, phenylbutazone, diclofenac
Cytostatic and immunosuppressive drugs:
 Most compounds of this group
Antithyroid drugs:
 Carbimazole, thiamazole, thiouracil
Psychotropic drugs:
 Imipramine, clozapine, mianserine, chlorpromazine, thioridazine
Anticonvulsants:
 Carbamazepine, valproic acid
Miscellaneous:
 Ticlopidine, thiazide diuretics, cimetidine

serum antibodies reacting with the drug or with metabolites can be demonstrated. Some cases of agranulocytosis occur without a preceding leukopenia (idiosyncratic reaction). In many cases, a dose dependency was shown. For example, penicillin-related agranulocytosis is more frequent after prolonged and high-dose therapy. Renal failure or folic acid deficiency predispose, at least for some drugs, to agranulocytosis.

In most cases, the clinical signs of agranulocytosis start as an acute infectious episode, with high fever, sore throat, and mouth or gingival ulcers. The lymph nodes of the neck are often enlarged and painful. The spleen may be enlarged or of normal size. In the blood smear, the granulocytes are severely reduced or absent, the absolute number of monocytes and lymphocytes may be decreased or is normal. The red blood cells and platelets are normal. The bone marrow aspirate shows a normal erythropoiesis and megakaryopoiesis. The myelopoiesis is severely reduced, showing a typical block of maturation at the promyelocyte stage. Bacterial infections often derive from the oropharyngeal cavity. After prolonged neutropenia, fungal infections are also possible. The laboratory investigations often show an increased sedimentation rate, C-reactive protein, and other markers of infection.

The first therapeutic measure is to discontinue all potentially offending drugs. The patient should be hospitalized and kept in a germ-reduced environment. A selective decontamination of the gastrointestinal tract is recommended. All infections should be carefully investigated and treated without delay. Chapter 3 gives details about the treatment of infections in neutropenic patients. In most cases of drug-induced agranulocytosis, a spontaneous regeneration of the myeloid cells occurs after 5–9 d. In a few cases the recovery is delayed for up to 20 d. Often, the patients develop a leukocytosis with a left shift which subsides after a few days. Corticosteroids are not indicated in the treatment of the usual drug-induced agranulocytosis. The hematopoietic growth factors (G-CSF, GM-CSF) hasten the recovery of neutrophils and should be given in cases of protracted leucopenia (for details, *see* Chapter 2). A renewed exposure to the incriminated drug should be avoided.

As far as the prophylaxis of drug-induced agranulocytosis is concerned, any drug treatment should be critically evaluated. Blood counts should be controlled at regular intervals after the administration of drugs with a known risk of agranu-locytosis (e.g., clozapine, but also antithyroid drugs). The prognosis of drug-induced agranulocytosis is generally good, but older patients with co-incident morbidity are at risk from sepsis.

5. CYCLIC NEUTROPENIA

In this rare disorder, infectious episodes occur in 19- to 23-d cycles. The common infections, most often accompanied by high fever, are bacterial skin infections, cellulitis, septicemias, and tonsillitis. Immediately before the fever begins, the circulating neutrophils decrease to values below 200/µL; they gen-erally recover after 4–5 d. Some cases have dominant inheritance, whereas in some cases a new mutation is observed. The diagnosis is usually made in early childhood; however, some cases become manifest only at the adult age. The pathophysiological basis of cyclic neutropenia is a defect of the hematopoietic stem cell. In many cases, germline mutations of the *ELA-2* gene (different from mutations seen in SCN) were identified. Some patients also have cyclic varia-tions of platelets and reticulocytes. The treatment of cyclic neutropenia has much improved since G-CSF was introduced into clinical practice more than 10 yr ago. Subcutaneous G-CSF normalizes the neutrophil count of patients with cyclic neu-tropenia; however, cyclic variations persist. The recommended dose of G-CSF is approx 3–5 µg/kg; however, some patients need much lower doses or only an intermittent treatment to normalize the neutrophil counts. The treatment with G-CSF is indicated if the patient has frequent or severe infections. As in other cases of neutropenia, the prophylaxis and treatment of infections is essential.

6. DIFFERENTIAL DIAGNOSIS OF EOSINOPHILIA

An eosinophilia (relative number of eosinophils ≥5%, absolute number >500/µL) is a frequent sign of allergic reactions, asthma, skin disorders, angioedema, and parasitoses such as trichinosis and ascariasis. Many tropical disorders (e.g., filariasis) have an eosinophilia of 20–30%. Further disorders with eosinophilia are IgA deficiency, Addison's disease, disorders of autoimmunity, vasculitis (especially Churg-Strauss syndrome), and eosinophilic gastroenteritis. The pathophysiology of eosinophilia is the production of interleukin (IL)-5 mediated by activated T-lymphocytes. Patients treated with the cytokines GM-CSF, IL-2, and IL-3 often develop eosinophilia. A paraneoplastic eosinophilia is sometimes observed in Hodgkin's lymphomas and some leukemias and lymphomas (especially of the T-cell phenotype). The malignant clone of some myeloproliferative disorders may also differentiate into eosinophils.

Idiopathic hypereosinophilic syndrome (IHES) is by definition an unexplained eosinophilia of more than 1500/μL that lasts longer than 6 mo. This rare disorder predisposes to organ complications which are due to the infiltration or degranulation of eosinophils in various tissues. IHES is observed almost exclusively in men and, if left untreated, has a poor prognosis. Complications such as intracavitary thrombosis, endocardial fibrosis, and pulmonary and neurological disturbancies are seen. Treatment should be started if the number of eosinophils increases rapidly or if organ complications are imminent. Recently, a specific chromosomal (submicroscopic) deletion was identified in at least half of patients with IHES. This deletion on chromosome 4 (del(4)(q12q12) creates the *FIP1L1-PDGFR*α fusion gene. Because clonality is proven in such patients, they should be reclassified as having chronic eosinophilic leukemia. Interestingly, patients with the fusion gene respond well to low doses of the tyrosine kinase inhibitor imatinib. Most patients treated so far have reached a molecular remission, but similarly to chronic myelogenous leukemia, resistance to imatinib may develop during treatment. Patients without the fusion gene generally have a transient or incomplete response to imatinib. Patients who fail imatinib may control their eosinophil counts with prednisone or hydroxyurea. Case reports have shown the efficacy of α-interferon, 2 chlorodeoxyadenosine, and cyclosporine A. As supportive treatment, antihistaminics should be given.

The eosinophilia-myalgia syndrome is a multisystem disorder that was reported several years ago and which was found to be caused by contaminants in some L-tryptophan preparations used as nutritional supplements. The clinical signs of the eosinophilia-myalgia syndrome were contractures of the skeletal muscles, scleroderma-like skin lesions, and damage to the heart and lung.

7. DIFFERENTIAL DIAGNOSIS OF BASOPHILIA

A basophilia (>50 basophils/μL) can occur during many infections, in allergic reactions, as a sign of thyrotoxicosis, in systemic mastocytosis, and in myeloproliferative syndromes. A clear basophilia in chronic myelogenous leukemia is a sign of acceleration or impending blast crisis.

8. DIFFERENTIAL DIAGNOSIS OF MONOCYTOSIS

A monocytosis (>1000/µL) is observed during some infections like tuberculosis, kala-azar, subacute bacterial endocarditis, disorders of autoimmunity, and some malignancies. A relative monocytosis is common during recovery from cytostatic therapies and after bone marrow transplantation. If monocytes are increased to a larger extent, a differential diagnosis to some leukemias must be made (especially acute monoblastic leukemias and chronic myelomonocytic leukemia). In these cases, special stains and bone marrow and cytogenetic studies must be performed.

SUGGESTED READING

Berliner N, Horwitz M, Loughran TP. Congenital and acquired neutropenia. *Hematology (Am Soc Hematol Educ Program)* 2004;63–79.

Cools J, Stover EH, Wlodarska I, Marynen P, Gilliland DG. The FIP1L1-PDGFRα kinase in hypereosinophilic syndrome and chronic eosinophilic leukemia. *Curr Op Hematol* 2004; 11:51–57.

Welte K, Boxer LA. Severe chronic neutropenia: pathophysiology and therapy. *Semi Hematol* 1997;34:267–278.

Young NS. Agranulocytosis. *JAMA* 1994;271:935–939.

8 The Myeloproliferative Syndromes

Ronald Paquette, MD, Erhard Hiller, MD, and Reinhold Munker, MD

1. INTRODUCTION

The myeloproliferative syndromes encompass four major clinical entities: chronic myelogenous leukemia (CML), polycythemia vera (PV), essential thrombocythemia (ET), and idiopathic myelofibrosis (IM). These disorders are clonal myeloid stem cell disorders characterized by the autonomous proliferation of the clone, which results in the overproduction of one or more hematopoietic cell lineages. The clinical presentation and natural history of each disorder is distinct, but the features of the disorders often overlap (e.g., CML with myelo-fibrosis or PV with thrombocytosis).

2. CHRONIC MYELOGENOUS LEUKEMIA

CML occurs predominantly in adults with a median age of approx 50 yr. It has an incidence of 1–2 per 100,000 people in the West but it is less common in Asia. Unlike the other myeloproliferative disorders, CML is a malignant process with a well characterized cytogenetic abnormality.

From: *Contemporary Hematology: Modern Hematology, Second Edition*
Edited by: R. Munker, E. Hiller, J. Glass, and R. Paquette © Humana Press Inc., Totowa, NJ

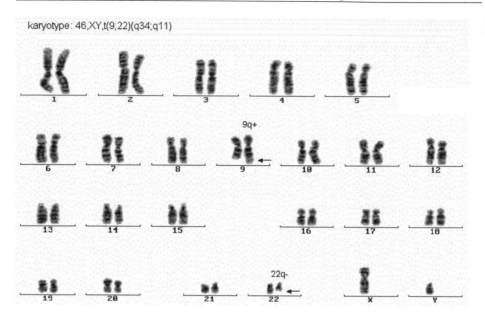

Fig. 8.1. Chronic myelogenous leukemia. Karyotype showing t(9;22).

2.1. Basic Biology

CML is a clonal stem cell disorder with a classic cytogenetic abnormality, the Philadelphia chromosome (Ph1), which results from a reciprocal translocation between chromosomes 9 and 22 (Fig. 8.1). At the molecular level, this translocation fuses the *BCR* gene to the *ABL* gene on chromosome 9, resulting in a chimeric gene that encodes a unique fusion protein (usually 210 kD) with enhanced tyrosine kinase activity. Rarely, patients with CML have a variant translocation resulting in a smaller BCR-ABL protein (190 kD). This BCR-ABL species is typically found in Ph1-positive acute lymphoblastic leukemia. Approximately 90% of patients with CML are found to have the Philadelphia chromosome by routine cytogenetics. In most of the remaining patients, the Ph1 chromosome is absent but the BCR-ABL translocation can be detected by flourescent *in situ* hybridization (FISH) or by reverse-transcription (RT)-PCR. Disease progression in CML is associated with the acquisition of one or more additional copies of the Ph1, or additonal cytogenetic abnormalities such as trisomy 8. The BCR-ABL protein and its constitutive tyrosine kinase activity is central to CML pathogenesis, as it affects numerous signaling cascades that activate cell growth, inhibit apoptosis, and downregulate the expression of genes encoding adhesion molecules.

2.2. Clinical Manifestations

There is usually an insidious onset of symptoms due to CML, usually occurring over several months. Alternatively, the diagnosis may be made after a routine blood test for unrelated reasons. Symptoms may relate to the hypermetabolic state associated with a large tumor burden, such as fevers and night sweats. Splenomegaly may cause a feeling of upper abdominal fullness or early satiety. Splenic infarcts may cause pain in the left lateral abdomen. Marked hyperleukocytosis (white blood cell [WBC] >100,000/μL) can cause neurological symptoms (such as decreased alertness, confusion, or seizures), visual changes, or, in rare cases, painful erection (priapism). On physical examination, splenomegaly is common, and the spleen may be massively enlarged. Less commonly, there can be hepatomegaly. The presence of lymphadenopathy suggests extramedullary disease progression to the acute phase (blast crisis). Patients in blast crisis often have systemic symptoms with fever, night sweats, fatigue, and bone pain. The clinical manifestations of blast crisis are similar to those of acute leukemia.

2.3. Laboratory Abnormalities

In patients with chronic phase CML, the WBC count is invariably increased and may be higher than 200,000/μL. The platelet count is frequently increased; thrombocytopenia suggests accelerated or blast phase CML. The hemoglobin concentration is usually normal. The peripheral blood smear is consistent with the diagnosis of CML when the differential includes the spectrum of myeloid cells including metamyelocytes, myelocytes, promyelocytes, and occasional blasts, in addition to segmented neutrophils and band forms. In the bone marrow, the cellularity is typically 90–100% and it demonstrates marked myeloid hyperplasia with a myeloid:erythroid ratio of 20:1 or higher. The number of blast cells in the bone marrow may be increased, but is below 15%. The leukocyte alkaline phosphatase (LAP) test result is characteristically low in CML, in contrast to leukemoid reactions, for which there is an elevated LAP score. As a consequence of the increased cell turnover, the lactate dehydrogenase (LDH) and uric acid are often increased.

The accelerated phase of CML is associated with increasing numbers of immature cells (promyelocytes and blasts) in the peripheral blood and bone marrow and decreasing platelet count. The WBC count may rise and splenomegaly may worsen on a previously effective dose of medication. The percentage of basophils in the blood may increase to more than 20%. In the bone marrow, the number of blast cells and promyelocytes increases to more than 20% but less than 30%. The criteria used to define the chronic, accelerated, and blast phase of CML are listed in Table 1.

Table 1
Diagnostic Criteria for Stages of Chronic Myelogenous Leukemia

Feature	Chronic	Accelerated	Blast
Blasts in BM or blood	<15%	15–29%	≥30%
Blasts + promyelocytes in BM or blood	<30%	≥30%	
Basophils in blood	<20%	≥20%	
Platelet count (unrelated to treatment)	>100,000		<100,000

BM, bone marrow.

Although blast crisis most commonly progresses from chronic-phase CML, patients may present in this stage of disease. Similarly, blast-crisis CML may rapidly evolve from chronic-phase disease without progressing through the accelerated phase. Blast-crisis CML is similar clinically to acute leukemia, with greater than 30% blasts in the blood or bone marrow, anemia, and thrombocytopenia. Extramedullary blast crisis may occur in the lymph nodes or other soft tissues. The blast cells have a myeloid phenotype in 80% of cases and a lymphoid phenotype approx 20% of the time. It is quite common for the flow cytometry to reveal biphenotypic features. Additional cytogenetic abnormalities may be present in addition to the Philadelphia chromosome (e.g., a duplication of the Phl chromosome, an isochromosome 17q, or trisomy 8).

2.4. Treatment

There are two prinicpal therapeutic options available: medical therapy with imatinib and allogeneic stem cell transplantation (SCT). Because of the issues discussed as follows, guidelines regarding the timing of transplantation in patients with CML are controversial at this time. Any newly diagnosed CML patient who is a potential transplant recipient should be referred to a transplant center to discuss this issue in detail. Imatinib mesylate is the first "targeted therapy" for leukemia. The drug was initially selected for study in CML because it was found to compete with adenosine triphosphate (ATP) for binding to the tyrosine kinase domain of the BCR-ABL protein. When imatinib occupies the ATP-binding site of BCR-ABL, it cannot bind ATP, it maintains an inactive conformation, and it has no tyrosine kinase activity. Imatinib was initially evaluated in patients who were not responding to interferon (IFN)-α, the most effective medical therapy for CML at the time. The study demonstrated that imatinib 400 mg/d was remarkably effective in this patient population that otherwise had a poor prognosis. Normalization of the peripheral blood counts (complete hematological response) was observed in 95% of patients. Half of the patients required less than 1 mo to achieve a complete hematological response and 86% reached this endpoint within 3 mo. Approximately 60% of patients had a greater than 65% reduction in the number of Ph1 chromosome-positive cells in the bone marrow (major cytogenetic response) and 40% had no Ph1 positive cells in the bone marrow (complete cytogenetic response) after 1 yr of therapy. As a result, in May 2001 imatinib was approved by the Food and Drug Administration (FDA) for the treatment of CML that was unresponsive to IFN therapy. A randomized trial of imatinib vs IFN-α plus cytarabine (standard therapy at the time) for newly diagnosed CML patients demonstrated markedly superior results for imatinib, with 85% of patients achieving a major cytogenetic response and 74% a complete cytogenetic response at 1 yr compared with 22% and 8%, respectively, for IFN-α plus cytarabine. Virtually all imatinib-treated patients who achieved a major cytogenetic response with imatinib did so within the first year of treatment. The risk of disease progression to accelerated or blast phase was approx 3% for the imatinib arm vs 8% for the combination arm after 18 mo of treatment. Therefore, imatinib has emerged as the medical treatment of choice for CML. Although the randomized study used an imatinib dose of 400 mg/d, it may not be the most effective dose. A single-arm study administering 400 mg of imatinib twice daily to newly diagnosed CML patients demonstrated a major cytogenetic response rate of 96% and a complete cytogenetic response rate of 90%. A randomized trial will be required to definitively identify the optimal imatinib dose. Despite these excellent results, limited clinical information as well as laboratory data suggest that imatinib is not curative. Only rarely have patients been taken off drug, even in cases of a complete cytogenetic response. Prolonged follow-up will be required to determine the durability of response to imatinib.

Depth of response to imatinib is an important prognostic variable. Several response landmarks have been identified by the clinical trials performed to date. The first chronological landmark after the initiation of imatinib is the achievement of a complete hematological response (normalization of peripheral blood counts). Most newly diagnosed patients will reach this endpoint within the first month of treatment, and virtually all patients who will respond do so within the first 3 mo. The next important landmark is the achievement of a major cytogenetic response. Approximately 70% of major cytogenetic responders reach this endpoint within 3 mo, and 90% do so by 6 mo. The third endpoint is the achievement of a complete cytogenetic response. At least 90% of patients who reach this endpoint do so within the first year of treatment. Although cytogenetic response is important, standard chromosomal analysis evaluates only 20 cells. FISH for the BCR-ABL translocation typically evaluates 200 cells. The quantitative PCR (Q-PCR) assay for the BCR-ABL translocation can detect up to a 4.5-log reduction in transcript levels. This assay is typically performed on peripheral blood and is much more sensitive than standard cytogenetic studies to assess disease response. Among CML patients who achieved a complete cytogenetic response, those who also had a 3-log or greater reduction in BCR-ABL transcript copy by Q-PCR number by 1 yr had 0% risk of disease progression after one additional year of follow-up compared with a 5% risk if less than a 3-log reduction was achieved; patients without a complete cytogenetic response had a 15% risk of disease progression. These data have helped to define the methods of following imatinib-treated patients and identifying those individuals with an inadequate response to therapy and, hence, increased risk of disease progression. Peripheral blood FISH and Q-PCR for BCR-ABL should be performed every 3 mo for imatinib-treated patients. Patients who fail to achieve a complete hematological response by 3 mo, a major cytogenetic response by 6 mo, or a complete cytogenetic response by 1 yr should be considered for alternative therapy, especially allogeneic SCT, when appropriate clinically. When a complete cytogenetic response is achieved, Q-PCR is the only method of measuring the size of the leukemic clone. A greater than twofold increase in Q-PCR levels unrelated to imatinib dose modification is suggestive of acquired imatinib resistance and early disease progression.

Acquired resistance to imatinib is often due to point mutation of BCR-ABL that results in an amino acid subtitution in the kinase domain of the encoded protein. The various amino acid substitutions identified to date interfere with the ability of imatinib to interact with the ATP-binding site and induce BCR-ABL into an inactive structural conformation. Imatinib resistance is manifested clinically as progressive loss of hematological or cytogenetic response that is unrelated to drug dosing. Because the degree of residual imatinib sensitivity varies between mutants, some resistance can be overcome by imatinib dose escalation. However, the benefit of imatinib dose escalation may be only transient. Second-generation tyrosine kinase inhibitors are currently being evaluated in clinical trials. These compounds have activity against most of the mutant BCR-ABL proteins that are resistant to the effects of imatinib. Alternative treatment approaches including allogeneic SCT should be considered for patients with *de novo* or acquired imatinib resistance. Recently, a new class of SRC-ABL inhibitors was developed. These molecules are pyrido[2,3-d] pyrimidines and bind both to the SRC kinase and the ATP-binding site in ABL. Such molecules are also active in most imatinib-resistant CML cell clones. One such compound (dasatinib) has oral bioavailability and has 2-log increased activity as an ABL kinase inhibitor compared with imatinib. More importantly, the activity is retained in 14 of 15 imatinib-resistant BCR-ABL mutants. This activity was confirmed in a mouse model of imatinib-resistant CML and in preliminary clinical studies.

The principal toxicity of imatinib is hematological, which is actually a reflection of its therapeutic efficacy. Neutropenia and thrombocytopenia are commonly observed after imatinib is initiated because the drug reduces the leukemic clone that produces all of the neutrophils, red cells, and platelets. The blood counts are gradually restored as the leukemic clone is reduced and normal hematopoietic cells grow in the bone marrow. Treatment should be transiently interrupted if severe peripheral blood cytopenias occur (neutrophil count <1000/μL, platelet count <50,000/μL) and re-instituted when the blood counts improve (neutrophil count >1500/μL, platelet count >75,000/μL). Fluid retention is a common side effect, but it is rarely severe. Skin rash can be managed with antihistamines and topical steroids in most cases. In rare cases, a systemic rash can be severe enough to require drug discontinuation and systemic steroids. The drug can usually be re-introduced at a lower dose once the rash has resolved. Transaminase elevations can be severe in rare cases and co-administration of acetaminophen may exacerbate this toxicity. Liver function tests should be monitored routinely, and treatment should be withheld if they exceed five times the upper limit of normal. Although dose reduction for toxicity is occasionally required, attempts should be made to re-escalate dosing after resolution of side effects because response to treatment appears to be dose-dependent.

Allogeneic SCT offers the only chance of cure for CML. Approximately 60–65% of the patients undergoing related-sibling SCT survive at least 5 yr. Survival is approx 50–55% if an unrelated donor is used. The results of SCT are best when the recipient is younger and when the transplant is performed within 12 mo of diagnosis. The effectiveness of SCT in eradicating CML depends to a large extent on a potent antileukemic activity mediated by the donor T-lymphocytes present in the stem cell product (graft-vs-leukemia [GVL] effect). Because the GVL effect occurs in the setting of chronic graft-vs-host disease (cGVHD), patients with cGVHD have a lower risk of disease relapse. If CML relapses after allogeneic SCT, a remission can be effectively re-induced by infusing additional lymphocytes collected from the original stem cell donor. The use of less intensive (nonmyeloablative) conditioning prior to allogeneic SCT is a promising method of reducing the toxicity of the transplant procedure for older patients with CML. Transplantation is discussed in more detail in Chapter 4.

The dramatic success of imatinib therapy has affected the clinical decision-making regarding the timing of allogeneic SCT. Imatinib offers a high rate of complete cytogenetic response with minimal toxicity, but it is not a cure and its long-term efficacy is unknown. Allogeneic SCT is a cure, but it carries with it the chance of early morbidity and mortality. It is not known if a trial of imatinib prior to allogeneic SCT will adversely affect the outcome of the transplant procedure. Because these issues are complex and are progressively evolving, any potential transplant candidate should be referred to a transplant center to discuss the therapeutic options in detail at the time of diagnosis. Potential transplant recipients who opt for an initial trial of imatinib rather than SCT must be monitored closely for response to treatment, as discussed previously, to identify those patients who are unlikely to benefit from imatinib therapy and thus should be transplanted instead. Indicators of inadequate imatinib response include failure to achieve a complete hematological response by 3 mo, a major cytogenetic response by 6 mo, or a complete cytogenetic response by 1 yr. Another indication for transplantation would be loss of complete cytogenetic response. For treatment algorithm, *see* Fig. 8.2.

The preceding discussions regarding the timing of allogeneic SCT and use of imatinib therapy for chronic-phase CML may also be applicable for patients with accelerated-phase disease. Blast-crisis patients are generally not transplanted unless they can be converted back into chronic phase disease because they almost invariably relapse in spite of the transplant. Patients who present with accelerated or blast phase of CML can benefit from imatinib therapy, but the response rates are lower and long-term disease control is less likely. Survival is superior for accelerated phase patients who are initially treated with imatinib 600 mg/d compared to 400 mg/d. The dose of 800 mg/d was not evaluated for this patient population, but extrapolation of preliminary data from chronic phase patients suggests this dose may be preferable for patients with accelerated phase disease. Blast-crisis patients should also initially receive 800 mg/d in divided doses. These patients frequently develop severe peripheral blood cytopenias on imatinib. The development of severe neutropenia or thrombocytopenia should be evaluated by bone marrow biopsy. Imatinib should only be held if the marrow is hypocellular without evidence of residual blasts, otherwise the cytopenias are usually attributable to the underlying disease and treatment should continue. The potential benefit of combining imatinib with chemotherapy for blast-crisis patients has not been carefully evaluated to date. Ideally, blast-crisis patients should be enrolled in clinical trials that address this issue. Blast-crisis patients who are potential candidates for allogeneic SCT should be treated to maximum response and then transplanted promptly. Because relapse occurs rapidly, especially for lymphoid blast-crisis patients, donor evaluation should be intiated at the time of diagnosis.

3. POLYCYTHEMIA VERA

PCV is a clonal, acquired disorder of the pluripotent hemopoietic stem cell. All three lineages of hemopoiesis are involved; however, the major manifestation is seen in erythropoiesis. Many cases of PCV also have an increased number of granulocytes or platelets.

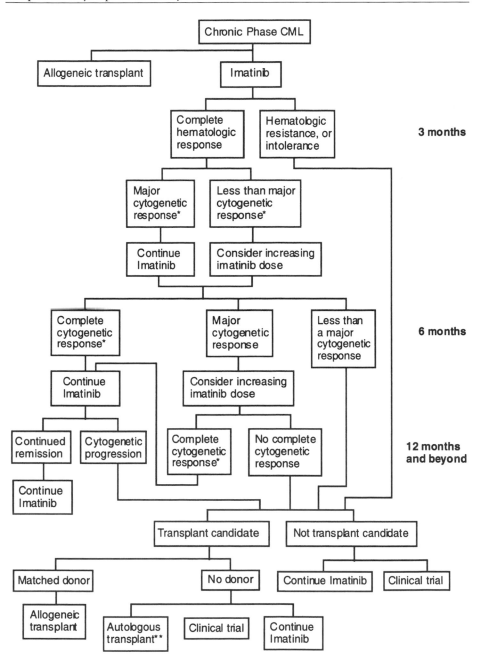

*Consider autologous stem cell harvest. **If stem cells were harvested in complete remission

Fig. 8.2. Proposed treatment algorithm for chronic-phase chronic myelogenous leukemia.

3.1. Basic Biology

In PCV, the erythroid progenitors proliferate in the absence of erythropoietin. The serum levels of erythropoietin are low in patients with PCV, whereas in patients with secondary polycythemias (e.g., with pulmonary disease or congenital heart disease), the erythropoietin levels are high. A defective expression of the thrombopoietin receptor by platelets from PCV was described. This translated into a defective signal transduction by JAK2 and STAT5 and may be a cause for the unregulated proliferation of megakaryocytes in PCV. The majority of patients with PCV do not have cytogenetic abnormalities. Interestingly, the increased expression of a gene named PRV-1 or CD177 was found on granulocytes (not progenitor cells) of patients with PCV compared with normal persons. Recently, a recurrent somatic missense mutation (JAK2V617F) was identified in granulocyte DNA samples in 121 of 164 patients with PCV. Of these 121 patients, 41 were homozygous and 80 had heterozygous mutations. Similar mutations were also found in some patients with ET or IM, but not in normal persons. An in vitro analysis showed that JAK2V617F is a constitutionally active tyrosine kinase. Incubation with a small molecular inhibitor leads to reduced proliferation of progenitor cells from patients with PCV, ET, and IM, implying that the JAK2 tyrosine kinase is a potential target for treatment in such patients.

3.2. Clinical Manifestations

PCV is a rare disorder with an estimated incidence of 0.5–0.8 new cases per year per 100,000 people. The disease is most common in the medium and older age groups. PCV is often asymptomatic in the beginning and may be discovered as an incidental finding (increased hemoglobin or hematocrit values). When symptoms are present, they are usually related to an increased blood volume and increased blood viscosity. The skin and visible mucous membranes are plethoric (dark red) and the lips and the tips of the fingers appear cyanotic. Some patients experience a burning pain in the fingers and toes (erythromelalgia). Many have bothersome pruritus, especially after a hot bath. At least half of the patients present with splenomegaly. The enlarged spleen may cause discomfort in the upper left abdomen and, in some cases, splenic infarctions cause severe pain. The increased blood viscosity reduces the oxygen supply to the brain resulting in vertigo, headaches, and even visual disturbances. Vascular changes can also be recognized in the fundus (purple color with dilated vessels). Patients with PCV often develop an arterial hypertension. A serious complication is the formation of arterial or venous thromboses, or bleeding episodes, especially when platelets are elevated. Apoplexia, angina pectoris, deep venous thrombosis, and pulmonary emboli may complicate this disorder. The vascular complications are responsible for the increased morbidity and mortality in PCV. Rare but disastrous complications include thrombosis of the splenic or portal veins, the Budd-Chiari syndrome, and mesenteric infarctions. The bleeding tendency (hematomas, bleeding of the skin and mucous membranes) in PCV is caused by functional defects of the platelets together with the increased blood viscosity. Patients with PCV also are prone to gastric ulcers, which may lead to massive gastrointestinal bleeding.

3.3. Diagnosis

In addition to an elevated hemoglobin and hematocrit, patients with PCV often have an increased platelet count, neutrophil count, and an increased LAP score. The serum vitamin B_{12} levels are usually increased as a result of the increased neutrophils, which produce increased levels of vitamin B_{12}-binding protein. An increased red blood cell mass is invariably present. In this study, blood is drawn from the patient, red cells are quantitated and labeled with ^{51}Cr, then reinjected. Blood is later redrawn, and the extent to which the labeled red cells were diluted by those in the circulation permits the calculation of the red blood cell mass. Among patients with a red blood cell mass, PCV must be distinguished from causes of secondary polycythemia.

The bone marrow cytology shows an increased cellularity with a predominance of erythropoiesis. Megakaryocytic hyperplasia is often present and may appear dysplastic. The bone marrow biopsy often shows fibrosis, which increases during the course of the disease. Iron studies often detect a decrease in iron stores even at diagnosis because of the increased production of red cells. Below are the diagnostic criteria for PCV (criteria of the Polycythemia Vera Study Group).

- Major criteria
  - A1.   Raised red cell mass (>125% of normal)
  - A2.   Absence of secondary polycythemia
  - A3.   Palpable splenomegaly
  - A4.   Marker of clonality (e.g., del {20q})
- Minor Criteria
  - B1.   Thrombocytosis
  - B2.   Neutrophil leukocytosisB3. Splenomegaly demonstrated by ultrasound or isotope study
  - B4.   Independent BFU-E-growth, or low serum erythropoietin

The diagnosis of PCV can be made if A1, A2, and A3 or A4 are present or if A1 + A2 + two B criteria are present.

3.4. Differential Diagnosis

A secondary polycythemia or erythrocytosis is generally due to the increased production of the hormone erythropoietin. This happens in disorders with tissue hypoxia in which the kidneys are stimulated to produce erythropoetin. The effect of erythropoietin is mediated by the hypoxia-inducible factor (HIF)-1. Other genes turned on by hypoxia are angiotensin-II and insulin-like growth factor (IGF)-I binding proteins.

Diseases with hypoxia are chronic lung disorders, sleep apnea syndromes, cyanotic heart disease, and certain hemoglobinopathies with altered oxygen affinity of the hemoglobin molecule. Persons living at high altitudes also develop a reactive erythrocytosis due to the chronic hypoxia. The causes of tissue hypoxia are usually evident or can be diagnosed with pulmonary function studies, blood gas analysis, or cardiac imaging studies.

A paraneoplastic polycythemia (associated with ectopic production of erythropoietin) is observed in certain kidney tumors, hepatomas, uterine myomas, cerebellar hemangiomas, and other rare tumors. Some nonmalignant kidney lesions (e.g., polycystic kidney disease) also stimulate the production of erythropoietin. As a diagnosis of exclusion, in rare instances no cause for the increased red cell production can be found (idiopathic erythrocytosis). Rarely, familial or congenital polycythemias are observed. In some but not all families, a gain-of-function truncation of the erythropoietic receptor is responsible. In the Chuvash polycythemia (observed in some ethic groups in Russia), a mutation of the VHL protein leads to impaired interaction with HIF-1, which results in defective oxygen sensing.

Some individuals have spurious erythrocytosis (Gaisböck's syndrome) due to a decreased plasma volume. This abnormality has been observed in hypertensive smokers. It is distinguished from PCV and secondary causes of polycythemia by a normal red blood cell mass study. There is no indication for treatment, although in extreme cases low-dose aspirin may prevent thromboembolic complications.

3.5. Treatment

The standard treatment for PCV is phlebotomy. The goal of phlebotomy is to reduce the hematocrit and blood viscosity in order to prevent thrombotic complications. In a patient with a newly diagnosed PCV, phlebotomies (450 mL each) should be made two or three times weekly until the hematocrit is in the range of 40–45%. When this value is reached, phlebotomies should be made as necessary to maintain the hematocrit in this range. This may be once a month or once every 3 mo. Repeated phlebotomies result in iron deficiency, which may cause symptoms like angular cheilosis. A recent randomized, placebo-controlled study demonstrated that aspirin 100 mg daily significantly decreased the combined incidence of cardiovascular events including myocardial infarction, stroke, deep venous thrombosis, and pulmonary embolism in PCV patients who were receiving standard phlebotomy. There was no significant increase in bleeding events associated with aspirin adminstration. Therefore, low-dose aspirin should be administered to PCV patients without a clinical contraindication to such therapy.

A second treatment option for patients with PCV is a cytotoxic treatment with hydroxyurea. Hydroxyurea is indicated if phlebotomies fail to control the increase in red cell volume or if an excessive thrombocytosis (>700,000/μL) occurs. The usual dose for hydroxyurea is 1–2 g/d. Subcutaneous IFN-α has been shown to be effective in the control of PCV and may be indicated for patients who do not tolerate hydroxyurea or in younger patients who fear a possible mutagenic risk of hydroxurea. The use of radioactive phosphorus or alkylating agents for PCV have been abandoned because of the high risk of leukemic transformation induced by these agents. Patients with PCV should avoid dehydration or other conditions that predispose to vascular complications. Patients with thrombocytosis (>700,000/μL) should receive a low-dose platelet anti-aggregating agent if there is no hemorrhagic tendency. If present, a hyperuricernia should be treated with allopurinol. Anagrelide is an effective drug for the treatment of thrombocytosis in PCV (see "Essential Thrombocythemia"). Selected younger patients with poor prognosis PCV are candidates for a human leukocyte antigen (IILA)-matched allogeneic SCT.

4. ESSENTIAL THROMBOCYTHEMIA

Thrombocythemia is present if the platelets are constantly elevated to more than 600,000/μL. A reactive thrombocytosis is, in most cases, self-limited and occurs after a major blood loss, after surgery, after splenectomy, or it may be paraneoplastic in some cases. Thrombocythemia can occur as part of other myeloproliferative syndromes (e.g., PCV, chronic myelogenous leukemia, or osteomyelofibrosis [OMF]) or may occur as the only manifestation of a myelo-proliferative syndrome (ET). ET is the rarest entity among the myeloprolifera-tive syndromes (incidence about 0.1 cases/100,000). Because the life expectancy of patients with ET is close to normal, the prevalence of ET is several-fold higher than the annual incidence.

4.1. Basic Biology

The etiology of the sustained thrombocytosis and megakaryocytic hyper-proliferation characteristic of ET is unknown. No specific cytogenetic abnor-malities or molecular markers have been associated with the disorder, and its diagnosis is one of exclusion. In ET, about half the patients have a clonal prolif-eration of hematopoietic progenitors, similarly to the other myeloproliferative disorders. In vitro, these patients show a spontaneous proliferation of early eryth-roid and/or megakaryocytic progenitors (burst-forming units-erythroid [BFU-E], colony-forming unit-megakaryocyte [CFU-Meg]). In contrast to the normal DNA content found in reactive thrombocytosis, the DNA content (ploidy) of the megakaryocytic progenitors is increased in ET.

4.2. Clinical Manifestations

ET may be asymptomatic and discovered when a routine blood count is performed. Bleeding manifestations and a predisposition to thromboembolic events are the main clinical findings. However, the incidence of these complications, and especially the incidence of major thrombotic events, remains controversial in ET. Recurrent gastrointestinal bleeding and epistaxis are the most common bleeding manifestations. Thrombotic complications are more common in elderly patients and are rare in young patients, even when platelet counts are quite high. Both venous and arterial thrombosis may develop, and vessels in unusual sites may be involved (e.g., the hepatic veins, mensenteric vessels, the veins of the penis resulting in priapism, and the splenic vein). The digital vessels of the fingers and toes may be occluded by a disturbed microcirculation, especially if the number of platelets is excessive. In the majority of cases, however, a benign course over a period of years can be documented despite high platelet counts. The same patients may have an arterial or venous thrombosis months or years later. Splenomegaly is found in a number of patients. Thrombotic events appear more frequent in patients with clonal hematopoiesis.

4.3. Diagnosis

Platelet count in ET is consistently increased above 600,000/μL (in many cases >10^6/μL). By definition, another myeloproliferative syndrome or a reactive thrombocytosis are excluded. The Philadelphia chromosome is not present in ET, and the red cell mass is normal. Bone marrow aspiration often results in a dry tap as a result of secondary fibrosis, and the bone marrow biopsy shows a megakaryocyte hyperplasia. There is no evidence for myelodysplastic syndrome. The serum interleukin (IL)-6 levels are normal in most cases, whereas in reactive thrombocytosis, an increase is frequently seen. This high platelet count can cause "pseudohyperkalemia" as a result of potassium released from platelets in vitro during the process of coagulation. This can be prevented by measuring potassium in an anticoagulated blood sample.

4.4. Treatment

ET is treated to prevent thromboembolic complications. In younger patients without a history of bleeding and without an excessive increase in platelets, low-dose acetyl salicylic acid (100 mg daily) is an adequate treatment. In other cases, after a complication, or with platelets above 900,000/μL, the platelet count should be controlled with hydroxyurea, IFN, or anagrelide. Hydroxyurea is given orally (0.5–1.5 g daily). IFN is injected subcutaneously (3–5 $\times$ 10^6 U three times weekly). IFN is particularly useful when managing ET during pregnancy. Anagrelide acts as a specific antagonist of megakaryocyte production and is also active for thrombocytosis occurring in other myeloproliferative syndromes. The drug (1–2 mg daily po) is generally well tolerated. Side effects usually associated with higher doses include fluid retention, tachycardia, or headache. Recently, data from a large study in Great Britain comparing anagrelide and hydroxyurea as treatment for high-risk ET were presented. Both treatment arms received low-dose aspirin. The study was stopped after 7 yr because patients in the anagrelide arm developed more complications (arterial thrombosis, major bleeding, and transient ischemic attacks). The incidence of leukemogenesis was similar in both treatment arms. Therefore, hydroxyurea should be considered as standard treatment for ET with anagrelide being reserved as second-line treatment. Platelet pheresis is a treatment that rapidly lowers excessive platelet counts in emergencies but it should not be used without other treatment modalities.

4.5. Prognosis

The prognosis of treated ET is mostly favorable with a median survival of 8–15 yr. The disease in some patients transforms into other myeloproliferative syndromes such as OMF or PCV but rarely into acute leukemia.

5. IDIOPATHIC MYELOFIBROSIS

IM (or agnogenic myeloid metaplasia) is characterized by fibrosis and sclerosis of the bone marrow. Extramedullary hematopoiesis takes place in the spleen resulting in splenomegaly, which may become massively enlarged. IM is a rare disorder occuring predominantly in persons over the age of 60 yr. Findings similar to those in IM can be observed during the progression of the other myeloproliferative syndromes (especially PCV and ET).

5.1. Basic Biology

IM is a clonal stem cell disorder. Several cytokines (e.g., platelet-derived growth factor and transforming growth factor-β) are produced excessively by megakaryocytes, induce the proliferation of the mesenchymal cells, and stimulate the deposition of collagen, laminin, and fibronectin in the bone marrow. Extramedullary hematopoiesis develops as a secondary phenomenon. Cytogenetic abnormalities [trisomy 8, trisomy 9, del (12p), del (13q), and others] are found in at least one-third of the cases of IM at diagnosis. At later stages, especially if a transformation or acceleration has occurred, the frequency of clonal cytogenetic aberrations is higher. In the peripheral blood of patients with IM, high numbers of circulating myeloid progenitor cells have been observed. This may correlate with an earlier transformation into acute myeloid leukemia. Angiogenesis is considered to be increased in IM.

5.2. Clinical Manifestations

Myelofibrosis may be present months or years before the diagnosis is made. Symptoms are often caused by a progressive enlargement of the spleen that lead to pain or upper abdominal fullness. In advanced cases of IM, the spleen may be felt down to the pelvis. Most patients develop anemia and complain of fatigue and general weakness. Progressive marrow fibrosis and splenomegaly often leads to worsening anemia and thrombocytopenia, and occasionally neutropenia. Patients often become transfusion dependent. Progressive weight loss is common because of early satiety. The course of the disease is inexorably progressive. Occasionally, IM evolves into acute myeloid leukemia.

5.3. Diagnosis

Typical findings for IM are a substantial bone marrow fibrosis, marked splenomegaly, and leukoerythroblastic blood smear due to presence of immature WBCs and nucleated red cells in the circulation. Anisocytosis, poikilocytosis, and teardrop-shaped erythroid cells are seen on the blood smear. Most patients are anemic because of ineffective erythropoiesis and hypersplenism. Patients initially have elevated platelet counts, which decline over time. Almost all patients have leukocytosis. A bleeding diathesis may be present as a result of functional abnormalities of the platelets.

5.4. Differential Diagnosis

Other myeloproliferative disorders, especially PCV and ET commonly evolve into IM. Patients with chronic myelogenous leukemia often develop some degree of marrow fibrosis. Myelodysplastic syndrome may be accompanied by myelofibrosis. Marrow fibrosis also may be present in Hodgkin's lymphoma, hairy cell leukemia, metastatic carcinoma, and tuberculosis. Rarely, myelofibrosis indistinguishable from IM may be associated with a positive antinuclear antibody (ANA) test. These patients may not fulfill adequate clinical criteria for a diagnosis of systemic lupus erythematosus, but the myelofibrosis can respond dramatically to glucocorticoids. For this reason an ANA should be checked to exclude this possibility. Acute megakaryocytic leukemia is a cause of "acute myelofibrosis" accompanied by pancytopenia, but not splenomegaly.

5.5. Treatment

Treatment of IM is mainly supportive. Anemic patients may require transfusions. Occasionally androgens may benefit anemic patients. Hydroxyurea may be useful to reduce the white blood count, platelet count, and spleen size, but it may induce or exacerbate anemia. Anagrelide can be used to manage isolated thrombocytosis. Thalidomide plus prednisone can occasionally improve splenomegaly. Etanercept (a soluble tumor necrosis factor [TNF]-α receptor) was found to palliate constitutional symptoms in patients with IM. A splenectomy may be beneficial if refractory anemia, thrombocytopenia, or intractable symptoms are due to massive splenic enlargement. Because it is not possible to predict how much a patient's hematopoiesis is being carried out in the spleen preoperatively, peripheral blood counts may worsen after splenectomy if the spleen is the primary site of blood cell production. The surgical risk may be considerable in patients with IM, particularly in those who are elderly. Splenic irradiation is typically of minimal and transient benefit. Patients with hyperuricemia should receive allopurinol to prevent symptomatic gout. Allogeneic SCT may be considered in young patients who have an HLA-matched sibling or unrelated donor. Because patients can survive for many years with minimal intervention, guidelines governing the timing of transplantation for IM have not been defined. In the future, reduced-intensity transplants may offer a chance for cure with less acute complications than full-intensity allogeneic transplants.

6. OTHER MYELOPROLIFERATIVE SYNDROMES

Several rare syndromes have features of the aforementioned entities, but do not fit exactly into one or the other disease categories.

Juvenile myelomonocytic leukemia (JMML) occurs in children and is negative for the Philadelphia chromosome. Instead, mutations of several genes have been identified that lead to constitutive activation of the RAS signaling pathway, which is normally activated in response to growth factors. Mutations affecting the *PTPN11* gene that encodes the Src homology 2 domain-containing protein phosphatase (SHP-2) occur in approximately one-third of cases. Activating mutations of a RAS gene occur in approximately one-fourth of patients. The *NF1* gene, which encodes a protein that negatively regulates RAS activity, has inactivating mutations in an additional minority of patients. Because mutations of these three genes have similar effects on the cell, the mutations are mutually exclusive. Clinically, the patients have hepatomegaly, splenomegaly, and lymphadenopathy in most cases. The myeloid progenitors in the bone marrow grow in culture without added growth factors. JMML responds poorly to cytotoxic drugs but retinoids have some activity. Cure can only be achieved with allogeneic SCT.

Chronic neutrophilic leukemia is a rare myeloproliferative syndrome, where only mature granulocytes are increased. The Philadelphia chromosome is negative.

Chronic myelomonocytic leukemia also has features of the myeloproliferative syndromes but is categorized (according to the French-American-British classification) among the myelodysplastic syndromes.

SUGGESTED READING

Carella AM, Lerma E, Corretti MT, et al. Autografting with Ph-mobilized hematopoietic progenitor cells in chronic myelogenous leukemia. *Blood* 1999;93:1534–1539.

Hansen JA, Gooley TA, Martin PJ, et al. Bone marrow transplants from unrelated donors for patients with chronic myelogenous leukemia. *N Engl J Med* 1998;338:962–968.

Hughes TP, Kaeda J, Branford S, et al. Frequency of major molecular responses to imatinib or interferon alfa plus cytarabine in newly diagnosed chronic myeloid leukemia. *N Engl J Med* 2003;349:1423–1432.

Kantarjian H, Talpaz M, O'Brien S, et al. High-dose imatinib therapy in newly diagnosed Philadelphia chromosome-positive chronic phase chronic myeloid leukemia. *Blood* 2004;103:2873–2878.

Landolfi R, Marchioli R, Kutti J, et al. Efficacy and safety of low-dose aspirin in polycythemia vera. *N Engl J Med* 2004;350:114–124.

Lee SJ, Anasetti C, Horowitz MH, et al. Initial therapy for chronic myelogenous leukemia: playing the odds. *J Clin Oncol* 1998; 16:2897–2903.

Levine RL, Wadleigh M, Cools J, et al. Activating mutation in the tyrosine kinase JAK2 in polycythemia vera, essential thrombocythemia, and myeloid metaplasia with myelofibrosis. *Cancer Cell* 2005;7:387–397.

Moliterno AR, Hankins D, Spivak JL. Impaired expression of the thrombopoietin receptor by platelets from patients with polycythernia vera. *N Engl J Med* 1998;338:572–580.

Nimer SD. Essential thrombocythernia: another "heterogeneous disease" better understood? *Blood* 1999;93:415–416.

O'Brien SG, Guilhot F, Larson RA, et al. Imatinib compared with interferon and low-dose cytarabine for newly diagnosed chronic-phase chronic myeloid leukemia. *N Engl J Med* 2003;348:994–1004.

Prchal JT. Polycythemia vera and other primary polycythemias. *Curr Opin Hematol* 2005;12:112–116.

Shah NP, Tran C, Lee FY, et al. Overriding imatinib resistance with a novel ABL kinase inhibitor. *Science* 2005;305:399–401.

Talpaz M, Shah N, Kantarjian H, et al. Activity of the ABL kinase inhibitor desatinib in imatinib-resistant Philadelphia chromosome positive leukemias. *New Eng J Med* 2006;354:2531–2541.

Tefferi A. Myelofibrosis: update on pathogenesis and treatment. In: *Hematology 2004: American Society of Hematology Education Program Book*. Washington, DC: American Society of Hematology, 2004:151–153.

9 Acute Myelogenous Leukemias

Reinhold Munker, MD

1. INTRODUCTION

Acute myelogenous leukemias (AMLs) are aggressive hematological neoplasms that require, in most cases, urgent treatment. Despite intensive treatment with cytostatic drugs, only a minority of patients can be cured at present. In adults, about 80% of all acute leukemias belong to the group of AML. The term "acute nonlymphocytic leukemia" is often used interchangeably for AML. The incidence of AML is about three to four new cases per 100,000 persons. AML is rare in children and young adults; the incidence of AML increases with advancing age, the median age being between 60 and 70 yr.

2. ETIOLOGY, BIOLOGY, AND PATHOPHYSIOLOGY OF AML

In most cases of AML, no etiological agent can be identified, but for some patients a genetic or acquired predisposition to develop AML is likely or proven. For example, some constitutional cytogenetic aberrations have been linked to the development of AML. A 10-fold increase in the incidence of AML has been observed in children with Down syndrome. Patients with Fanconi anemias, Bloom syndrome, and ataxia telangiectasia have an elevated risk of developing AML. Splenectomy increases the risk of subsequent leukemia in Hodgkin's

From: *Contemporary Hematology: Modern Hematology, Second Edition*
Edited by: R. Munker, E. Hiller, J. Glass, and R. Paquette © Humana Press Inc., Totowa, NJ

lymphoma. Exposure to benzene or ionizing radiation increases the risk of AML. Both myelodysplastic and myeloproliferative disorders often terminate in AML ("blastic transformation"). Approximately 15% of all AML cases are treatment-related, and can present in two different ways. The more common form of treatment-related AML results from exposure to alkylating agents. This type of AML has a medium latency period of 3–6 yr and usually proceeds through a myelodysplastic phase. Cytogenetics usually reveals a deletion of all, or of the long arm, of chromosomes 5 or 7. A second, less common type of therapy-related AML is associated with exposure to etoposide or other topoisomerase II inhibitors. This form of AML has a shorter latency period and does not have a myelodysplastic phase. Molecular markers of these cases involve a rearrangement of the *MLL/ALL-1* gene located on chromosome 11q23.

In AML, a myeloid stem cell (or an early progenitor cell) is transformed. This stem cell expands and proliferates in the blood and bone marrow and suppresses normal hematopoiesis. A characteristic finding in AML is the *leukemic bulge* (the appearance of immature leukemic cells in blood and bone marrow without terminal maturation). Blasts of myeloid leukemias proliferate under the influence of myeloid growth factors, some of which are produced by the leukemic cells themselves (autocrine growth of tumor cells).

Consistent with the clonal transformation of myeloid stem cells, AML blasts express cytogenetic abnormalities in 50–70% of cases (by classic cytogenetics). AML cells harboring specific cytogenetic abnormalities may demonstrate unique biological and clinical manifestations. Common cytogenetic abnormalities and their prognostic impact are discussed later. Segments from two different genes are fused and give rise to a chimeric gene consisting of the 5' end of one gene and the 3' end of the other gene. From these genes, a new leukemia-associated messenger RNA is transcribed and a new protein is synthesized. For example, virtually all cases of acute promyelocytic leukemia harbor a translocation between chromosomes 15 and 17. Cells with t(15;17) have a fusion of retinoic acid receptor *(RAR)*α and *PML* genes. The encoded fusion protein is a dominant negative inhibitor of the normal RARα protein and thereby causes the arrest of myeloid maturation at the promyelocyte stage. The inhibition of terminal differentiation is mediated by the association of the fusion protein with the nuclear co-repressor–histone deacetylase complex. Other common cytogenetic aberrations giving rise to fusion genes are t(8;21) and inversion 16 [inv(16)]. The t(8;21) results in the fusion of the *AML1* gene (which encodes the subunit α of the core-binding factor) on chromosome 21 with the *ETO* gene on chromosome 8. The novel chimeric gene produces a transcript that can be detected by reverse-transcription (RT)-PCR. The protein product of this gene is important in maintaining the leukemic phenotype. A schematic drawing of t(8;21) that involves the subunit α of the core-binding factor is reproduced in Fig. 9.1. t(8;21) is considered a good-

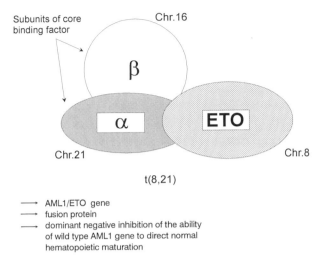

Fig. 9.1. The translocation t(8;21) involves the subunit α of core-binding factor.

risk translocation. Interestingly, granulocytic sarcomas (chloromas) are some-what more common in patients with t(8;21). The *AML1* gene is also involved in the t(3;21)(q26;q22) associated with therapy-related myelodysplastic syndome (MDS). As a consequence, *AML1* is fused with *EVI1*, *EAP*, or *MDS1* genes. In these cases, the *AML1* promoter drives the expression of a fusion transcript that contains the *AML1* DNA-binding domain but lacks the transactivation domain. Inv(16)(p13;q22) results in the fusion of the core-binding factorβ (CBFβ) sub-unit at 16 q22 to the smooth-muscle myosin heavy-chain gene at 16p13. CBFβ is the heterodimeric partner of the human *AML1* gene involved in t(8;21). Together, they form the transcription factor designated as core-binding factor. In addition to translocation events, mutations of cellular proto-oncogenes, especially *N-ras*, also play a role in the pathogenesis of AML. Patients with normal cytogenetics still constitute a large group of all patients with AML. Recently, rearrangements and mutations of several genes were identified that are common in this group of patients and that can even be used prognostically. The *FLT3* gene encodes mem-brane receptor protein tyrosine kinase, which is involved in the regulation of proliferation, differentiation, and apoptosis of hematopoietic stem and progeni-tor cells. It was found that an internal tandem duplication of this gene occurs in approx 30–40% of patients with normal cytogenetics AML. This internal tandem duplication spans exons 14 and 15 and creates an in-frame transcript that is translated into a constitutively activated protein. In addition, mutations and overexpression of the *FLT3* gene have been reported as potentially leukemogenic pathways. Most clinical studies have shown that internal tandem duplications of the *FLT3* gene in patients with normal cytogenetics are a marker of poor prognosis, resulting in early relapse and/or death from leukemia. The *MLL* gene is the human homolog of the *Drosophila trithorax* gene, located at chromosome band 11q23. It was recently found that submicroscopic rearrangements of *MLL* can be found in patients with normal cytogenetics AML. These rearrangements were shown to result from partial tandem duplications spanning exons 5–11 or 12. These tandem duplications are found in 5–20% of cases, may co-exist with other submicroscopic mutations, and correlate with a short remission duration. The CCAAT enhancer-binding protein α (*CEBPA*) gene is, in its normal state, involved in myeloid differentiation. Mutations of this gene can be detected in 4–15 % of patients with AML, more commonly in subtypes M1 and M2. Interestingly, mutations of *CEBPA* seem to confer a better prognosis. The brain and acute leukemia cytoplasmic (*BAALC*) gene is located on the chromosome segment 8q22.3 and encodes a protein with no known homology to any other known protein. The overexpression of *BAALC* appears to confer a poor prognosis.

These recent advances in understanding the molecular biology of AML have already led to a more accurate classification of AML and will lead to improved treatment.

In addition to morphology, immune markers, cytogenetic, and molecular markers, gene expression profiling has been found to be a useful research tool in delineating subtypes of AML and making prognostic predictions. Gene expression profiles in supervised cluster analysis recognize the established prognostic subsets, such as cases with t(8;21), inv(16), or 11q23 abnormalities. Novel classes of genes or signatures can be recognized within the established subgroups. Patients with normal cytogenetics or high-risk, good cytogenetic markers especially will benefit from a more accurate risk assessment. For example, gene expression profiling permits recognition of *CEBPA* mutations in several different subgroups of AML. The findings of gene expression profiling in different platforms (which may not be be translated in other array systems) depend on uniform sample processing, and the prognostic value of many subsets must be confirmed in patients from different ethnic backgrounds. However, because new treatments for AML are being developed, it appears possible to target treatments for AML on individual genetic profiles. An example for a gene expression profile of 285 cases of AML is given in Fig. 9.2.

3. CLINICAL MANIFESTATIONS

In *de novo* AML, the onset of symptoms usually occcurs within days or weeks of presentation. The patients suffer from fatigue, shortness of breath, fever, and, in some cases, bone pain. About 30% of patients have major infection at diagnosis (cellulitis, pneumonia, or septicemia). The clinical examination reveals the signs of failing hematopoiesis: the patients are often anemic and consequently are pale and have dyspnea on exertion. The patients are often neutropenic and virtually all are thrombocytopenic, presenting with petechial bleeding, gum bleeding, or other signs of bleeding or easy bruising. About 10% of patients have skin infiltrates (flat elevated plaques or nodules), and some patients develop extramedullary tumors (chloromas). In cases of AML with monocytic differentiation, the gingiva is often hyperplastic. Many patients have a moderate splenomegaly. In contrast to acute lymphoblastic leukemias (ALLs), enlarged lymph nodes are an infrequent feature of AML and the CNS (meningeosis) is rarely involved. Further complications such as acute renal failure are seen in cases with high white cell count at diagnosis (leukostasis, hyperuricemia, tubular damage). Cases with leukostasis (leukemic thrombi in the microcirculation) also may develop pulmonary infiltrates or CNS ischemia. Some forms of AML, such as acute promyelocytic leukemias (APLs), are especially prone to bleeding complications.

4. DIAGNOSIS AND CLASSIFICATION OF AML

The diagnosis of AML is apparent when the white cell count is increased (sometimes in excess of 100,000 cells/μL) and only abnormal myeloid blasts are found in the peripheral blood. These blasts are generally large, have ample cytoplasm, and few to numerous azurophilic granules. In some cases of AML, the white cell count at diagnosis is normal or decreased (leukopenia). In all cases of AML, by definition, more than 20% of leukemic blasts can be found in the bone marrow aspirate. Morphological evaluation of Wright-stained blood and bone marrow cells is the first step for the diagnosis of acute leukemias, followed by cytochemical, immunological, cytogenetic, and molecular studies. Cyto-chemical stains permit the distinction of myeloid and lymphoid leukemias and are the basis of the French-American-British (FAB) classification of acute myeloid leukemias. AML blasts are reactive to stains for peroxidase, Sudan black, and nonspecific esterase. The blasts of ALLs are negative for these stains, but show a coarse positivity for periodic acid-Schiff reagent. The distinction of acute myeloid and ALL is important because of the different prognosis and different treatment. A pathognomonic sign for AML is the presence of Auer rods in leukemic blasts. Auer rods derive from pathological lysosomes and are frequent in the AML subtypes M2, M3, and M4. Figure 9.3 (see also Color Plate 4) shows typical blasts of APL (FAB-type M3) with numerous cytoplasmic granules and Auer rods. In Fig. 9.4 (see also Color Plate 5), a peroxidase stain of AML blasts is shown. Figure 9.5 (see also Color Plate 6) shows a fluorescence in situ hybridization (FISH) with painting probes for chromosomes 5 and 17 in a case of APL (molecular cytogenetics). A bone marrow biopsy has the advantage of quantifying the density and pattern of

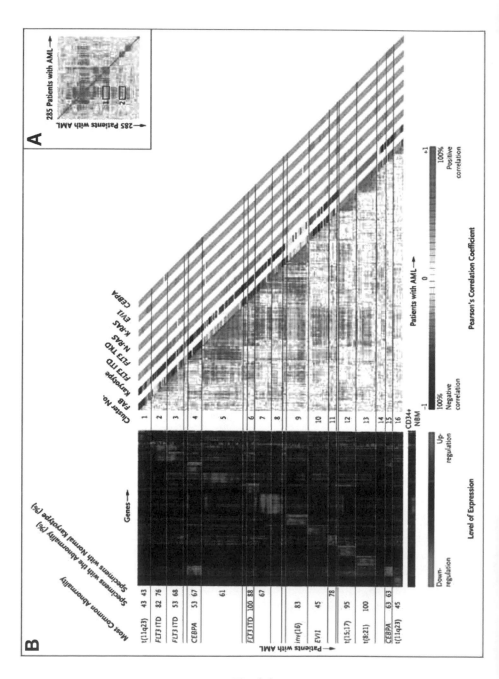

Fig. 9.2

infiltration by leukemic blasts. Some, but not all, surface markers can also be studied on biopsy specimens. In some cases, a bone marrow aspiration does not give a sufficient sample of the leukemic blasts. This may occur in hypoplastic leukemias or with myelofibrosis. In these cases, a bone marrow biopsy will provide an adequate diagnostic sample. A brief description of the subtypes of AML according to the FAB classification is given in Table 1. The World Health Organization has recently established a new classification, which incorporates cytogenetic risk profiles (Table 2).

Surface markers as defined by the cluster designation (CD) nomenclature generally confirm the diagnosis of AML. AML blasts generally express HLA-DR, CD13, CD14, and CD33 and are negative for most lymphoid markers. CD14 is positive in AML with monocytic differentiation. The minimally differentiated blasts of AML M0 (and some other leukemias) express the progenitor antigen CD34, which has a negative prognostic impact. If a broad panel of monoclonal antibodies is used, lineage infidelity with aberrant marker combinations can be observed in up to 50% of cases. The expression of the lymphoid marker CD7 in AML is considered as a sign of poor prognosis. Leukemias that express both bona fide myeloid and lymphoid markers (mixed lineage leukemias) are rare and have a poor prognosis. The *MDR1* (multi-drug resistant phenotype) gene catalyze the efflux of cytostatic drugs like anthracyclines and vinca alkaloids. Leukemias overexpressing *MDR1* respond poorly to chemotherapy.

As mentioned, the molecular correlates of many cytogenetic aberrations are known, thus permitting studies of minimal residual disease with PCR.

4.1. Differential Diagnosis of AML

In most cases, the diagnosis of AML is clear-cut. In MDS and myeloproliferative syndromes, an increase of blasts can occur, but the number of blasts in the bone marrow is, by definition, below 20%.

4.2. Laboratory Features of AML and Further Laboratory Investigations

As a result of high cell turnover, lactate dehydrogenase and uric acid values are often increased. Besides thrombocytopenia, the plasmatic coagulation may

---

Fig. 9.2. *(opposite page)* Example of a gene expression profile of 285 cases of acute myelogenous leukemia using 2856 probe sets. In the left part, the expression of 40 top genes is correlated with each of 16 individual gene expression clusters. In the right part, all patients are correlated with gene expression signature and morphological, cytogenetic, and molecular markers. (Reproduced from Valk PJ, Verhaak RG, Beijen MA, et al. Prognostically useful gene expression profiles in acute myeloid leukemia.*N. Eng J Med* 2004;350:1617–1628, with permission.)

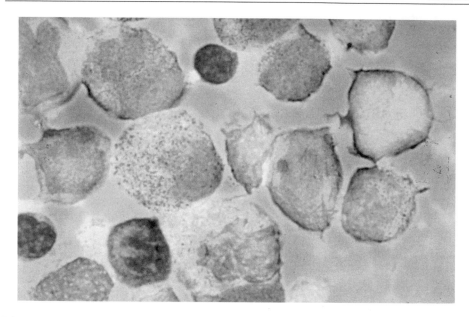

Fig. 9.3. Acute promyelocytic leukemia. Myeloid blasts with numerous cytoplasmic granules and Auer rods (acute myelogenous leukemia, French-American-British classification type M3).

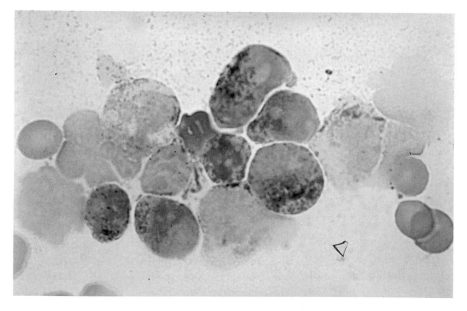

Fig. 9.4. Acute myelogenous leukemia. Peroxidase stain of myeloblasts.

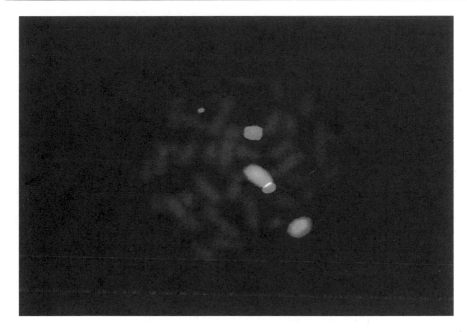

Fig. 9.5. Acute myelogenous leukemia. Blasts stained with painting probes for chromosomes 5 and 17, red-green cell with t(5;17).

be disturbed. In patients with myelomonocytic and monoblastic leukemias, the lysozyme in serum and urine may be increased. All patients with acute leukemias should be examined for clinical and laboratory signs of infection (*see* Chapter 3). Because many patients with acute leukemias are candidates for bone marrow or stem cell transplantation (SCT), the human leukocyte antigen (HLA)-type should be determined as early as possible and potential donors should be sought.

5. PROGNOSTIC FACTORS IN AML

Unfavorable prognostic features are: unfavorable cytogenetics (Table 3), age greater than 60 yr, poor performance status, major infections at diagnosis, leukocyte count greater than 50 000/μL, FAB-types M0, M5, M6, or M7, a disturbance of the plasmatic coagulation, and secondary leukemias.

Favorable prognostic features are: favorable cytogenetics, younger age, Auer rods, normal growth pattern in bone marrow cultures, and complete remission after one cycle of induction chemotherapy. More prognostic factors based on molecular markers and gene expression patterns are currently being delineated. An example of a new marker is the internal tandem duplication of the *FLT3* gene.

Table 1
French-American-British (FAB) Classification of Acute Meylogenous Leukemia

FAB-type	Morphological features	POX	ANAE	Frequency
M0	Undifferentiated Lymphoid markers negative, reactive with some myeloid markers (CD33, CD13), ultrastructural peroxidase	0	0	<5%
M1	Myeloid, no maturation Poorly differentiated blasts with rare azurophilic granules	±	0	15–20%
M2	Myeloid with maturation Myeloblasts, promyelocytes, occasionally eosinophils and basophils, often Auer rods	++	0	25–30%
M3	Promyelocytic Two variants: hypergranular (90%) and atypical microgranular (10%)	+++	0	10%
M4	Myelomonocytic Leukemic myeloblasts and mono- blasts, variant: M4Eo with abnormal eosinophils	++	++	15%
M5	Monoblastic Leukemic monoblasts (two variants: M5a, M5b)	0	+++	2–9%
M6	Erythroleukemia More than 50% abnormal erythropoietic cells, >30% myelo- blasts among all nonerythroid cells	0	0	<5%
M7	Megakaryoblastic Usually associated with myelo- fibrosis, platelet markers present	0	0	2–10%

POX, peroxidase; ANAE, α-naphthyl acetate esterase

Table 2

World Health Organization Classification of Acute Myelogenous Leukemia (AML)

1. *AML with recurrent cytogenetic translocations*
   AML with t(8;21)(q22;q22)
   AML with abnormal bone marrow eosinophils: inv(16)(p13;q22) or t(16;16)(p13;q11)
   Acute promyelocytic leukemia: t(15;17)(q22;q11) and variants
   AML with 11q23 (*MLL*) abnormalities
2. *AML with multilineage dysplasia*
   With/without a prior myelodysplastic syndrome
3. *AML and myelodysplastic syndromes, therapy related*
   Alkylating agent-related
   Topoisomerase type II inhibitor-related
   Other types
4. *AML not otherwise categorized*
   Includes most AMLs categorized in the French-American-British classification,
   excludes AMLs in groups 1–3
   Acute panmyelosis with myelofibrosis
5. *Acute biphenotypic leukemias*

Table 3

Common Cytogenetic Abnormalities in Acute Myelogenous Leukemia (AML) and Their Prognostic Impact

Cytogenetic marker	Association with FAB-type	Prognostic impact
t(8;21)	AML M2	Good
Inv(16)	AML M4 Eo	Good
t(15;17)	AML M3	Good
Normal karyotype	Various	Intermediate
–Y, +6, del(12p), t(9;11)	Various	Intermediate
11q23	AML M4, M5	Poor
Trisomy 8	Various	Poor
Inv(3)	AML M1, M4	Poor
Del5/5q– or 7/7q–	Various	Poor
Multiple aberrations	Various	Poor

FAB, French-American-British classification.

Table 4
Treatment Protocols for Acute Myelogenous Leukemia

Drug combinations	Dosage	Schedule
3 + 7 Protocol		
Daunorubicin	45–60 mg/m^2	d 1–3 , i.v.
Cytosine arabinoside	200 mg/m^2	d 1–7 , i.v.
Induction for APL (AIDA, GIMENA)		
All-*trans*-retinoic acid	45 mg/m^2	d1–30, orally
Idarubicin	12 mg/m^2	d 2, 4, 6, 8, i.v.
High-dose Ara-C-		
Anthracycline		
Daunorubicin	45 mg/m^2	d 7–9, i.v.
Cytosine-arabinoside	3000 mg/m^2 (every12 h)	d 1–6, i.v.
High-dose Ara-C-(consolidation)		
Cytosine-arabinoside	3000 mg/m^2 (every12 h)	d 1,3,5, i.v.
AMSA-Ara-C		
Cytosine-arabinoside	2 g/m^2	d 1–6, i.v.
Amsacrine	120 mg/m^2	d 5–7, i.v.
Gemtuzumab-ozogamicin	9 mg/m^2	d 1, 14, i.v.

ICE, Interluekin-1β-converting enzyme; EORTC, European Organisation for Research and Treatment of Cancer; AIDA, ATRA plus idarubicin; GIMEMA, Gruppo Italiano Malattie Ematologiche dell'Adulto; APL, acute promyelocytic leukemia; AMSA, acridinylamine methanesulfon-m-anisidide.

6. TREATMENT STRATEGIES

6.1. Induction Treatment

The first aim of treatment in acute leukemias is to induce a complete remission. The standard induction protocol is the combination of an anthracycline with cytosine arabinoside (3 + 7 protocol; *see* Table 4). With minor variations, this protocol has been the basis for the treatment of AML for the last 25 yr and has been able to induce remission in 60–80% of patients with newly diagnosed AML. Because of comorbidity or reduced performance status, not all patients qualify for full-dose treatment; therefore, the overall complete remission rate of unselected patients is closer to 50–60%. In patients who do not reach complete remission, or who show an insufficient early effect on bone marrow blasts, the induction should be repeated. The criteria for a complete remission are defined as less than 5% blasts in the bone marrow, no blasts in the peripheral blood, adequate granulocyte (>1500/μL) and platelet (>100,000/μL) counts. After the induction of complete remission, a consolidation treatment should follow. Using this strategy, a median duration of remission of 12–15 mo can be expected. Depending on the biological characteristics of the leukemic cells and patient selection, between 10% and more than 50% of patients in complete remission will survive 5 yr or longer. In the past, other drugs (e.g., 6-thioguanine, vinca alkaloids, or etoposide) were added to the 3 + 7 protocol without an improved outcome. Approximately half of patients who fail the induction regime fail because of resistant disease; the other half fail because of major complications (e.g., infection, hemorrhage, multi-organ failure). Some studies indicate that idarubicin instead of doxorubicin may improve the outcome of induction chemotherapy. More recently, high-dose cytosine arabinoside was tested in the setting of induction treatment. Although the percentage of complete remissions or the overall survival did not improve with high-dose cytosine arabinoside, the duration of complete remissions was improved. This approach has toxic complications, especially in older patients, and cannot be considered as a standard approach.

6.2. Complications of Treatment

After the induction treatment, the patients remain granulocytopenic for at least 15–20 d and are susceptible to bacterial, fungal, and viral infections (*see* Chapter 3). The disturbances of coagulation and the thrombocytopenia predispose the patients to bleeding and need support with platelet concentrates and other blood products. It was shown that myeloid growth factors (granulocyte colony-stimulating factor [G-CSF] or granulocyte/macrophage colony-stimulating factor [GM-CSF]) given after chemotherapy shorten the period of neutropenia, especially in older patients, without decreasing the rate of complete remissions. Because the use of myeloid growth factors in AML does not improve the overall prognosis, however, a selective approach should be taken, giving growth factors to older patients with a high risk of neutropenia-related infections.

6.3. Consolidation Treatment

A consolidation treatment is administered to patients who have reached complete remission. Two (to four) courses of consolidation are considered as standard. Depending on the risk factors for AML, 20–25% of the patients will survive for more than 4 yr. The fraction of patients who become long-term survivors increases with intensive consolidation treatment. In a randomized study, high-dose cytosine arabinoside (3 g/m^2) was compared with standard-dose cytosine arabinoside (100–400 mg/m^2). In patients 60 yr old or younger, 44% remained in complete remission in the high-dose treatment group vs 24–29% in the standard dose group. Neurological toxicity precludes the use of high-dose cytosine arabinoside in older patients. The effect of high-dose cytarabine is especially marked in patients with favorable cytogenetic features. In a long-term follow-up of these patients, 78% were in continuous remission when treated with high-dose cytarabine. Patients treated with intermediate- or standard-dose cytarabine had 57 and 16% continuous complete remissions, respectively. In the other cytogenetic groups, no major influence of the cytarabine dose on the long-term rate of complete remissions (approx 20%) could be demonstrated.

6.4. Role of Allogeneic Bone Marrow Transplantation

Allogeneic bone marrow transplantation (BMT) or allogeneic SCT is a treatment with curative potential in AML. The antileukemic effect of transplantation is mediated by the conditioning regimen and by the antileukemic effect of donor cells. The long-term disease-free survival depends on the timing of transplantation: more than 50% of patients transplanted in first complete remission can expect cure, vs 25–35% in second remission. Even in refractory AML, 15–20% of patients will enter remission. The pool of donors for allogeneic BMT has increased as unrelated, but histocompatible, donors can also be used with success. At present, the searched for appropriate donors for patients with AML should first include family members. If no match can be found, the registries should be searched for matched unrelated donors. A further alternative is cord blood registries (*see* Chapter 4). For standard-risk patients who have a donor and do not have a contra-indication to an allogeneic transplant, the transplantation should be performed in first complete remission. In patients with good risk features [e.g., APL, leukemias with t(8;21)], the transplantation should be deferred until the second remission. Patients with refractory leukemia should also be referred for a donor search, because these patients have a chance (5–8%) of long-term survival free of disease. Patients in first remission who do not have an allogeneic donor, or who are reluctant to undergo an allogeneic transplant should undergo intensive consolidation or autologous transplantation (*see* following section).

6.5. Role of Autologous Transplantation

Remission bone marrow or stem cells can be harvested, preserved in liquid nitrogen, and reinfused into the patient after further chemotherapy. Autologous transplantation eliminates the complications and toxicities of allogeneic transplantation, but relapse is inevitable because of the presence of leukemic stem cells in the graft. There is hope that in vitro manipulation of the graft ("purging") may eliminate clonogenic leukemic cells. In one multi-center study, autologous transplantation was compared with allogeneic transplantation and intensive consolidation treatment. The results of autologous transplantation were nearly comparable with those of allogeneic transplantation and were better than intensive consolidation treatment. The projected rate of disease-free survival at 4 yr was 55% for allogeneic transplantation, 48% for autologous transplantation, and 30% for intensive chemotherapy. The relapse rate was highest in the intensive-chemotherapy group and lowest in the allogeneic transplant group, whereas the rate of early deaths was highest after allogeneic transplantion and lowest after intensive chemotherapy. However, at 4 yr, the overall survival after complete remission was comparable in all three groups (59% yr for allogeneic, 56% for autologous transplantation, and 46% for intensive chemotherapy) because of the rescue of relapses after chemotherapy by autologous transplantion. Autologous transplantation can also be performed in patients up to the age of 65 yr. These favorable results of autologous transplantation may not be generalizable for all adult patients with AML who lack an HLA-identical donor. In a randomized comparison, a postinduction course of high-dose cytarabine provided equivalent disease-free survival and slightly better overall survival when it was compared with autologous marrow transplantation. In any case, intensive consolidation treatment (given as high-dose chemotherapy or autologous transplantation) provides a chance for long-term survival in AML. Autologous transplantation generally has a shorter cytopenia than high-dose cytarabine. With optimal supportive treatment, autologous SCT is a well tolerated procedure, but it does not provide the graft-vs-leukemia effect offered by allogeneic transplantation.

6.6. Treatment of Relapsed or Refractory AML

In relapsed AML, a re-induction treatment with the original protocol can be considered if the duration of the first remission is more than 9 or 12 mo. In other cases and in primary refractory AML, second-line protocols that incorporate high-dose cytosine arabinoside, anthracycline, and other drugs are recommended. A second complete remission that is generally of short duration can be achieved in 30–50% of patients with these protocols. If an allogeneic donor has been found, the patients should be referred for BMT without delay.

6.7. Treatment of APL

Following the observation that APL responds to retinoids, the prognosis and the treatment of APL has changed dramatically. Earlier studied showed that even refractory cases of APL obtained complete remission with oral all-*trans*-retinoic acid (ATRA). The treatment of APL is the first example for a differentiation treatment of human cancer. At present, the optimal treatment for patients with APL is to combine retinoids with induction chemotherapy. In a randomized study it was shown that the inclusion of retinoic acid improved both disease-free and overall survival in patients with APL (disease-free survival at 4 yr around 70%). Retinoic acid has changed the prognosis of APL by reducing the likelihood of relapse. The standard dose of ATRA is 45 mg/m^2 per day (given orally). About 20–30% of patients treated with retinoic acid develop "retinoic acid syndrome" (unexplained fever, weight gain, pleural and pericardial effusions, interstitial pulmonary infiltrates). In this case, retinoic acid should be stopped and treatment with cytostatic drugs must be started. Steroids may also be necessary. Different from other types of AML, the prognosis of APL is improved if the patient receives maintenance chemotherapy. The optimal maintenance therapy is currently investigated in studies, but generally includes retinoic acid. Another agent with activity in APL is arsenic trioxide (>80% responses, many complete remissions) in patients who relapsed after chemotherapy and/or ATRA). Currently, the effect of arsenic incorporated into induction regimens for APL is being investigated. In APL, the disappearance of the *PML/RAR a* gene product corresponds to a stable remission, whereas the reappearance (tested by a sensitive PCR) heralds relapse in many cases. Patients who reach a second remission should be investigated for a SCT or BMT. It was found recently that patients who have a second molecular remission and who are able to mobilize PCR-negative stem cells actually have a better outcome (especially older patients) than patients who undergo an allogeneic transplant.

6.8. Treatment of Secondary Leukemias

Patients with secondary leukemias have little chance of obtaining a complete remission with current chemotherapy protocols. Therefore, these patients should undergo allogeneic BMT early, if they have a histocompatible donor. The transplantation may be done without further chemotherapy or after one cycle of chemotherapy for cytoreduction to decrease the risk of relapse after transplantation.

6.9. Treatment of AML in Older Patients, Antibody Conjugates

Older patients often have unfavorable cytogenetics and, as a result of comorbidity, may not be able to tolerate a full-dose induction chemotherapy. In older patients, AML is more often secondary to MDS. Patients in good performance status can and should be treated with intensive chemotherapy. However, even when older patients are treated with standard doses of chemotherapy, their rates of complete remission and of long-term survival are lower than those in younger patients. In most patients older than 65 yr with AML, the treatment goals are palliative. Patients should be treated for complications and infections and receive blood transfusions. Some older patients have a prolonged survival on supportive treatment. Selected patients may be candidates for a reduced-intensity allogeneic SCT. Patients with CD33-positive AMLs who are not candidates for aggressive chemotherapy or who have relapsed after a short remission may benefit from gemtuzumab-ozogamicin. This drug consists of a humanized monoclonal antibody directed against CD33 coupled to an antitumor antibiotic. Most myeloid leukemias are positive for CD33. Complete or partial remissions can be expected in about 30% of older patients with relapsed AML. Toxicities are more severe if patients with high white cell counts are treated. Therefore, in cases with high white cell counts, a pretreatment with oral chemotherapy or leukapheresis is recommended. Common side effects include acute infusion reactions, neutropenia, increases in bilirubin, and transaminases. Occuring less frequently is veno-occlusive disease. Patients who later undergo an allogeneic transplantation are at an increased risk of veno-occlusive disease. CD33 antibodies can also be conjugated to radioactive isotopes and other toxins. These conjugates have not yet been developed commercially. Older patients may be candidates for the treatment with new molecules like farnesyl transferase inhibitors, which do not have the side effects of traditional chemotherapy and may be lead to a clearance of blasts in selected cases.

6.10. New Treatment Strategies and Outlook

New treatment strategies based on the molecular aberrations found in most AML are currently under development. Farnesyl transferase inhibitors have shown activity in refractory AML. Inhibitors of histone deacetylases induce differentiation of AML blasts and are currently in clinical trials. As mentioned, activating mutations of the FLT3-receptor tyrosine kinase occur in about 30% of AMLs. Currently, four inhibitors of *FLT3* are in clinical trials. Further approaches that are in the early stages of clinical testing involve new agents that reverse MDR, tumor vaccines, immunotoxins directed against myeloid differentiation antigens, and monoclonal antibodies conjugated to radioisotopes.

Immunotherapy for AML offers the theoretical benefit of antileukemic response mediated by T-lymphocytes or natural killer cells without the complications and morbidity of graft-vs-host disease. As the cures observed after allogeneic transplantation underscore, the human immune system is definitely able to recognize and eliminate the blasts of AML. However, the immunotherapeutic approach needs development. Several groups have developed vaccines, based on peptides, proteins, and direct cell-mediated antigen-recognition.

The Wilms tumor antigen (WT1) is overexpressed in many cases of AML. Several groups have developed vaccines from WT1 peptides. Early clinical responses were seen in patients with low tumor loads. The clinical responses correlated with the activity or frequency of WT1-specific cytotoxic T-lymphocytes after vaccination. Further targets expressed on myeloid blasts and used as potential targets for immunotherapy are proteinase-3, PR-1, and MY4. Selected patients with refractory AML vaccinated against tumor-associated AML reached even molecular remissions.

SUGGESTED READING

Bloomfield CD, Lawrence D, Byrd JC, et al. Frequency of prolonged remission duration after high-dose cytarabine intensification in acute myeloid leukemia varies by cytogenetic subtype. *Cancer Res* 1998;58:4173–4179.

Burnett AK, Eden OB. The treatment of acute leukaemia. *Lancet* 1997;349:270–275.

Burnett AK, Goldstone AH, Stevens RMF, et al. Randomized comparison of autologous bone marrow transplantation to intensive chemotherapy for acute myeloid leukaemia in first remission: results of the MRC AML10 trial. *Lancet* 1998;351:700–708.

Caligiuri MA, Strout MP, Gilliland DG. Molecular biology of acute myeloid leukemia . *Semin Oncol* 1997;24:32–44.

Cassileth PA, Strout MP, Gilliland DG. Chemotherapy compared with autologous or allogeneic bone marrow transplantation in the management of acute myeloid leukemia in remission. *N Engl J Med* 1998;339:1649–1656.

Fenaux P, Chomienne C, Degos L. Acute promyelocytic leukemia: biology and treatment. *Semin Oncol* 1997;24:92–102.

Marcucci G, Mrózek K, Bloomfield CD. Molecular heterogeneity and prognostic biomarkers in adults with acute myeloid leukemia and normal cytogenetics. *Curr Op Hematol* 2005;12:68–75.

Mayer RJ, Davis RB, Schiffer CA, et al. Intensive postremission chemotherapy in adults with acute myeloid leukemia. *N Engl J Med* 1994;331:896–903.

Stock W, Thirman MJ. Pathobiology of acute myeloid leukemia. UpToDate® Version 14.2 (June 2006)(http://utdol.com).

Stone RM, O'Donnell M, Sekeres MA. Acute myeloid leukemia. *Hematology 2004: American Society of Hematolology Education Program Book.* Washington, DC: American Society of Hematology, 2004:98–117.

Tallman MS, Andersen JW, Schiffer CA, et al: All-*trans*-retinoic acid in acute promyelocytic leukemia. *N Engl J Med* 1997;337:1021–1028.

Tallman MS, Gilliland DG, Rowe JM. Drug therapy of acute myeloid leukemia. *Blood* 2005;106:2243.

Valk PJM, Delwel R, Löwenberg B: Gene expression profiling in acute myeloid leukemia. *Current Op Hematol* 2005;12:76–81.

10 Acute Lymphoblastic Leukemias

Reinhold Munker, MD
and Vishwas Sakhalkar, MD

CONTENTS

INTRODUCTION
MOLECULAR BIOLOGY OF ALL
CLINICAL MANIFESTATIONS
DIAGNOSIS AND CLASSIFICATION OF ALL
PROGNOSTIC FACTORS AND COMPLICATIONS IN ALL
TREATMENT STRATEGIES
SUGGESTED READING

1. INTRODUCTION

Acute lymphoblastic leukemias (ALLs) are a group of hematological neoplasias defined by cytomorphology, cytochemistry, immunological markers, and more recently, molecular markers. The prognosis of ALL has much improved in the last 30 yr, especially in the age group between 2 and 10 yr, where most patients can be cured by chemotherapy. The incidence of ALL is lower than for acute myelogenous leukemia (AML) (~1–2 cases per 100,000 inhabitants in Western countries per year). In contrast to AML, a bimodal age peak is found in ALL: most cases occur in children (with a peak incidence of 10 per 100,000 at 3 yr) and young adults followed by a second age peak beyond 60 yr. The peak is more pronounced in whites, higher socioeconomic strata, and industrialized nations in the Western hemisphere, and is mainly due to early pre-B-cell ALL. Although recent studies in the United States, the United Kingdom, and Italy seem to implicate an increased incidence of early pre-B-cell ALL as being responsible for an increase in incidence of B-lineage ALL, a very large study in Nordic countries did not mirror this finding. It could be partially explained by a concomi-

From: *Contemporary Hematology: Modern Hematology, Second Edition*
Edited by: R. Munker, E. Hiller, J. Glass, and R. Paquette © Humana Press Inc., Totowa, NJ

tant decrease in incidence of undifferentiated ALL due to improved methods of diagnosis. ALL is four times as common as AML in children. In the United States, about 3000–4000 new cases of ALL are diagnosed each year; of these, about 2500 are children.

2. MOLECULAR BIOLOGY OF ALL

The earliest event in ALL is the transformation and clonal proliferation of a lymphoid stem cell. The phenotype of ALL blasts is determined by the cell of origin and the degree of differentiation of this stem cell. In a number of cases, an aberrant gene expression leads to an incomplete or inadequate expression of differentiation markers. Similarly to AML, the blasts of ALL are incapable of terminal differentiation.

With sensitive cytogenetic analysis, most cases of ALL have cytogenetic aberrations (e.g., translocations, deletions, inversions), some of which are prognostically relevant (discussed later). With the techniques of molecular biology, most breakpoints involved in the cytogenetic aberrations have been cloned, and in some patients, submicroscopic lesions in the DNA of leukemic cells have been detected. Taken together, molecular studies have revealed a large heterogeneity of ALL. However, despite the advances of molecular biology, the mechanisms of leukemogenesis are only beginning to be understood.

Among B-lineage ALL, t(8;14) is pathognomonic for the surface immunoglobulin (Ig)-positive B-ALL with L3 morphology (this is considered to be the leukemic form of Burkitt's lymphoma). In some cases, other chromosomes (chromosome 2, chromosome 22) are fused with chromosome 8. Leukemias with these aberrations often present with an involvement of the CNS and/or abdominal lymph nodes. In B-ALL, the c-myc proto-oncogene is juxtaposed with Ig loci (IgH, IgK, or IgL), thereby expressing a dysregulated c-myc protein. In B-precursor ALL, several cytogenetic lesions are known. The t(1;19) fuses the E2A and PBX-1 genes and produces a fusion protein that activates transcription through the E2A transactivation domain. About 2–5% of children and up to 20% of adult cases with ALL have the Philadelphia chromosome (Phl, t9;22). As in chronic myelogenous leukemia (CML), the c-abl proto-oncogene on chromosome 9 is fused with the bcr gene on chromosome 22. In contrast to CML, a fusion transcript of 6.5 kb and a fusion protein of 190 kDa are produced in most cases of Ph1-positive ALL. Ph1 positivity has a negative prognostic impact in ALL. Some B-precursor ALLs have abnormalities of the long arm of chromosome 11 (11q23). In these cases, the MLL gene is rearranged. The function of the MLL protein (synthesized in cases with MLL rearrangement) is to maintain the expression of particular members of the HOX family. Mutated MLL proteins have a dominant gain of function effect and disrupt the normal expression of HOX proteins. Altered expression of HOX family members has also been found to induce leukemia in other model systems. In some cases of ALL, the tumor suppressor genes *p15* and *p16* are homogeneously deleted. Almost half of pediatric patients with early pre-B-cell ALL (25% of all pediatric ALL) have a unique chromosomal rearrangement, t(12;21)(p13;q22), which was identified by fluorescent *in situ* hybridization (FISH) in 1994. It was missed earlier because it involves rearrangement of chromosomal segments with an essentially identical banding pattern. This abnormality results from the fusion of *TEL* (now called *ETV6*) and *AML1* (*CBFA2*).

In T-lineage ALL, a number of chromosomal aberrations are also found. Examples are t(1;14), t(11;14), and t(7;9). In t(1;14) the *SCL* (or *TAL-1*) gene is dysregulated. In such cases, the T-cell antigen receptor alpha/delta is juxtaposed with either the *TTG1* or *TTG2* loci. Transgenic mice that overexpress the *TTG1* or *TTG2* genes develop T-cell lymphomas. In leukemic cells with t(7;9), a truncated form of the TAN-1 protein is expressed. The *TEL-AML1* transcription factor gene results from the translocation t(12;21). The TEL-AML1 fusion protein inhibits the transcription, which is normally initiated when AML1 binds to a core-enhanced sequence. The resulting protein complex regulates transcription. Like the normal AML1, the abnormal TEL-AML1 fusion protein can bind to the core-enhanced sequence, where instead of activating transcription, this results in closure of chromatin structure, which inhibits transcription. The major cytogenetic abnormalities encountered in ALL and the fusion genes caused by these genetic changes are described in Table 1.

Depending on whether the malignant cells are derived from early T- or B-cells, the genes for the T-cell receptor and Ig are rearranged in ALL. These rearrangements however, are not specific for a certain type of leukemia, as about 10% of T-ALLs and occasionally AMLs have rearranged Ig genes. The etiology of ALL is unknown in the vast majority of cases. In Down syndrome (DS) and other rare genetic syndromes, especially chromosomal breakage syndromes like Fanconi anemia, ataxia telangectasia, and Bloom syndrome, the incidence of ALL (as of other malignancies) is increased. A large study in Scandinavia during 1984–2001 involving 3494 children with acute leukemia revealed that 2.1% of the children with ALL had DS, the most common syndrome that causes a 10- to 20-fold increased incidence of ALL. All inherited/genetic causes combined are responsible for less than 5% of all cases of ALL. Patients with DS had similar age and sex distribution and no major differences in blood counts compared with non-DS children with ALL. None of the DS patients had T-cell leukemia. Outcome was inferior to that of non-DS children (in contrast to AML in DS) and treatment results did not improve over time. Recently, a syndrome similar to T-ALL was observed in 2 out of 11 children who underwent gene therapy for severe combined X-linked immunodeficiency. It was found that the retroviral vector

Table 1
Important Chromosomal Aberrations in Acute Lymphoblastic Leukemia

Translocation	Genes involved		Function	Frequency
t(9:22)	BCR	↓	Unknown	Adults 20–30%
(q34;q11)	ABL		Tyrosine kinase	Children 5%
t(1;19)	E2A		bHLH transcription factor	Adults 2%
(q23;pl3)	PBX1		Homeotic	Children 5%
t(11;v)	MLL	↓	Trithorax-like	3–7% (75% in infants
(q23;v)	Variable		Variable	
t(12;21)	TEL	↑	Ets-like transcription factor	Adults 3%
(p13;q22)	AML1		Runt-like transcription factor	Children 25%
t(17;19)	E2A		bHLH transcription factor	<1%
(q22;p13)	HLF		bZIP transcription factor	
t(8;14)	MYC		bHLH transcription factor	2–5%
(q24;q32)	IgH		Immunoglobulin enhancer	
t(8;14)	MYC	↑	bHLH transcription factor	<1%
(q24;q11)	TCRα		T-cell receptor enhancer	
t(1;14)	TAL1/SCL	↑	bHLH transcription factor	<1%
(p32;q11)	TCRδ		T-cell receptor enhancer	
t(11;14)	TTG2	↑	LIM protein	1%
(p15;q11)	TCRδ		T-cell receptor enhancer	
t(7;9)	TAN1		Notch-like	<1%
(q34;q34)	TCRβ		T-cell receptor enhancer	

↑, Prognostically favorable; ↓, prognostically unfavorable.
bHLH, basic helix-loop-helix; bZIP, basic leucine zipper.
Modified from Sallan et al. Educational brochure, American Society of Hematology, 1997.

had integrated near the promoter of the *LMO2* gene, leading to aberrant transcription and expression. Indeed, *LMO2* is one of genes activated in T-ALL. As a secondary event, one of these cases had acquired a mutation of the *TAL1* gene in the leukemic blasts.

A very simple classification of ALL is based on DNA histograms (hyperdiploid [25% of pediatric patients, 7% of adult patients], pseudodiploid, and, rarely, hypodiploid) and is a prognostic indicator in pediatric studies of ALL, with worsening prognosis in hyperdiploid cases. The major cytogenetic categories observed in different age groups are schematically depicted in Fig. 10.1.

The acute T-cell leukemia caused by human T-lymphotropic virus (HTLV)-1 is a special case of ALL (*see also* Chapter 22). In these leukemias, HTLV-1 is integrated into the genome of T-cells and encodes transforming proteins like rex and tax.

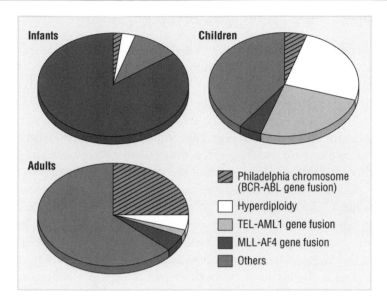

Fig. 10.1. Relative incidence of cytogenetic respectively molecular features in acute lymphoblastic leukemia with major prognostic and therapeutic significance in different age groups (*see* text). (Reproduced from Greaves, M. Childhood leukaemia. *BMJ* 2002;324:283–287, with permission.)

2.1. Concept of Minimal Residual Disease

Many patients in complete remission relapse as a result of a low number of leukemic cells in the bone marrow or other sanctuary sites that cannot be recognized by the usual morphological methods (minimal residual disease). These leukemic cells, however, can be recognized by methods like flow cytometry or PCR.

Although the surface markers on leukemic cells are not leukemia-specific, some leukemias have aberrant marker combinations that are suitable for the analysis of minimal residual disease. It is evident that further improvements in the treatment of ALL will depend on the ability to influence or eliminate minimal residual disease. The sensitivity of immunological studies can be enhanced by combining these studies with genotypic analysis (e.g., FISH). More recently, studies using PCR also attempt to quantify the number of leukemic cells expressing leukemia-associated transcripts. PCR reactions can be established not only for the leukemia-associated translocations encountered in ALL or AML but also for clonotypic changes in individual patients with ALL. Examples are the gene for IgH in leukemias of B-cell derivation and the gene for the T-cell receptor in blasts of T-lineage.

3. CLINICAL MANIFESTATIONS

As for all acute leukemias, the signs and symptoms of ALL result from the infiltration of the bone marrow and other organs by malignant blasts. Consequently, anemia, neutropenia, and thrombocytopenia result. The signs of anemia are pale skin and mucous membranes, and easy fatigability; signs of neutropenia are infections, especially abscesses and pneumonias. Thrombocytopenia is indicated by gum bleeding, petechial bleeding, sometimes retinal bleeding, and easy bruising. Hematomas are less frequent. Children often have bone and joint pain, and sometimes a painful enlargement of the spleen. In comparison with AML, the cytopenias in ALL are often less steep and extramedullary manifestations are more frequent. Characteristic signs of ALL are enlarged lymph nodes and a swelling of the spleen or liver. In many cases, ALL of the T-phenotype presents with an enlarged mediastinum. The mediastinal tumor may cause such symptoms as venous engorgement or compression of the airways. About 5–10% of patients with ALL already have an involvement of the CNS at diagnosis. Characteristic signs are headaches, meningeal irritation, or a paralysis of the cranial nerves due to infiltration and somnolence, or stroke due to increased blood viscosity leading to ischemia. Other organ manifestations like infiltration of skin, testes, or kidneys are less frequent.

4. DIAGNOSIS AND CLASSIFICATION OF ALL

Diagnosing ALL is easy if the white cell count is increased with immature lymphoid blasts in the peripheral blood and if platelets and neutrophils are decreased. The blasts of ALL have large, rounded, and indented nuclei and scant, darker blue cytoplasm. In contrast to the blasts found in AML, no cytoplasmic granules or Auer rods are present. (Fig. 10.2, Color Plate 7; a typical ALL lymphoblast is shown.) The blasts of B-ALL are larger and often vacuolated (Fig. 10.3, *see* Color Plate 8). Some patients with ALL have a normal or decreased white cell count, but if the blood smear is carefully inspected, there are always blasts. The next essential step in the diagnosis of an acute leukemia is a bone marrow biopsy with aspiration, which is usually performed at the iliac crest. The cytochemical profile of ALL blasts is shown in Table 2: the blasts of ALL are negative for peroxidase, Sudan black, or chloroacetate esterase; approx 80% are positive for the periodic acid-Schiff (PAS) stain (often large cytoplasmic aggregates of PAS). Acid phosphatase may also be positive.

In many cases, the bone marrow aspiration shows a dense infiltration with leukemic blasts (>50–90%). In a few cases, the infiltrate of leukemic cells is so dense that no aspiration is possible (dry tap). In such cases, a bone marrow biopsy will establish the diagnosis of acute leukemia. The differentiated immunological

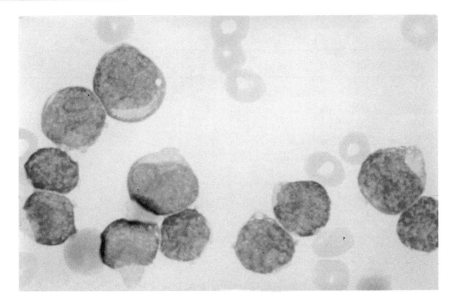

Fig. 10.2. Acute lymphoblastic leukemia (French-American-British [FAB]-type L2).

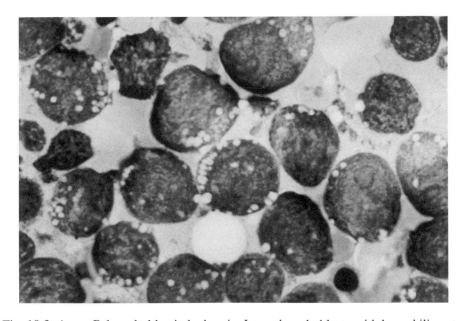

Fig. 10.3. Acute B-lymphoblastic leukemia. Large lymphoblasts with basophilic cytoplasm and vacuoles.

Table 2
French-American-British (FAB) Classification of Acute Lymphoblastic Leukemias

FAB type	Morphological features	POX	PAS	Acid phosphatase
L1	Small homogeneous with scanty cytoplasm, moderate basophilia, inconspicuous nuclei	0	+/++	0/+
L2	Larger, heterogeneous cells, variable cytoplasm, basophilia, prominent nucleoli	0	+/++	0/+
L3	Larger, homogeneous cells with dark basophilic cytoplasm, prominent vacuoles, prominent nucleoli	0	+/++	0/+

POX, peroxidase; PAS, periodic acid-Schiff.

and cytochemical differentiation of the blasts can be performed from blood. It is of special importance to differentiate between ALL and AML, because the treatments and prognoses are different. Leukemic blasts should always be phenotyped for the expression of differentiation antigens (B, T, natural killer [NK], and myelomonocytic markers) using a panel of monoclonal antibodies. In addition, ALL subtypes are defined by immunological markers. Certain cytoplasmic markers are also helpful to differentiate ALL, including cytoplasmic Ig for early B-ALL, cytoplasmic CD3 for T-ALL, and the enzyme terminal transferase (TdT) reactive in most ALL. TdT is expressed in all cases of ALL with the exception of B-ALL (Table 3); however, it can also be found in some cases of typical AML. Occasionally, the bone marrow shows less then 25% blasts with ALL morphology, despite extramedullary manifestations such as enlarged lymph nodes and a mediastinal mass. These cases are classified as lymphoblastic lymphomas with bone marrow involvement. Because of the diagnostic and prognostic relevance of cytogenetics (as mentioned), ALL blasts should always be examined in a cytogenetic laboratory. Some cooperative groups base treatment strategies in ALL on the presence or absence of certain molecular markers. Therefore, the DNA and RNA of leukemic cells should be isolated at diagnosis.

When a case of ALL is newly diagnosed, a chest X-ray should be performed in order to recognize a mediastinal tumor (typical of T-ALL) and to exclude pneumonic infiltrates. If the chest X-ray shows an enlarged mediastinum, a computed axial tomography (CAT) scan (or a magnetic resonance tomography [MRT] scan) of the mediastinum should also be requested to measure the exact dimensions of the mediastinal tumor. As mentioned in Chapters 3 and 8, possible

Table 3
Immunological Classification of Acute Lymphoblastic Leukemias (ALLs)

Type of ALL	HLA-DR	TdT	CD10	CD19[a]	CyIg	SIg	CD7	CyCD3	Frequency	
									Adults	Children
Pro-B-ALL	+	+	0	+	0	0	0	0	4–10%	7%
Common ALL	+	+	+	+	0	0	0	0	50–60%	70%
Pre-B-ALL	+	+	+	+	+	0	0	0	≈10%	≈15%
B-ALL	+	0	+/–	+	+/–	++	0	0	3–4%	2–3%
Early T-ALL	0	+	0/+	0	0	0	+	+	7–10%	≈1%
T-ALL[b]	0	+	0/+	0	0	0	+	+	15–20%	≈10%
							(+CD1a, CD2, CD3)			

CD, cluster of differentiation (*see* Appendix 2); CyIg, cytoplasmic immunoglobulin; SIg, surface immunoglobulin; CyCD3, cytoplasmic CD3.

[a] As accessory markers for B-lineage, CD79a and/or CD22 are useful.

[b] The subtype of thymic (cortical) ALL is characterized by the CD1a and has a better prognosis in adult patients

infections should be investigated in a patient with acute leukemia before the chemotherapy is started.

Patients with ALL should have a lumbar puncture to exclude or confirm an involvement of the CNS with leukemia. The sediment should be carefully screened for the presence of leukemic blasts. All treatment protocols for ALL include a prophylaxis to the CNS by administering drugs (e.g., methotrexate) to the intrathecal space. In case of a thrombocytopenia (<50,000/μL), a platelet concentrate should be transfused before the lumbar puncture.

4.1. Laboratory Features of ALL

The blood and bone marrow findings were mentioned previously. Signs of increased cell turnover are increased uric acid, lactate dehydrogenase, and, less frequently, a hypercalcemia. Evidence of disseminated intravascular coagulation is rare in ALL.

4.1.1. THE FRENCH-AMERICAN-BRITISH CLASSIFICATION OF ALL

The French-American-British (FAB) group distinguishes three categories of ALL according to morphological criteria (Table 2). With the exception of the type L3, which correlates with the immunological type of B-ALL and which can be considered as a leukemic form of Burkitt's lymphoma, the FAB types of ALL furnish little prognostic information. Type L1 is more frequent in children with ALL, whereas L2 is more frequent in adults.

According to immunological criteria, at least six categories of ALL can be distinguished (Table 3). A positive reaction is scored if more than 10–15% of the blasts bear the antigen investigated. None of the markers as defined by the cluster of differentiation (CD) nomenclature is leukemia-specific. Some or all can be found on proliferating cells or regenerating bone marrow. Some combinations are leukemia-associated. However, the diagnosis of ALL or of acute leukemia in general should only be made if the population of leukemic cells can also be identified by cytomorphology.

Gene expression profiling was found helpful to subdivide cases of ALL according to the phenotypes, genotypes, and the oncogenic pathways involved. For example, cases involving the *HOX11L2*, *LYL1*, and *HOX11* genes are characterized by high levels of MYC expression and the loss of p16^{INK4a} and p14^{ARF}, whereas cases involving LYL1 are characterized by high levels of N-MYC expression and the deletion of other as-yet unidentified genes. Gene expression profiles on their own may have prognostic significance in ALL, but prospective studies must be performed in order to understand whether certain markers will mandate different treatments. Gene expression profiling has already identified novel leukemia-associated genes, which can be monitored in blood or bone marrow while the patient receives treatment.

The most frequent form of ALL is designated as Common-ALL (in adults 50–60% of all patients with ALL, in the pediatric age group more than 70%). The second most frequent form of ALL bears markers of T-cell lineage (T-ALL, 10–30% of all patients). A very immature form of B-lineage ALL is designated as early pre-B-ALL, whereas B-ALL has a more mature immunophenotype with the expression of surface Ig. The so-called acute undifferentiated leukemia has become rare. At present, more than 98% of all acute leukemias can be either classified as lymphoid or myeloid. With more sensitive typing methods, an increasing number of acute leukemias have been found to bear both lymphoid and myeloid markers ("leukemias of mixed lineage"). This phenomenon is also described as "lineage infidelity" and is related to the leukemic transformation. At least in the pediatric age group, mixed lineage leukemias appear to have an unfavorable prognosis. Some bona fide ALLs express myeloid markers (e.g., CD33) without being positive for myeloperoxidase (a specific myeloid marker). This phenomenon does not appear to have clinical relevance. In Fig. 10.4, the combined findings in a case of ALL (immunophenotype, karyotype, and genotype) are shown.

In Japan and the Caribbean, a form of acute T-cell leukemia associated with a human retrovirus (HTLV-1) is endemic. This acute T-cell leukemia (ATL) manifests itself with lymph node swelling, hypercalcemia, skin lesions, and a hepatosplenomegaly. Most cases have an aggressive clinical course (see Fig. 15.5 and Color Plate 19).

5. PROGNOSTIC FACTORS AND COMPLICATIONS IN ALL

Unfavorable prognostic features are leukocyte count greater than 50,000/µL, age less than 1 yr or greater than 40 yr, male sex (at least for children), meningeal involvement at diagnosis, slow remission induction (indicating drug resistance), and certain cytogenetic and molecular aberrations (BCR/ABL translocation, MLL rearrangement).

At present and as a result of the chemosensitivity of pediatric ALL, treatment intensity is, at least in children, among the most powerful positive prognostic factors.

Hyperdiploidy (increased number of chromosomes) is a favorable prognostic factor, at least in children. The presence of the TEL/AML1 fusion gene in the leukemic cell population also has a favorable prognostic impact. The L3 type of ALL (which corresponds to B-ALL) used to have the worst prognosis but has improved in recent years. In the present era of intensive induction and reinduction treatments, the pre-B- and T-phenotypes are less prognostically different. Early pre-B-ALL contributes to the bulk of pediatric patients, and a distinct category comprised of common ALL antigen (cALLa, CD10)-positive leukemias that are too immature to synthesize cytoplasmic Igs contribute to about 60% of all pediatric ALL. Although biologically diverse, they are more likely to have favorable prognostic characteristics such as hyperploidy and have excellent prognosis, resulting in a cure rate of about 90%, prompting therapeutic trials with less intensive chemotherapy for this group of patients.

Despite the prophylaxis administered to all patients with ALL, up to 10% develop a meningeal involvement. Risk factors are a high initial blast count and the immunophenotypes B-ALL and T-ALL. If the diagnosis of meningeal leukemia is unclear, suspicious cells in the cerebrospinal fluid (CSF) should be immunophenotyped. In some cases, meningeal leukemia is associated with the formation of blastic tumors in the CNS; therefore, a CAT scan or MRT of the brain should be obtained. *See* Fig. 10.4 for a case example.

Up to 15% of boys with ALL develop an isolated testicular relapse. Testicular relapses should be treated with a bilateral irradiation and the reinduction of chemotherapy.

6. TREATMENT STRATEGIES

Marked improvement in survival, from 30% in 1970 to more than 80% in pediatric ALL at present, has been achieved mainly by intelligent yet empiric intensive multi-agent chemotherapy with universal CNS prophylaxis. This remarkable success story (brought about by multi-center randomized clinical trials without new drugs) has served as a paradigm for treatment of other cancers. A finding in many studies, however, is that in the United States, non-white children have significantly lower cure rates (especially in 1- to 9-yr age group)—72–74% compared with 82% in white children.

6.1. Induction Treatment

This phase aims at rapidly lowering the leukemic burden and decreasing the incidence of emergence of resistance to chemotherapy. A minimum of three drugs is required to achieve durable long-term remission. The present treatment protocols for induction combine corticosteroids, vincristine, and asparaginase or anthracyclines. Addition of antimetabolites (such as methotrexate and cytosine-arabinoside), epipodophyllotoxins, and alkylators (e.g., cyclophosphamide) to the four drugs benefits patients with high-risk ALL, albeit with higher short-term morbidity and no significant increase in mortality. The protocols induce a complete remission in more than 95% of pediatric patients and in 70–80% of adults with ALL. The induction treatment is generally given over 2 mo.

6.2. Consolidation Treatment

If a remission is reached with the induction treatment, a consolidation treatment is given. Consolidation employs multiple cytostatic drugs, including drugs not used in the induction (e.g., methotrexate or epipodophyllotoxins plus cytarabine). The rationale of the consolidation treatment is to reduce minimal

A 39-yr-old female presents with a white cell count of 403 000/μL (98% blasts with lymphoid morphology), a platelet count of 71 000/μL and a hemoglobin of 9.2 g/dL. The blasts are positive for PAS and negative for peroxidase.

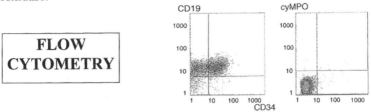

The blasts are positive for CD19, HLA-DR, TdT, most are positive for CD34, and are negative for cytoplasmic myeloperoxidase, and negative for myeloid surface markers

Immunological Diagnosis: **Early pre-B-ALL**

A cytogenetic study is performed, the translocation t(4;11)(q21;q23) is found (breakpoints are marked with a line)

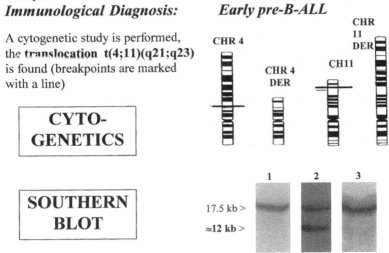

DNA is extracted and hybridized with an Ig-JH-probe, an extra band is found at approx 12 kb (clonal rearrangement of immunoglobulin genes) Lane 1: germ line control, lane 2: diagnostic bone marrow, lane 3: bone marrow in morphological remission (a faint band corresponding to clonal DNA persists).

Fig. 10.4. Diagnostic findings in acute lymphoblastic leukemia: combination of immunophenotype, karyotype, and genotype in a case of CD10⁻ ALL.

residual disease as much as possible. Many study groups vary the treatment according to the risk of relapse. In patients in the low-risk category, the treatment intensity is decreased. This avoids an unnecessary toxicity. Many protocols also include a reinduction treatment, repeating a modified induction protocol after 5 or 6 mo. Patients with special risk features (e.g., a high white cell count), receive an intensified consolidation treatment. Their regimens would consist of

Table 4
Treatment Protocols for Adult Acute Lymphoblastic Leukemia (ALL)

I. GMALL Protocol for ALL[a]
A. Induction Chemotherapy

Part 1	Predniso(lo)ne 3×20 mg/m^2 (days 1–28)
	Vincristine 2 mg (days 1, 8, 15, 22)
	Daunorubicin 45 mg/m^2 (days 1, 8, 15, 22)
	L-Asparaginase 5000 U/m^2 (days 15–28 every other day)
Part 2	Cyclophosphamide 1000 mg/m^2 (days 29, 43, 57)
	Cytosine-arabinoside 75 mg/rn^2 (days 31–34, 38–41, 45–48, 52–55)
	6 Mercaptopurine 60 mg/m^2 (days 29–57)
Intrathecal prophylaxis	15 mg methotrexate (d 0, 31, 38, 45, 52)
Prophylactic irradiation of CNS	if complete remission is reached after d 28

B. Consolidation Treatment
If complete remission after (A) and adequate regeneration of hematopoiesis
Week 13 and week 17 (+ further CNS prophylaxis)

C. Reinduction Chemotherapy (weeks 21–26)

Part 1	Prednisolone 3×20 mg/m^2 (d 1–28)
	Vincristine 2 mg (days 1, 8, 15, 22)
	Doxorubicin 25 mg/m^2 (days 1, 8, 15, 22)

(continued)

intensified chemotherapy immediately after induction (early intensification), followed by intensified chemotherapy following a short less-intensive phase (delayed intensification). The UK ALL group has shown improved results in high-risk children by using a third round of intensified chemotherapy in between the phases of early and delayed intensification. Children with BCR-ABL and infants have a worse prognosis and Ph1-positive patients are candidates for an allogeneic stem cell transplantation (SCT) or bone marrow transplantation (BMT) after reaching remission.

6.3. Continuation or Maintenance Treatment

ALL generally requires a prolonged maintenance treatment for cure. Many protocols administer monthly vincristine, and prednisone or dexamethasone, methotrexate weekly, and daily mercaptopurine. In pediatric protocols, maintenance is given for 2 yr in females and 3 yr in males (mainly to prevent testicular relapse) counted from the end of induction. In rare individuals with a deficiency of thiopurine S-methyltransferase (the enzyme that inactivates mercaptopurine) the drug causes a severe cytopenia, but can be safely given at lower doses. Hence many protocols either monitor drug metabolite levels and/or tailor drug dosage to peripheral leukocyte and platelet counts. Examples for standard-risk protocols for adults with ALL are shown in Table 4.

Table 4 (Continued)

Part 2	Cyclophosphamide 1000 mg/m^2 (day 29) Cytosine arabinoside 75 mg/m^2 (days 31–34, 38–41) Thioguanine 60 mg/m^2 (days 29–42)

Further CNS prophylaxis (methotrexate, cytosine arabinoside, and dexamethasone)

D. Second Consolidation Chemotherapy (after week 29)
Two alternating cycles of cyclophosphamide/cytosine arabinoside and teniposide/arabinoside

E. Maintenance Therapy (until month 30)
Oral 6-mercaptopurine (daily) and methotrexate (weekly), further CNS prophylaxis (methotrexate, cytosine arabinoside, and dexamethasone, every 2 mo)

II. HyperCVAD Protocol for Adult ALL
Part 1 Cyclophosphamide 300 mg/m^2 i.v. over 3 h every 12 h for six doses on days 1–3, mesna, vincristine 2 mg i.v. on days 4 and 11, doxorubicin 50 mg/m^2 i.v. on day 4, dexamethasone 40 mg/d on days 1–4 and 11–14
Part 2 Methotrexate 200 mg/m^2 over followed by 800 mg/m^2 i.v. by continuous infusion over 24 h, leucovorin 15 mg starting 24 h after completion of MTX infusion and given every 6 h for eight doses (until MTX levels are less than 0.1 µM), cytarabine 3 g/m^2 i.v. over 2 h every 12 h for four doses on day 2 and 3, methylprednisolone 50 mg i.v. twice daily on days 1–3 (a total of eight alternating cycles is given; for details on CNS prophylaxis and maintenance treatment *see* original literature)

III. CALGB Induction Regimen
Induction regimen: cyclophosphamide 1200 mg/m^2, daunorubicin 45 mg/m^2 for 3 d i.v. on days 1–3, vincristine 2 mg iv. on days 1,8,15, and 22, Prednisone 60 mg/m^2 d p.o. on d 1–21, l-asparaginase 6000 U/m^2 i.v. on d 5,8,11,15,18, and 22
(For consolidation, CNS prophylaxis, and late intensification *see* original protocol description, a maintenance is given with vincristine, prednisone, and 6-mercaptopurine, total treatment lasts 24 mo.)

IV. Example for a Pediatric Protocol (POG 9905 for standard-risk ALL, shortened version)
- Induction: all regimens (weeks 1–5)
- Dexamethasone, vincristine, L-asparaginase, intrathecal methotrexate
- Consolidation: regimens A and B (weeks 5–24) for low-risk patients (risk determined by age, white blood cell count at diagnosis, molecular markers, DNA index, and response to therapy)
- Intravenous methotrexate, intrathecal methotrexate, 6-mercaptopurine, dexamethasone, vincristine
- Consolidation: regimens C and D (weeks 5–32) for high-risk patients
  Intravenous methotrexate, L-asparaginase, intrathecal methotrexate, 6-mercaptopurine, dexamethasone, vincristine, daunomycin, cyclophosphamide, cytosine arabinoside, 6-thioguanine
- Intensive continuation: all regimens
  HD-MTX, 6-mercaptopurine, intrathecal methotrexate, vincristine, dexamethasone
- Continuation: all regimens
Methotrexate p.o., 6-mercaptopurine, intrathecal methotrexate, vincristine, dexamethasone (total duration of 2.5 yr in complete remission)

---

[a]Low-risk category, modified from German multi-center adult ALL study group. MTX, methotrexate; CALGB, Cancer and Leukemia Group B.

6.4. Prophylaxis of Meningeal Leukemia

CNS prophylaxis of leukemia is an integral part of all protocols for pediatric and adult ALL. Systemic therapy plays an integral role in prevention of relapse in CNS. High-dose systemic therapy, especially corticosteroids, cytarabine, and methotrexate, when given in conjunction with intrathecal chemotherapy, helps decrease intensity of CNS radiation, especially in high-risk pediatric ALL (T-cell, presence of high white blood cell [WBC] counts, age >10 yr, or overt CNS leukemia at diagnosis), who contribute about 40% of the cases. This strategy eliminates need for CNS irradiation in low-risk pediatric patients if additional intrathecal injections are added during consolidation and maintenance. CNS radiation may be responsible for poor intellectual development, multiple neuroendocrine abnormalities, and second malignancies. Systemic L-asparaginase also decreases CSF asparagine levels and may help control CNS disease.

Generally, intrathecal methotrexate is administered at diagnosis and at different times (12–15 injections, up to 23 injections in pediatric patients depending on intensity of systemic therapy and type of disease) during the consolidation and maintenance therapy. Some protocols also give irradiation to the brain (12–18 Gy depending on the age group especially those with high-risk features). The treatment of meningeal leukemia consists of two or three weekly intrathecal injections of 15 mg methotrexate, 40 mg cytosine arabinoside, and 4 mg dexamethasone (in adults) or 24 mg hydrocortisone (in children). When no more blasts can be seen in the CSF, five more intrathecal injections should be given. Intraventricular injections via an Ommaya port are an alternative treatment to intrathecal injections. Ommaya devices are implanted by neurosurgeons. All intrathecal injections have to be performed under absolute sterility. For the definitive treatment, a consolidation by irradiation (24 Gy to the whole brain and the neuraxis) is recommended.

6.5. Supportive Treatment and Prevention of Early Complications

Patients with ALL, as with other acute leukemias, need an intensive supportive treatment. Infections should be investigated and treated aggressively. Patients with ALL are at risk for pneumocystis pneumonia infections; therefore, most centers give a prophylaxis with oral trimethoprim-sulfamethoxazole (TMP-SMX, 2 or 3 d/wk, orally). Patients who do not tolerate TMP/SMX can be treated with aerosolized pentamidine or dapsone. ALL blasts are very sensitive to chemotherapy and steroids. Therefore, the possibility of a tumor lysis syndrome should always be considered during the induction chemotherapy. The laboratory features of a tumor lysis syndrome are an increase in uric acid, potassium, phosphate, and decreased calcium. If no prophylaxis is made, tumor lysis syndrome may lead to acute renal failure. The prophylaxis consists of an adequate hydration (at 2000 mL/m^2 in children or 3 L/d isotonic fluids in adults). Electrolytes should be balanced and allopurinol should be given. The urine should be alkalized with sodium bicarbonate to maintain urine pH between 7.0 and 7.5, as uric acid precipitates at pH less than 5.0, and phosphate precipitates at a pH greater than 7.5. Hyperkalemia, hypocalcemia, and hyperphosphatemia due to electrolyte release from dying leukemic cells can be life-threatening. Uric acid stones can precipitate renal failure. Recombinant fungal urate oxidase (Rasburicase) acts more rapidly against hyperuricemia than allopurinol, but can cause hemolysis or methemoglobinemia in patients with glucose-6-phosphate dehydrogenase deficiency. Acute renal failure is treated by hemodialysis. Extreme leukocytosis (leukocytes >200,000/L) should be ameliorated rapidly by leukapheresis to prevent or treat CNS complications. Adding cytokines (e.g., granulocyte colony-stimulating factor) has ameliorated the short-term complications of neutropenia during ALL treatment, but has by itself no major prognostic impact in ALL. Fever and presumed or diagnosed infections necessitate starting broad-spectrum antibiotics including addition of antifungal therapy for continued fever until definitive therapy can be instituted. Complications of thrombocytopenia and anemia are prevented by prophylactic transfusions of irradiated (to prevent graft-vs-host disease) and filtered blood products. Administration of filtered blood products lowers risk of allosensitization, cytomegalovirus (CMV) infections, and febrile and possibly allergic reactions.

6.6. Cure Rates and Late Complications in ALL

With the strategies outlined, about 80% of pediatric patients appear to be cured. In the adult patient group, the cure rate is lower (about 20–40% long-term, relapse-free survivors). Along with the relatively good prognosis of pediatric ALL, the problem of late effects has emerged. A retrospective analysis found an incidence of second malignancies of 1.5% 10 yr after diagnosis. Children who had irradiation to the brain had an increased risk of CNS tumors, endocrine abnormalities, and significant intellectual handicaps; hence, some newer protocols have eliminated CNS irradiation in all cases except CNS ALL. In the total group of patients with ALL, non-Hodgkin's lymphomas and other cancers were found. Patients treated with inhibitors of topoisomerase II are at a risk of developing secondary myeloid leukemias (mean latency period 3 yr). Other late effects are endocrine disturbances, obesity, short stature, and osteoporosis. The administration of growth hormone ameliorates the growth deficit. Some children with ALL who had cranial irradiation develop neuropsychological problems, usually 1–3 yr or more after chemotherapy. The administration of anthracyclines, especially at high cumulative doses, may lead to a cardiomyopathy. Cardio-protective substances (e.g., dexrazoxane) are under development.

6.7. Treatment of Relapsed or Refractory
ALL and Indications for BMT

The prognosis of refractory ALL is poor. Clofarabine, a purine nucleoside antimetabolite is now approved by the Food and Drug Administration for relapsed or refractory pediatric ALL after at least two prior regimens. The recommended dose is 52 mg/m^2 daily for 5 d. It inhibits synthesis and repair of DNA, and thus acts on multiplying and quiescent leukemic cells. Alternative protocols with high-dose cytosine arabinoside or monoclonal antibodies targeted against T- or B-cell differentiation antigens have some clinical efficacy. The strategies for relapses depend on the time of relapse. Relapses that occur early after the maintenance is discontinued should be treated with alternative protocols. Relapses occurring several years after the end of the maintenance phase should be treated with the initial regime and then consolidated with a different protocol. All patients with ALL who relapse are candidates for BMT or SCT. Therefore, the search for a histocompatible donor should begin early. Certain high-risk patients (e.g., those with a high likelihood of relapse, a high WBC count, Ph1-positivity, or an MLL rearrangement) should be referred for BMT (if a donor is found) after they have entered complete remission. In an international study in patients with ALL aged 15–45 yr, allogeneic transplantation was compared with intensive chemoconsolidation. The 5-yr, relapse-free survival was 38% in the chemotherapy group and 44% in the transplant group (not statistically different). In the chemotherapy group, almost all deaths were caused by relapses; in the transplant group the main cause of death was transplant-related complications. Allogeneic transplants are recommended for all patients in second remission who have a matched donor, as these patients have a low likelihood of cure. For children with relapsed ALL, the transplantation of cord blood stem cells also appears feasible. Children that relapse during therapy or within 6 mo of completion of chemotherapy are less likely to respond to chemotherapy and hence are clearly benefited by an SCT, especially if a matched sibling donor is available. The earlier the relapse during chemotherapy, the worse the prognosis. It is therefore logical that failure to induce a remission probably carries the worst prognosis in pediatric ALL. Autologous transplantation does not have a clear indication in the treatment of ALL. Even if the autologous graft is incubated with monoclonal antibodies or toxins, most patients treated with this approach so far have relapsed.

6.8. Treatment of B-ALL

Patients with B-ALL (FAB group L3) do not enter into the standard ALL protocols, but are treated with special protocols that feature high-dose cyclophosphamide and high-dose methotrexate and omit a longer maintenance treatment. The response and cure rates of B-ALL have improved in recent years (the rates of complete remissions are about 70% and the long-term, leukemia-free survival approaches 50%). Some studies have added ifosfamide or etoposide to the drugs given for B-ALL.

6.9. Treatment of ALL in Older Patients

Patients with ALL who are older than 50 to 65 yr generally have a poor outcome. This is due to comorbidities, but also due to the biological character-istics of the leukemic cells, with a higher percentage of patients having poor prognosis karyotypes. In published case series, a remission rate of 43–58% and an early death rate of 16–24% were reported. The overall survival for these patients was only in the range of 7–12 mo. Patients who are in good performance status benefit from intensive chemotherapy, but it is unclear which maintenance che-motherapy is best at prolonging remission. To improve the prognosis for older patients, new approaches are needed. Successful examples for targeted therapies are imatinib for bcr/abl-positive leukemias and rituximab for CD20-positive leukemias.

6.10. Use of Monoclonal Antibodies in the Treatment of ALL

Recently, monoclonal antibodies have become available for clinical use and are widely used in the treatment of non-Hodgkin's lymphomas. In mature B-ALL and Burkitt's lymphomas, the initial results of the combination of chemotherapy and a CD20 antibody (rituximab) are promising. Longer follow-up will determine if such antibodies have also activity in other types of B-lineage ALL and if they will improve the long-term cure rates. Other antibodies (directed against CD19, CD22, CD25, and CD52) are currently under development or in clinical trials. Occasional patients with B-lineage ALL co-express the myeloid marker CD33. Such patients are candidates for a treatment with antibodies or toxins directed against CD33.

6.11. Current Treatment Approaches for Ph+ (BCR/ABL+) ALL

Imatinib was found to have single agent activity in relapsed or refractory Ph+ ALL. At a dose of 400–800 mg p.o., at least half of patients had a clinical response that lasted on average 2–3 mo. In many patients, blasts in the peripheral blood cleared, although no major response was seen in bone marrow blasts. Imatinib induced responses even in patients who relapsed after an allogeneic transplant. Based on these encouraging results, clinical trials were started for newly diag-nosed patients with Ph1+ ALL, combining imatinib given orally with standard chemotherapy. Preliminary results from these studies show that this combination is safe and highly effective, at least at short-term follow-up. Historically, Ph1+ ALL has a chance of complete remission with aggressive chemotherapy of only

50–60%. The preliminary results of the combination of chemotherapy with imatinib show complete remission rates of 80–90%. Some of these patients may then undergo an allogeneic SCT with a chance for cure.

6.12. Future Perspectives

As ALL is a rare disease, the achievement of excellent cure rate makes it increasingly difficult, statistically and even ethically, to test the effectiveness of newer strategies and modalities for treatment. Extensive cooperation within large research groups across continents is needed to generate sufficient data to appreciate subtle improvements in outcome measures.

Multiple new drugs, inhibitors of signaling cascades, targeting surface receptors, oncogenes, angiogenesis, and apoptotic pathways are presently under development. The successful use of imatinib has encouraged similar new treatment approaches. Because many breakpoints of leukemia-associated genes have been cloned, a specific genetic therapy with antisense constructs, small interfering RNAs, and ribozymes is a logical approach. An alternative path of research directs the immune system against the leukemic cells, making the leukemic cells a target for autologous or allogeneic killer cells. In good-risk pediatric patients, the treatment intensity has already been curtailed to minimize long-term toxicities. Pharmacogenetics, pharmacogenomics, gene arrays, and proteomics will be used to tailor the treatment intensity in individual patients and help discover novel proteins that would target and modulate hitherto unreachable molecular targets to render resistant cells susceptible to chemotherapy. Genes that are already known to influence the outcome and treatment intensity in ALL are thiopurine methyltransferases and thymidylate synthase. Study of presence or absence of mutations in these and other enzymes that are critical for metabolism of certain drugs may help individualize the intensity of chemotherapy.

Gene expression profiling has identified specific subgroups of patients who have increased sensitivity (such as L-asparaginase sensitivity in TEL-AML1 subtype and hyperdiploidy), or resistance to chemotherapeutic agents (such as methotrexate in T-cell ALL due to lesser expression of folylpolyglutamate synthetase). This method is easier than the in vitro drug sensitivity testing. Although it is unlikely that gene expression profiling will replace the established risk stratification methods base on age, sex, counts, and cytogenetics, it will soon complement it.

SUGGESTED READING

Gökbuget N, Hoelzer D. Treatment with monoclonal antibodies in acute lymphoblastic leukemia: current knowledge and future prospects. *Ann Hematol* 2004;83:201–205.
Greaves, M. Childhood leukaemia. *BMJ* 2002;324:283–287.

Hoelzer D, Gökbuget N. Treatment of elderly patients with acute lymphoblastic leukemia. In: Perry MC, ed. American Society of Clinical Oncology Educational Book. American Society of Clinical Oncology, 2005; p 533–539.

Horowitz WM, Messerer D, Hoelzer D. Chemotherapy compared with bone marrow transplantation for adults with acute lymphoblastic leukemia in first remission. *Ann Int Med* 1991;115:13–18.

Larson RA, Stock W, Hoelzer DF, Kantarjian H. Acute lymphoblastic leukemia in adults. Educational Brochure, American Society of Hematology, 1998.

Le Beau M, Larson RA. Cytogenetics in acute lymphoblastic leukemia. UpToDate® Version 14.2 (June 2006)(www.utdol.com).

Pui CH, Relling MV, Downing JR. Acute lymphoblastic leukemia. *N Engl J Med* 2004;350:1535–1548.

Pui CH, Evans WE. Treatment of acute lymphoblastic leukemia. *N Engl J Med* 2006;354:166–178.

Zeller B, Gustafsson G, Forestier E, et al. Acute leukaemia in children with Down syndrome: a population-based Nordic study. *Br J Haematol* 2005;128:774–782.

11 Myelodysplastic Syndromes

Ronald Paquette, MD
and Reinhold Munker, MD

CONTENTS

1. DEFINITION

Myelodysplastic syndromes (MDS) are a heterogeneous group of clonal disorders characterized by one or more peripheral blood cytopenias and dysplasia of at least one lineage (classically three lineages) in the bone marrow. The approximate incidence is two to four cases for a population of 100,000 annually.

2. ETIOLOGY

In the elderly population in which MDS typically occurs, its etiology is poorly understood. MDS occurs infrequently before the age of 50 but its incidence increases rapidly thereafter. Prior exposure to chemotherapeutic agents, ionizing radiation, or benzene are well established risk factors in a minority of cases. Alkylating agents and etoposide are the drugs that most frequently cause MDS, and the risk is proportional to the duration of exposure. MDS also can arise in patients with pre-existing Fanconi anemia or aplastic anemia.

From: *Contemporary Hematology: Modern Hematology, Second Edition*
Edited by: R. Munker, E. Hiller, J. Glass, and R. Paquette © Humana Press Inc., Totowa, NJ

Table 1
Cytogenetic Abnormalities in Myelodysplastic Syndromes

Alteration	Prognostic significance[a]
5q–[b]	Favorable
–5, –7, or 7q–	Adverse
+8	Adverse
20q–	Neutral
11q–	Neutral
–Y	Neutral
–17 or 17p–	Adverse
Translocation of 3q26	Adverse
Translocation of 11q23	Adverse
Multiple	Adverse

[a]Compared with a normal karyotype.
[b]As sole abnormality.

3. PATHOPHYSIOLOGY

The vast majority of MDS cases are acquired. The development of MDS is due to accumulated DNA damage in the hematopoietic stem cell. This damage may take the form of chromosomal gains or losses, translocations, or point mutations. The most common cytogenetic abnormalities observed in MDS are shown in Table 1. Most single cytogenetic abnormalities, with the exception of monosomy 5 or 7 or the deletion of 7q, are not associated with an adverse prognosis. These cytogenetic changes are frequently observed as a complication of prior alkylating chemotherapy. Cases of MDS harboring *11q23* translocations can be observed as early as 2 yr following exposure to etoposide, and are associated with a high risk of disease progression to acute myelogenous leukemia (AML).

The critical genes affected by most of the cytogenetic abnormalities are unknown at present. An exception is the *p53* gene, which is a tumor suppressor gene residing on the short arm of chromosome 17. The p53 protein prevents entry of a cell into S phase or triggers programmed cell death (apoptosis) in response to DNA damage. In the absence of functional *p53*, cells can continue to proliferate even with extensive DNA damage, leading to the accumulation of additional chromosomal abnormalities. Alterations of *p53* are observed in 5–10% of

MDS cases. MDS patients with monosomy 17 or a deletion of *17p* often have an inactivating mutation of the remaining *p53* gene, and thus have no functional p53. The *MLL* oncogene resides on *11q23*, the chromosomal region that is rearranged in MDS patients with a history of etoposide exposure. The functions of the normal MLL protein and the fusion proteins encoded by the genes resulting from MLL translocations are unknown. One form of refractory anemia with ringed sideroblasts (RARS) is inherited as an X-linked disorder. It results from mutation of the erythroid-specific 5-aminolevulinate synthase gene, which impairs the activity of the encoded enzyme.

The most common molecular abnormalities in MDS are point mutations of the *Ras* genes. The *H-*, *K-*, and *N-Ras* genes encode signal transducing proteins that act downstream of growth factor receptors. The RAS proteins have the ability to bind and hydrolyze guanosine triphosphate (GTP). When the RAS proteins bind GTP, they signal cells to proliferate; after they hydrolyze the GTP to guanosine diphosphate (GDP), the RAS proteins become inactive. The GTPase activating protein (GAP) increases the GTPase activity of the RAS protein. Mutations of the *Ras* genes diminish the intrinsic GTPase activity of the encoded RAS proteins, and decrease their sensitivity to GAP, causing RAS to be in a constitutively active state. In this way, *Ras* mutations lead to increased levels of cell proliferation. In MDS, these point mutations predominantly affect the *N-* and *K-Ras* genes. Mutations of other genes that affect the RAS signaling pathway have been described in MDS. The neurofibromatosis type 1 (*NF1*) gene encodes a GAP protein. The *NF1* mutations diminish the ability the encoded protein to activate GTPase activity, thus increasing the amount of time that the RAS proteins are GTP-bound and active.

In addition to abnormalities in DNA integrity, alterations in DNA methylation may also be present in MDS. These epigenetic changes can affect gene expression. The cumulative effect of genetic and epigenetic abnormalities is to alter cell cycle regulation, programmed cell death (apoptosis), and growth factor signaling pathways. The manner in which these cellular processes are altered differs depending on the stage of MDS. In MDS subtypes with fewer than 5% myeloblasts, there is a high frequency of cells undergoing apoptosis. Hematopoiesis is ineffective because of the increased rate of cells dying in the bone marrow. In MDS subtypes with increased numbers of myeloblasts, the rate of apoptosis is decreased and hematopoiesis is ineffective as a result of impaired differentiation of the blasts into mature blood cells. These differences in biology between MDS subtypes suggest that the therapeutic approach should be different depending on the nature of problem. Anti-apoptotic agents would theoretically benefit low-risk MDS, whereas cytotoxic therapy would be more appropriate when increased blasts are present.

4. CLINICAL AND LABORATORY MANIFESTATIONS

The symptoms experienced by patients with MDS are related to the type and severity of the peripheral blood cytopenias. Patients commonly present with symptoms of fatigue and decreased exercise tolerance due to anemia. Less often, patients will have bleeding, easy bruisability, or recurrent bacterial infections as an initial complaint.

Physical examination may reveal pallor, peripheral edema, and if the anemia is severe, evidence of heart failure. Petechiae may be present on the lower extremities or the buccal mucosa if severe thrombocytopenia is present (i.e., the platelet count is less than 20,000/μL); ecchymoses may be observed. Splenomegaly may be present, especially in patients with chronic myelomonocytic leukemia (CMML).

Laboratory tests may reveal an isolated decrease of one peripheral blood count or multiple cytopenias. The anemia may be microcytic, normocytic, or macrocytic, but it is typically reticulocytopenic (corrected reticulocyte count <1%). Leukopenia due to a decrease in the absolute neutrophil count may be present. Occasionally, the white blood count may be elevated with a left-shifted myeloid series and nucleated red blood cells may be present in the peripheral blood (leukoerythroblastic picture). An absolute monocytosis (monocytes >1000/μL) is present in CMML. Thrombocytopenia may be present, although the platelet count may be elevated in patients with refractory anemia (RA) and an isolated 5q− abnormality, or in some cases of RARS.

The peripheral blood smear often demonstrates cellular morphological abnormalites. The neutrophils may be hypogranular, and the nucleus may have a bilobed appearance (pseudo-Pelger-Huet abnormality). Myeloblasts may be present in the peripheral blood, and they may contain Auer rods. Leukoerythroblastic abnormalities, including a left-shifted myeloid series (with circulating metamyelocytes, myelocytes, promyelocytes, and myeloblasts), nucleated red blood cells, and giant platelets may be present. The red cells may be microcytic or macrocytic, and teardrop forms may be present. Chemistry tests typically are normal except the lactate dehydrogenase, which is elevated as a result of increased rate of cell death in the bone marrow.

The bone marrow biopsy usually is hypercellular for the age of the patient. However, approx 15% of patients have a hypocellular marrow (cellularity <25%). The presence of peripheral blood cytopenias in spite of bone marrow hypercellularity reflects the high rate of intramedullary cell death and ineffective hematopoiesis. The hallmark of MDS is the presence of tri-lineage dysplasia in the marrow. The erythroid series usually is megaloblastic in appearance, with prominent nuclear-cytoplasmic asynchrony. The erythroid cells may have additional abnormalities including bi-nuclearity or nuclear budding. Figure 11.1 (*see* Color Plate 9) gives an example for the dysplastic changes in erythropoiesis.

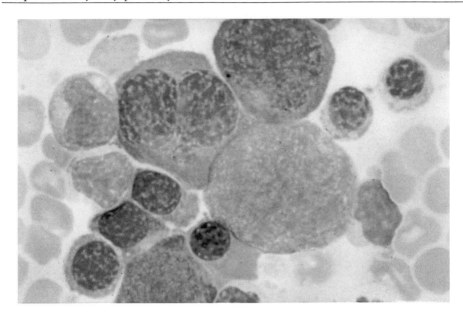

Fig. 11.1. Myelodysplastic syndrome. Dysplastic changes in erythropoiesis.

Ringed sideroblasts, erythroid precursors with iron-laden mitochondria surrounding the nucleus, may be increased and they exceed 15% of the nucleated
bone marrow cells in patients with RARS. An example of ringed sideroblasts in
a case of MDS is shown in Fig. 11.2 (*see* Color Plate 10). Megakaryocytes
frequently are small (micromegakaryocytes) with decreased nuclear ploidy
(mono- or binucleated). The myeloid series usually is left-shifted and increased
myeloblasts are present in more advance stages.

Patients with MDS have been categorized into five types based on the blood
and bone marrow abnormalities discussed previously, and the percentage of
myeloblasts present in the bone marrow (Table 2).

Because of the variability of the clinical presentation of MDS, the differential
diagnosis depends on the laboratory abnormalities present. If pancytopenia is
present, the differential diagnosis is as shown in Table 1. Vitamin B_{12} or folate
deficiency should be ruled out if the patient presents with a macrocytic anemia
or the bone marrow has a megaloblastic appearance. The differential diagnosis
of microcytic anemia should be considered if the patient instead has low red
blood cell indices. Chronic myelomonocytic leukemia must be differentiated from
other causes of monocytosis such as tuberculosis, subacute bacterial endocarditis,
systemic lupus erythematosus, rheumatoid arthritis, Hodgkin's lymphoma, or
other malignancies. Monocytosis can also be observed in the M4 or M5 subtypes
of acute AML, Philadelphia chromosome-negative (atypical) chronic myeloid

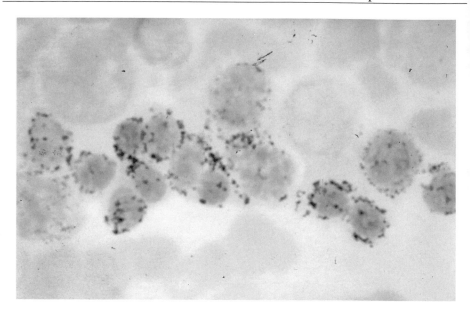

Fig. 11.2. Myelodysplastic syndrome. Ringed sideroblasts (coarse perinuclear iron staining).

leukemia (CML), and other myeloproliferative disorders. CMML can be differentiated from atypical CML by a higher frequency of circulating immature myeloid cells (10–20% of the leukocytes) and more profound granulocytic dysplasia in the bone marrow of the latter entity.

5. PROGNOSIS

The most important variables associated with the survival and risk of developing AML are the percentage of bone marrow myeloblasts and the number and types of cytogenetic abnormalities present. The number of peripheral blood cytopenias is of secondary prognostic importance. An International Prognostic Scoring System (IPSS) has been devised to estimate the clinical course of patients with MDS (*see* Tables 3 and 4).

6. MDS IN CHILDREN AND YOUNG ADULTS

Myelodysplasia is uncommon in the pediatric age group. In about one-third of children, a predisposing condition like Schwachman-Diamond syndrome, Fanconi anemia, or neurofibromatosis is found. Juvenile myelomonocytic leukemia (JMML) occurs only in infants and young children, and is associated with aberrant *Ras* signaling and an abnormal sensitivity of the blasts to granulocyte-macrophage colony-stimulating factor (GM-CSF). In most cases, mutations of

Table 2
Classification of Myelodysplastic Syndromes:

A. FAB Classification of Myelodysplastic Syndromes

Subtype	Blood myeloblasts	BM myeloblasts	Other features
RA	<1%	<5%	
RA with RS	<1%	<5%	RS > 15% BM cells
RAEB	<5%	5–20%	
CMML	< 5%	< 20%	AMC > 1000/mL

B. WHO Classification of Myelodysplastic Syndromes

Myelodysplastic syndromes

RA with or without RS	Erythroid-only dysplasia (<5% blasts)
Refractory cytopenia with multi-lineage dysplasia	Two or three lineage dysplasia (<5% blasts)
RAEB-1	Blasts 5–9%
RAEB-2	Blasts 10–19%
5q– syndrome	<5% blasts
Myelodysplastic syndromes, unclassifiable	Dysplasia, not meeting above criteria

Myelodysplastic/myeloproliferative syndromes

CMML
Atypical chronic myelogenous leukemia
JMML

FAB, French-American-British; BM, bone marrow; RA, refractory anemia; RS, ringed sideroblasts; RAEB, refractory anemia with excess blasts; CMML, chronic myelomonocytic leukemia; AMC, absolute monocyte count; WHO, World Health Organization; JMML, juvenile myelomonocytic leukemia.

PTPN11, RAS, or NF1 can be identified. A high proportion of children with MDS have bone marrow cytogenetic aberrations, and the most common is monosomy 7. Unfavorable prognostic factors are a low platelet count, elevated hemoglobin F, and complex cytogenetic aberrations. JMML has shown transient responses to multi-agent chemotherapy, clofarabine, and *cis*-retinoic acid, but, as in all cases of pediatric MDS an allogeneic stem cell transplant is the treatment with the best long-term outcome.

7. TREATMENT

Because the majority of patients with MDS are elderly, supportive care is the treatment of choice for many patients. The objective is to maintain the quality of life for the patient. Blood transfusions frequently are required for symptomatic

Table 3
International Prognostic Scoring System for Myelodysplastic Syndromes

Prognostic variable	Score value				
	0	0.5	1.0	1.5	2.0
BM blasts (%)	<5	5–10	—	11–20	21–30
Karyotype	Good	Intermediate	Poor	—	—
Cytopenias	0/1	2/3	—	—	—

Karyotypes: Good = normal, -Y, 5q-, 20q-; Poor = complex (≥3;three abnormalities) or chomosome 7 abnormalities; Intermediate = other abnormalities.
BM, bone marrow. Adapted from Greenberg et al., 1997.

Table 4
Survival and Risk of Leukemia for International Prognostic Scoring System (IPSS) Risk Groups

Risk group	Score[a]	Median survival (yr)	Risk of leukemia
Low	0	5.7	19%
INT-1	0.5–1.0	3.5	30%
INT-2	1.5–2.0	1.2	33%
High	> 2.0	0.4	45%

[a]see Table 3 for IPSS score values.

anemia and antibiotics are administered for bacterial infections. Chronic red blood cell transfusions lead to iron overload. In patients who will require ongoing transfusional support, iron chelation should be considered after 20 U of packed red cells have been administered or when the serum ferritin level exceeds 1000 ng/mL. Desferoximine by subcutaneous or intravenous infusion has traditionally been used for this purpose. Recently, deferasirox (Exjade®) was approved for transfusion-associated iron overload. It is administered orally, at a dose of 20 mg/kg/d. Renal and hepatic function should be monitored closely. Platelet transfusions typically are reserved for individuals who are actively bleeding or those who have experienced life-threatening bleeding below a certain platelet count.

Hematopoietic growth factors may benefit a minority of patients with MDS. A trial of erythropoietin administration may be useful in treating anemia in approx 20–40% of patients with MDS. Erythropoietin is most likely to benefit individuals who are not transfusion-dependent and who have a serum erythropoietin level of less than 200 U/L. Erythropoietin has been administered in a variety of doses and schedules, but 10,000 U three times a week or 40,000 U once a week by subcutaneous injection are often used. Darbepoietin is a recombinant erythropoietin with a larger half-life due to the addition of two glycosylation sites. It has efficacy similar to that of erythropoietin but can be given less frequently (200 μg weekly or 500 μg every 2 wk). Administration of granulocyte colony-stimulating factor (G-CSF) in doses capable of normalizing or doubling the neutrophil count (beginning at 1 μg/[kg · d] by subcutaneous injection) in combination with erythropoietin may improve the chances of an erythroid response. However, the impact of G-CSF on survival has not been evaluated.

Although neutropenia predisposes many patients with MDS to the risk of serious bacterial infections, the chronic use of myeloid growth factors including G-CSF or GM-CSF has not been shown to improve survival or prevent infections in patients with MDS. Therefore, long-term administration of myeloid growth factors is not recommended. The use of G-CSF or GM-CSF in a neutropenic MDS patient with an active infection may be of benefit, but this has not been demonstrated in a clinical trial.

The drug 5-azacytidine (Vidaza®) was recently approved by the Food and Drug Administration (FDA) for the treatment of MDS. 5-azacytidine is a hypomethylating agent that may reactivate tumor suppressor or cell cycle regulatory genes that are turned off in the MDS clone as a result of methylation of regulatory regions upstream of the genes. 5-Azacytidine also has cytotoxic activity. In a randomized, controlled trial 5-azacytidine dosed 75 mg/(m2 · d) subcutaneously for 7 d every 28 d was compared with supportive care in patients with >5% bone marrow loss, transfusion-dependent anemia, or severe peripheral blood cytopenia. Clinical improvement (at least a 50% reduction in transfusion requirements) was observed in 60% of patients receiving 5-azacytidine compared with 5% of patients receiving supportive care after 4 mo. Several of the 5-azacytidine-treated patients (7%) achieved a complete response. The risk of leukemic transformation or death was significantly reduced. The major side effects of 5-azacytidine, nausea and vomiting, were controlled by pretreatment with a serotonin receptor antagonist. Neutropenia was also a common toxicity. A related hypomethylating agent, 5-aza-2'-deoxycytidine (decitabine), has orphan drug status in Europe. It is administered intravenously at a dose of 15 mg/(m2 · d) for 3 d every 6 wk. It has been reported to induce responses in approx 20% of patients with MDS, but it can cause severe and delayed myelosuppression. As a result, its use is primarily being evaluated in advanced MDS (e.g., MDS-refractory anemia with excess blasts [RAEB], RAEB in transformation [RAEB-T]).

Other novel therapies have been studied recently for MDS. The drug thalidomide, which can suppress the production of proapoptotic cytokines, has been reported to improve anemia in approx 20% of patients with MDS. However, the drug is not well tolerated by elderly patients with MDS because it frequently causes fatigue, sedation, constipation, fluid retention, dizziness, and peripheral neuropathy and more potently inhibits TNF-α. A structurally related compound that lacks the neurotoxicity of thalidomide is lenalidomide (formerly CC5013). This oral drug has produced encouraging results in clinical trials and was recently approved by the FDA for treatment of MDS patients with 5q⁻ cytogenetic abnormality. Transfusion-dependent, low- and intermediate-risk patients with MDS with 5q⁻ abnormality were treated on a phase II trial of lenalidomide therapy 10 μg daily for 21 or 28 days per 28-day cycle. Approximately 67% of the patients became transfusion-independent with lenalidomide. In addition, cytogenetic responses were observed in 74% of patients; 44% had a complete cytogenetic response. These remarkable results were very stable with chronic drug administration. Myelosuppression was the most common and severe toxicity, and most patients required dose reduction during the course of the trial. Arsenic trioxide (Trisenox®) is a drug that is FDA approved to treat acute promyelocytic leukemia. Trials demonstrated that approx 25% of MDS patients with anemia will experience improvement in hemoglobin levels with arsenic. Antithymocyte globulin, which is routinely used to treat aplastic anemia, was reported to render approximately one-third of patients with MDS red blood cell transfusion-independent. Platelet and neutrophil responses also were observed. Responses occurred in patients with RA and RAEB subtypes, but not in those with RARS. Other clinical features that were associated with a higher likelihood of response were younger age and the presence of thrombocytopenia.

Chemotherapy with AML treatment regimens has been explored in MDS. Although complete remissions have been achieved in 40–60% of selected patients, the risk of treatment-related mortality can be high in the elderly and remission durations typically are short. The impact of aggressive chemotherapy on survival in MDS has not been investigated. Unlike AML, chemotherapy is not curative for MDS. Patients with a high risk of developing AML may be considered for aggressive chemotherapy, but it has not been demonstrated that withholding treatment until AML develops is worse than treating those patients early. Therefore, it is unclear which, if any, subgroups of patients with MDS may benefit from this approach to treatment.

Allogeneic stem cell transplantation (SCT) is the only curative modality for MDS, but because the vast majority of patients are elderly, most are not eligible for this form of treatment. The major risks of SCT in patients with MDS are treatment-related toxicity, acute graft-vs-host disease, and disease relapse. Early transplant-related mortality following an allogeneic SCT is approx 40% and disease-free survival is 30–40% for patients with MDS. Patients who have increased numbers of myeloblasts in the bone marrow (RAEB or RAEB-T) have a very high risk of disease relapse (50–70%) following SCT, whereas those without increased blasts (RA or RARS) have a low risk of relapse (<5%). Attempts to reduce the risk of relapse in high-risk patients by administering AML induction chemotherapy prior to performing the SCT have not resulted in improved survival. Therefore, patients with MDS who potentially could do well for several years with supportive care alone are most likely to be cured following SCT, but they may be subjected to a high risk of early morbidity and mortality with the transplant. In contrast, patients with MDS who are at greatest risk from dying from their disease also are most likely to have a poor outcome following SCT. Retrospective analyses have failed to demonstrate a survival benefit for SCT in patients with low and Int-1 IPSS scores because of the early excess mortality from the procedure.

One approach to reduce the morbidity and mortality from allogeneic SCT has been to administer less-intensive chemotherapy in doses that are not capable of eliminating all of the recipient's bone marrow (nonmyeloablative transplant). In this approach, the drugs used prior to transplant in the conditioning regimen are potently immunosuppressive to permit the transplanted donor cells to engraft and, over time, to replace the recipient's hematopoietic cells. This approach relies on the potential ability of the donor immune system, rather than the conditioning chemotherapy, to eradicate the MDS clone. Although nonmyeloablative SCT is a promising approach for patients with MDS, there currently are inadequate data to determine the indications for the use of this treatment.

SUGGESTED READING

Bennett JM, Catovsky D, Daniel MT, et al (for the French-American-British (FAB) Co-operative Group). Proposals for the classification of the myelodysplastic syndromes. *Br J Haematol* 1982;51:189–199.

Beran M, Shen Y, Kantarjian H, et al. High-dose chemotherapy in high-risk myelodysplastic syndrome. Covariate-adjusted comparison of five regimens. *Cancer* 2001;92:1999–2015.

Greenberg P, Cox C, LeBeau MM, et al. International scoring system for evaluating prognosis in myelodysplastic syndromes. *Blood* 1997;89:2079–2088.

Harris NL, Jaffe ES, Diebold J, et al. World Health Organization classification of neoplastic diseases of the hematopoietic and lymphoid tissues: report of the Clinical Advisory Committee Meeting – Airlie House, Virginia, November 1997. *J Clin Oncol* 1999;17:3835–3849.

List AF, Kurtin S, Roe DJ, et al. Efficacy of lenalidomide in myelodysplastic syndromes. *N Engl J Med* 2005;352:549–557.

McKenna RW. Myelodysplasia and myeloproliferative disorders in children. *Am J Clin Pathol* 2004;122:S58–69.

Molldrem JJ, Leifer E, Bahceci E, et al. Antithymocyte globulin for treatment of the bone marrow failure associated with myelodysplastic syndromes. *Ann Intern Med* 2002;137:156–163.

Silverman LR, Demakos EP, Peterson BL, et al. Randomized controlled trial of azacitidine in patients with the myelodysplastic syndrome: a study of the cancer and leukemia group B. *J Clin Oncol* 2002;20:2429–2440.

12 Aplastic Anemias

Ronald Paquette, MD
and Reinhold Munker, MD

CONTENTS

1. DEFINITION

The aplastic anemias are characterized by peripheral blood pancytopenia, bone marrow hypocellularity, and absence of a clonal hematological process. They have an incidence of approximately two patients per million population in the West and four per million in Asia.

2. ETIOLOGY

Aplastic anemia can be either inherited or acquired (*see* Table 1). The majority of the congenital aplastic anemias have an autosomal recessive inheritance pattern. Patients with inherited bone marrow failure states often have associated physical and developmental abnormalities including growth retardation, skeletal malformations, and skin pigmentary changes. Because of the variability of the clinical manifestations, these disorders may be diagnosed at any time from birth to adulthood.

From: *Contemporary Hematology: Modern Hematology, Second Edition*
Edited by: R. Munker, E. Hiller, J. Glass, and R. Paquette © Humana Press Inc., Totowa, NJ

Table 1
Etiology of Aplastic Anemia

Inherited
Fanconi anemia
   Diamond-Blackfan anemia
   Dyskeratosis congenita
   Kostmann's syndrome
   Shwachman-Diamond syndrome
   Thrombocytopenia absent radius syndrome

Acquired
   Idiopathic
      Drugs
      Chloramphenicol
      Nonsteroidal anti-inflammatory agents
      Sulfonamides
      Sulfonylureas
      Antithyroid drugs
      Anticonvulsants
      Gold salts
      Penicillamine
      Allopurinol
     Hepatitis
     Benzene
     Ionizing radiation
     Cytotoxic chemotherapy

The etiology of most cases of acquired aplastic anemia usually cannot be determined, and therefore is considered idiopathic. At least two-thirds of patients have no clear antecedent precipitating cause. Drugs, as a group, are the most frequently implicated as a cause of aplastic anemia. Many drugs have been associated with at least one case of aplastic anemia. However, because aplastic anemia is rare, an etiological association between any drug and this disorder is difficult to establish. Only a few classes of drugs have been shown to be statistically associated with the development of aplastic anemia in epidemiological studies. Chloramphenicol, an antibiotic now rarely used in the West, can cause either dose-dependent bone marrow suppression or idiosyncratic aplastic anemia. Although the nonsteroidal anti-inflammatory agents (NSAIDS) indomethacin, diclofenac, and phenylbutazone have an association with the development of aplastic anemia, most NSAIDS have not been reported to cause this disorder. Sulfa derivatives including the sulfa antibiotics, the sulfonylureas, and furosemide all have been associated with aplastic anemia. Two drugs used to treat rheumatoid arthritis, gold and penicillamine, have been statistically associated with aplastic anemia. The antiseizure medication carbamazepine also has been implicated in this etiology of this disorder.

Approximately 2–5% of patients with aplastic anemia have a history of hepatitis occurring within several months prior to the development of pancytopenia. Typically, the hepatitis is resolving when patients present with abnormal blood counts. None of the hepatitis viruses identified so far, including hepatitis A, B, C, E, or G (GVB-C), have been shown to be causally associated with the development of aplastic anemia.

Benzene, an organic solvent with a variety of industrial uses, causes dose-dependent bone marrow failure. Occupational safety regulations have been enacted that strictly limit exposure to this compound. As a result, cases of aplastic anemia due to benzene exposure have progressively declined in the last few decades.

Radiation and cytotoxic chemotherapy are iatrogenic causes of bone marrow failure. In contrast, accidental exposure to ionizing radiation is a rare cause of aplastic anemia. Approximately 100–200 cGy of total body irradiation given as a single dose can cause pancytopenia, whereas 400–800 cGy can induce irreversible bone marrow failure.

3. PATHOPHYSIOLOGY

There are at least three mechanisms for the development of aplastic anemia. The inherited forms of aplastic anemia, especially Fanconi anemia, are caused by DNA instability. Some acquired forms of aplastic anemia are due to direct injury of hematopoietic stem cells by a toxic insult, such as ionizing radiation. The pathogenesis of the majority of acquired cases involves an autoimmune reaction against the stem cells.

Fanconi anemia is perhaps the most common of the inherited forms of aplastic anemia, all of which are rare. At least seven different genetic abnormalities can produce a Fanconi anemia phenotype. Cells from all types of the disease share a sensitivity to drugs that cross-link DNA. As a result of this sensitivity to DNA damage, patients with Fanconi anemia have a high risk of evolving myelodysplastic syndrome (MDS) and acute myelogenous leukemia (AML) following the initial aplasia. DNA damage activates a complex consisting of Fanconi proteins A, C, G, and F. This in turn leads to the modification of the FANCD2 protein. This protein interacts, for example, with the breast cancer susceptibility gene *BRCA1*. The exact sequence of how patients with Fanconi anemia develop aplastic anemia from mutagen sensitivity and DNA damage is still unknown.

Direct toxic injury to hematopoietic stem cells can be induced by exposure to ionizing radiation, cytotoxic chemotherapy, or benzene. These agents can cross-link DNA and induce DNA strand breaks leading to inhibition of DNA and RNA synthesis.

Immune-mediated destruction of hematopoietic stem cells probably is the major pathophysiological mechanism of aplastic anemia. Although the inciting events are unknown, it appears that cytotoxic T-lymphocytes are responsible for inhibiting stem cell proliferation and inducing stem cell death. Direct killing of the stem cells has been hypothesized to occur via interations between Fas ligand expressed on the T-cells and Fas (CD95) present on the stem cells, which triggers programmed cell death (apoptosis). T-lymphocytes also may suppress stem cell proliferation by elaborating soluble factors including interferon-γ.

4. CLINICAL MANIFESTATIONS

Symptoms at presentation in patients with aplastic anemia are due to pancytopenia. Moderate to severe anemia is manifested as fatigue and dyspnea on exertion. Neutropenia is associated with the development of bacterial or fungal infections. Bleeding or bruising due to thrombocytopenia also commonly occur. Physical examination may reveal pallor, mucosal bleeding, ecchymoses, or petechiae. The presence of hepatomegaly, splenomegaly, or lymphadenopathy suggests another diagnosis.

5. DIAGNOSIS AND CLASSIFICATION

The differential diagnosis of aplastic anemia includes causes of pancytopenia (Table 2). Aspiration and biopsy of the bone marrow are performed to obtain samples for routine histochemical stains, flow cytometry, and cytogenetic analysis. Depending upon the clinical setting (especially if splenomegaly is present), a tartrate-resistant alkaline phosphatase stain (to exclude hairy cell leukemia) or a reticulin stain (to exclude myelofibrosis) also should be considered. The bone marrow aspirate typically contains acellular or hypocellular spicules when aplastic anemia is present. Cellular elements may include a minimal number of residual myeloid or erythroid cells. Plasma cells and lymphocytes may be relatively increased in numbers but they do not represent clonal populations. The cellularity of the bone marrow biopsy usually has less than or equal to 10% cellularity. Figure 12.1 (Color Plate 11) shows the bone marrow findings in a case of severe aplastic anemia. For comparison, a normal bone marrow section is shown in Fig. 12.2 (Color Plate 12). Paroxysmal nocturnal hemoglobinuria (PNH), MDS, and AML also can present with a hypocellular marrow. The latter two disorders should be rigorously excluded with the use of flow cytometric

Table 2
Differential Diagnosis of Pancytopenia

Aplastic anemia
Paroxysmal nocturnal hemoglobinuria (PNH)
Myelodysplastic syndromes (MDS)
Acute leukemia
    Acute myelogenous leukemia
    Acute lymphoblastic leukemia
    Blast crisis of chronic myelogenous leukemia
Lymphoproliferative disorders
    Hodgkin's lymphoma
    Non-Hodgkin's lymphoma
    Multiple myeloma
    Hairy cell leukemia
Metastatic carcinoma
Myelofibrosis
Vitamin B_{12} or folic acid deficiency
Hypersplenism
Gaucher's disease or other storage pool diseases
Sepsis (especially pneumococcal)
Granulomatous disease involving the bone marrow
    Coccidiodomycosis
    Histoplasmosis
    Mycobacterium avium intracellularae
    Mycobacterium tuberculosis
Human immunodeficiency virus
Rheumatological disorders
    Rheumatoid arthritis
    Systemic lupus erythematosus

studies, immunohistochemical stains, and cytogenetic analysis. PNH may co-exist with aplastic anemia as an overlap syndrome in up to 20% of patients, but the clinical behavior of this entity is similar to that of aplastic anemia. The peripheral blood granulocytes should be analyzed for the surface expression of phosphati-dyl-inositolglycan (PIG)-linked molecules (CD55 and CD59, *see* Appendix 2); red blood cells from untransfused patients should also be analyzed for these markers. Children and young adults, especially those with suggestive physical findings, should have a blood sample sent for chromosome breakage analysis in order to exclude Fanconi anemia. Fanconi anemia is the most common of the rare inherited bone marrow failure syndromes (*see* above and Table 1). Fanconi anemia has autosomal recessive inheritance, presents with pancytopenia associated with

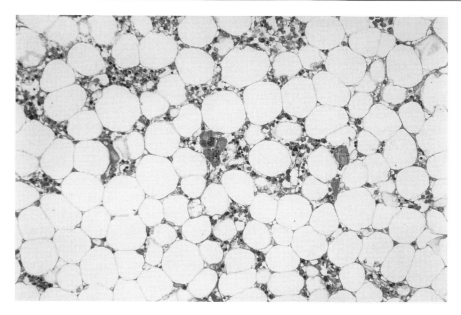

Fig. 12.1. Aplastic anemia, histological section.

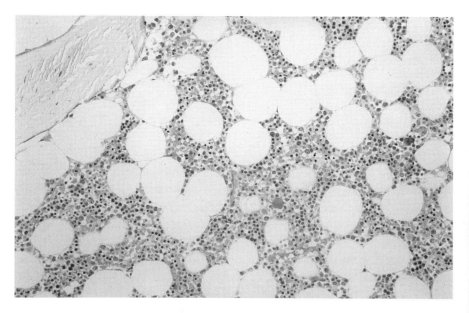

Fig. 12.2. Normal bone marrow, histological section.

physical abnormalities (skin pigmentation, malformations such as thumb aplasia and microcephaly, and hypogonadism). The age group when Fanconi anemia is usually discovered is in childhood, but occasionally young adults present with the stigmata of Fanconi anemia or have a positive chromosome breakage assay without the physical signs of Fanconi anemia. The pancytopenia of Fanconi anemia progresses in more than 90% of cases to full-blown aplastic anemia. Patients with Fanconi anemia are also prone to develop malignancies (AML, some solid tumors).

The classification of aplastic anemia is based on the severity of the peripheral blood abnormalities. Severe disease is characterized by any two of the following: absolute neutrophil count (ANC) less than 500/µL, corrected reticulocyte count less than 1% (or reticulocyte count <20,000/µL), and platelet count less than 20,000/µL. Very severe disease has the same criteria as severe disease except the ANC is less than 200/µL. Patients are considered to have moderate disease if they have a hypocellular bone marrow, do not fulfill severe disease criteria, and have at least two of the following: ANC less than or equal to 1200/µL, platelet count less than or equal to 70,000/µL, and hemoglobin less than or equal to 8.5 g/dL with an absolute reticulocyte count less than or equal to 60,000/µL.

6. TREATMENT

Acutely ill patients must first be stabilized by administering empiric broad-spectrum antibiotics for neutropenia fevers, or transfusing platelets for active bleeding. A critical early decision is whether or not the patient is eligible for allogeneic bone marrow transplantation (BMT). This is important because such patients have a lower risk of graft rejection if transfusion with blood products is minimized prior to transplantation. Urgent referral of such patients to a transplant center is essential. Unless transplantation is excluded as an option, all patients should be given cytomegalovirus (CMV) seronegative blood products until their CMV immune status is known. Seronegative transplant candidates should continue to receive CMV seronegative blood. This is done because CMV can cause serious infections following BMT. All blood products must be leukocyte reduced and irradiated in potential BMT recipients to minimize allosensitization and eliminate the potential risk of transfusion-related graft-vs-host disease (GVHD).

Related allogeneic BMT is the therapy of choice for Fanconi anemia and severe or very severe aplastic anemia in children and young adults. The upper age for which transplantation is the best initial option is controversial, and may range from 25 to 45 yr depending on the transplant center. The risk of mortality from GVHD increases with age, but delaying transplantation to treat with immunosuppression first increases exposure to blood products and subjects patients to risk of infection or bleeding. If transplantation is an option, patients and their siblings should have human leukocyte antigen (HLA)-typing performed as rapidly as possible. It is preferable to use bone marrow rather than peripheral blood progenitor cells (PBPCs) as the source of stem cells for transplantation in aplastic anemia. This is because PBPCs have a much higher T-lymphocyte dose and a higher risk of GVHD than bone marrow. Cyclophosphamide and antithymocyte globulin (ATG) are used to condition aplastic anemia patients prior to transplantation of related-donor bone marrow. Radiation therapy (total body irradiation) must be added to the conditioning regimen when using unrelated-donor bone marrow because of the increased risk of graft rejection. In contrast, reduced-intensity conditioning must be used for patients with Fanconi anemia because of their increased risk of toxic side effects (often with fludarabine and ATG). The goal of the conditioning therapy is to suppress the recipient's immune system in order to permit engraftment of the donor cells. Long-term survival following allogeneic BMT for severe aplastic anemia is approx 65–75% when related-donor bone marrow is used and 30–55% with unrelated-donor bone marrow. The most important favorable prognostic variables affecting survival are patient age less than 20 yr, time between diagnosis and transplant of less than 1 yr, and use of a related donor.

Immunosuppressive therapy is the initial treatment of choice for patients with moderate disease, patients without an HLA-identical sibling, and "older" patients. Immunosuppressive therapy consists of ATG or antilymphocyte globulin (ALG) plus cyclosporine. One standard ATG and cyclosporine regimen is provided in Table 3. A test dose of ATG is given subcutaneously prior to full dosing to exclude patients with anaphylaxis. High doses of glucocorticoids must be administered with the ATG/ALG to prevent the development of serum sickness, which usually occurs 10–14 d after starting ATG. Steroids should be tapered off within 3–4 wk after starting ATG as they do not improve the response rate and are associated with an increased infection risk. Cyclosporine should be continued until maximal response, then tapered very slowly over many months (to minimize relapse). Combined immunosuppressive therapy with ATG or ALG and cyclosporine yields a response rate of 65–80%. Cyclosporine as a single agent can be a useful treatment for aplastic anemia. As initial therapy, cyclosporine induces fewer remissions than ATG in patients with severe disease, but it can be useful when reinstituted in early relapse to prevent the need for retreatment with ATG. Cyclosporine may also be considered as initial therapy in patients without severe cytopenias. Because aplastic anemia is a rare disease, referral to a tertiary center for enrollment in active clinical trials is encouraged.

Hematopoietic growth factors, including granulocyte colony-stimulating factor, granulocyte-macrophage colony-stimulating factor, and erythropoietin should play only an adjunctive role in the treatment of acquired aplastic anemia. Although

Table 3
Antithymocyte Globulin (ATG) Protocol for Aplastic Anemia

ATG test dose:
   ATG 1:1000 dilution in saline 0.1 cc intradermally (i.d.) with control saline 0.1 cc i.d.
      in other arm. If no anaphylaxis occurs, ATG can subsequently be given.
Premedications for ATG (given 30 min prior to ATG):
   Acetaminophen 650 mg p.o.
   Diphenhydramine 50 mg p.o. or IVPB
   Hydrocortisone 50 mg IVPB
ATG Therapy:
   ATG 40 mg/kg in 1000 cc NS over 8–12 h daily for 4 d
Concomitant Medications:
   Prednisone 100 mg/m^2 p.o. q.d. beginning with ATG and continuing for 10–14 d;
      then, if no serum sickness develops, taper the dose over 2 wk.
   Cyclosporine 5 mg/(kg · d) p.o. divided BID until maximal response then taper by 1 mg/
      (kg ·mo), or more slowly. Patients aged 50 or older should receive 4 mg/(kg · d). Dose
      should be decreased for deterioration in renal function or elevated liver enzymes

these growth factors can improve the peripheral blood counts in some aplastic
anemia patients, they have not been shown to induce disease remission. In general, the likelihood of response to a hematopoietic growth factor is inversely
related to the severity of the peripheral blood cytopenia for which it is being
administered. The precise roles of these medications in the treatment of aplastic
anemia have not yet been clearly defined. The most clear-cut indication for the
use of the myeloid growth factors is in neutropenic patients with active infection.

Patients who fail to respond to an initial course of ATG/ALG plus cyclosporine
should be given a second treatment with immunosuppression. Approximately
20–50% of such patients may respond to a second course of treatment.

7. LATE COMPLICATIONS

Patients with aplastic anemia who respond to immunosuppressive therapy
face two major risks: disease relapse and the development of clonal hematopoietic disorders. Relapse of aplastic anemia most frequently occurs within the first
2 yr after immunosuppressive treatment; however, it may occur at any time.
Between 10 and 40% of patients suffer a disease relapse. Relapse has been
defined as a decrease of peripheral blood counts to levels that are less than half
of those at the time of stable response, to levels that meet the criteria for severe
disease, or to levels requiring reinstitution of transfusion support. Fortunately,
most relapsed patients respond to reinstitution of cyclosporine or administration

of another ATG course. A more ominous complication is the development of a clonal hematological process including MDS, and AML. There is a 12–15% risk of developing MDS or AML after 10 yr. Therefore, a patient with aplastic anemia who experiences falling blood counts after an initial response to immunosuppressive treatment must be evaluated for the latter two possibilities by performing bone marrow studies with cytogenetic analysis. The treatment of either of these disorders in the setting of previous aplastic anemia is similar to that of the *de novo* conditions.

A clonal population of granulocytes deficient in glycosyl phosphatidylinositol-linked proteins can be detected in approximately one-third of patients with aplastic anemia who have received immunosuppressive therapy. However, hemolytic anemia and clinically evident PNH occurs in perhaps 10% of these patients. Performing flow cytometry of granulocytes for CD55 and CD59 can be used to monitor the evolution of a PNH clone over time. The presence of a PNH clone in patients who fulfill the criteria for aplastic anemia does not alter the approach to treatment. However, if a large PNH clone develops (>50% of granulocytes are deficient for CD55 and CD59), and the platelet count is over 100,000/ μL, coumadin should be initiated (target INR 2–3) to reduce the risk of thrombosis in this disorder. At this time, there is no standard treatment for hemolytic PNH, but recent clinical trial results of a monoclonal antibody targeting the C5-complement component holds promise for future therapy.

SUGGESTED READING

Hall C, Richards S, Hillman P. Primary prophylaxis with warfarin prevents thrombosis in paroxysmal nocturnal hemoglobinuria (PNH). *Blood* 2003;102:3587–3591.

Marsh JC, Ball SE, Darbyshire P, et al; British Committee for Standards in Haematology. Guidelines for the diagnosis and management of acquired aplastic anaemia. *Br J Haematol* 2003;123:782–801.

Young NS, Maciejewski J. The pathophysiology of aplastic anemia. *N Engl J Med* 1997;336:1365–1372

13 Lymphocytosis, Lymphocytopenia, Lymphadenopathy, and Splenomegaly

Reinhold Munker, MD

CONTENTS

1. INTRODUCTION AND DEFINITIONS

Enlarged lymph nodes or an increase in the size of the spleen (splenomegaly) are seen during many infections, but can also be symptoms of many blood diseases. A lymphocytosis is present if the lymphocyte count in peripheral blood is increased to more than 4000/μL; a lymphopenia is present if the lymphocytes are decreased to less than 1000/μL. In general, a palpable spleen must be considered enlarged (splenomegaly). In order to measure the size of the spleen accurately, the spleen should be examined with ultrasound. The maximum normal size is approx $12 \times 10 \times 5$ cm, as determined by ultrasonic evaluation. It is also possible, using ultrasound, to recognize infiltrates of malignant lymphomas or splenic infarcts. High-resolution computed tomography (CT) is also able to determine the spleen size accurately. Lymphadenopathy is a term for enlarged and/or pathological lymph nodes. Lymph nodes must be considered enlarged or pathological if they present as chain of multiple lymph nodes or their size measures more than 1 cm. Other commonly used methods are CT and magnetic resonance imaging.

From: *Contemporary Hematology: Modern Hematology, Second Edition*
Edited by: R. Munker, E. Hiller, J. Glass, and R. Paquette © Humana Press Inc., Totowa, NJ

217

2. DIFFERENTIAL DIAGNOSIS OF A LYMPHOCYTOSIS

A reactive lymphocytosis is observed during many bacterial infections; for example, during pertussis (whooping cough), rickettsiosis, brucellosis, tuberculosis, and shigellosis, as well as during certain viral infections such as varicella, *Herpes zoster*, cytomegalovirus (CMV) infections, infectious mononucleosis, hepatitis, coxsackie virus, and adenovirus infections, rubella, and mumps. Children with pertussis frequently have a lymphocyte count of up to 40,000/µL. This is due to the action of pertussis toxin, which blocks the migration of lymphocytes through the capillaries. Infectious mononucleosis is characteristically accompanied by an increase of CD8[+] lymphocytes and is described separately (*see* Chapter 18). Lymphocytosis is commonly seen in children with exanthema subitum, a rash caused by human herpesvirus-6. Some patients with congenital immune deficiencies develop a reactive lymphocytosis. HIV-infected patients having an increased number of CD8[+]-positive lymphocytes appear to have a better prognosis and somewhat fewer opportunistic infections. Patients who are treated with the cytokine interleukin (IL)-2 develop an increase in the number of lymphocytes as a result of the proliferation of CD16[+] natural killer cells. A lymphocytosis with predominantly mature appearing small lymphoid cells observed in elderly patients is most frequently due to a B-chronic lymphocytic leukemia (*see* Chapter 18). Other malignant lymphomas like hairy cell leukemia or Sezary syndrome have circulating lymphoid cells in the blood, which usually have a characteristic morphology (for details, *see* Chapter 15).

In order to differentiate between a neoplastic or a nonmalignant-reactive lymphocytosis, immunological and molecular studies are often necessary. In the former case, only one type of immunoglobulin light chain and a monoclonal rearrangement of the immunoglobulin genes or of the T-cell receptor genes are detected. Persistent polyclonal B-lymphocytosis with circulating binucleated lymphoid cells and an increase of serum immunoglobin M is a rare condition observed in smokers and is generally benign. The T-gamma lympho-proliferative disorder is characterized by a monoclonal proliferation of CD8[+] and CD16[+] lymphoid cells, morphologically described as "large granular lymphocytes." These patients often have anemia and are neutropenic. The disease is indolent in most cases and infections are related to the degree of neutropenia. Some cases, however, show a rapidly progressive course.

3. DIFFERENTIAL DIAGNOSIS OF LYMPHOCYTOPENIA

A decrease of lymphocytes in the peripheral blood (lymphocytopenia or lymphopenia) is seen in certain immune deficiency syndromes (e.g., ataxia telangiectatica and others; *see* Chapter 17), in disseminated malignancies,

Hodgkin's lymphoma, active sarcoidosis, and in autoimmune disorders like lupus erythematodes and myasthenia gravis. Some cases of advanced AIDS and of severe aplastic anemia are accompanied by lymphopenia. Lymphopenia is frequently a secondary reaction to treatment with corticosteroids, extended field irradiation, or treatment with cytotoxic drugs. A rare cause of lymphopenia is the loss of lymph in intestinal lymphangiectasia and in disorders like Whipple's disease.

4. DIFFERENTIAL DIAGNOSIS OF LYMPHADENOPATHY

A reactive lymph node swelling (lymphadenopathy) is a frequent sign of a bacterial or viral infection. A pharyngitis or middle ear infection is often accompanied by a prominent lymphadenopathy, especially in children. Patients with erysipelas frequently develop enlarged lymph nodes in the draining lymphatic area. Infectious lymphadenopathies are often painful or sensitive to palpation, whereas neoplastic lymphadenopathies are indolent in most cases. An exception is syphilis in the secondary stage, which characteristically presents with a painless lymph node swelling. Lymph nodes tend to form fistulas in tuberculosis and actinomycosis. Further bacterial infections producing enlarged or sometimes painful lymph nodes are brucellosis, cat scratch disease, and tularemia. Lymphogranuloma inguinale is a venereal infection with a soft swelling of inguinal lymph nodes. Toxoplasmosis is caused by the protozoan toxoplasma gondii and can present with a generalized lymphadenopathy (for details, *see* Chapter 17, "Hematological Aspects of AIDS"). The so-called lymphadenopathy syndrome is an early stage of HIV infection. By definition, two or more extrainguinal lymph nodes are enlarged for more than 3 mo. During the later stages of HIV infection (AIDS, AIDS-related complex) multiple lymph nodes can also be enlarged. Infectious mononucleosis is characterized by an acute swelling of several lymph nodes and high fever (for details, *see* Chapter 18, "Infectious Mononucleosis and Other Epstein-Barr Virus Syndromes"). Rheumatic and autoimmune diseases, sarcoidosis, and some allergic reactions are also accompanied by enlarged lymph nodes.

Pseudolymphomas are, by definition, benign or nonmalignant; however, they have a tendency to transform into a non-Hodgkin's lymphoma in some cases. Castleman's disease is an example of a pseudolymphoma. Kikuchi-Fujimoto disease is a rare and self-limited disease characterized by lymph node swelling, fever, splenomegaly, and leucopenia. Histologically, the enlarged lymph nodes show patchy irregular areas of necrosis. The etiology of Kikuchi-Fujimoto disease is unclear.

The diagnostic procedures for enlarged lymph nodes depend on the clinical circumstances. First of all, all lymph node areas should be inspected and palpated

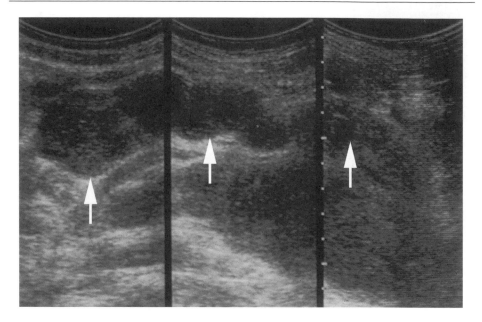

Fig. 13.1. Ultrasound image of mesenteric lymph nodes (bulky disease, patient with a large-cell lymphoma; arrows point to lymph nodes, transverse section).

carefully. The next step is to measure the exact dimensions of all lymph nodes by means of ultrasound and to document these findings. Figure 13.1 shows ultrasound findings in a patient who was found to have a large-cell lymphoma. Serologically, antibodies against HIV, Epstein-Barr virus (EBV), CMV, toxoplasmosis, and other infectious agents should be investigated. If the cause of the enlarged lymph nodes cannot be found within 2–4 wk, or if other signs of a malignant tumor are present, a lymph node should be biopsied and examined by a pathologist.

Because inguinal lymph nodes often have nonspecific reactive changes, an axillary or cervical lymph node should preferably be biopsied. Fresh unfixed material should also be sent to the pathologist for further immunophenotyping in case of a malignant lymphoma. If a malignant lymphoma is confirmed or strongly suspected, staging should be performed (including CT scans of thorax and abdomen [*see* Chapters 14 and 15], Hodgkin's lymphoma, and non-Hodgkin's lymphomas). Enlarged lymph nodes can also be secondary to metastatic carcinomas. Examples are nasopharyngeal tumors, breast cancer, and gastrointestinal cancers. The lymph node metastases of epithelial cancers are generally indurated and attached to the surrounding tissues. If a malignant tumor is suspected, but the histology of the lymph node biopsy shows only reactive changes, a second biopsy should be made in a different lymph node area.

5. DIFFERENTIAL DIAGNOSIS OF SPLENOMEGALY

An enlargement of the spleen (splenomegaly) is a common physical finding in such hematological neoplasias as leukemias, myeloproliferative syndromes, and lymphomas. In osteomyelofibrosis, a huge and indurated spleen is often observed. Patients with acquired and inherited hemolytic anemias often present with a splenomegaly due to the increased destruction and sequestration of red blood cells. During certain severe infections such as endocarditis, hepatitis, infectious mononucleosis, septicemia, toxoplasmosis, malaria, and fungal infections, the spleen also enlarges and can be felt in the left upper abdomen. In tropical countries, splenomegaly is a frequent symptom due to malaria, leishmaniasis, or schistosomiasis or chronic hemolytic anemias. In disorders like sarcoidosis, lupus erythematosus, or rheumatoid arthritis (Felty's syndrome), splenomegaly can be observed. Splenomegaly is also associated with portal hypertension (liver cirrhosis, chronic heart failure, portal vein thrombosis, portal vein aneurysm, or Budd-Chiari syndrome), and accumulative disorders like Gaucher's disease, amyloidosis, or splenic cysts. Patients who are treated with cytokines like IL-2 often develop a transient splenomegaly. A moderate splenomegaly is commonly found in patients with AIDS. As mentioned, ultrasound is a reliable method to measure spleen size and detect changes of splenic texture. Figure 13.2 shows the infiltration of the spleen with a low-grade non-Hodgkin's lymphoma.

The term hypersplenism means that patients who have an enlarged spleen often develop a thrombocytopenia, in many cases also a neutropenia and/or anemia due to the splenomegaly itself. Hypersplenism is related to the sequestration, and, in many cases, enhanced destruction of platelets, red cells, and granulocytes.

Splenectomy may be indicated in cases of certain symptomatic hemolytic anemias like hereditary spherocytosis, and refractory autoimmune thrombocytopenias; in some cases of hairy cell leukemia or other lymphomas; in cases of isolated splenic vein thrombosis; and rarely in other conditions. Rarely, enlarged spleen can be the only disease manifestation of a non-Hodgkin's lymphoma. In most cases, the surgical risk of splenectomy is small (0.1–1%) but may be considerable in advanced cases of osteomyelofibrosis or portal hypertension. For most non-malignant disorders, a laparoscopic splenectomy is preferable over a splenectomy by laparotomy. For experienced surgeons, laparoscopic splenectomies have fewer complications, need less pain medication and have a shorter stay in the hospital. Immediately after a splenectomy, leukocytosis and thrombocytosis develop, which normalize however within 5–10 d. Following splenectomy, Howell-Jolly bodies, which are red cells with DNA remnants (*see* Fig. 13.3 and Color Plate 13) usually removed by an intact spleen, can be seen in the peripheral

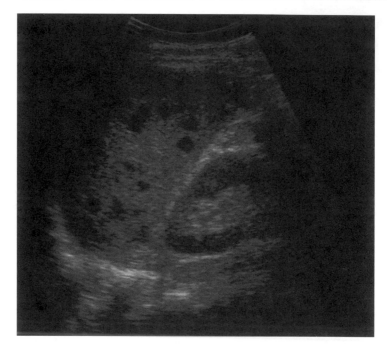

Fig. 13.2. Ultrasound image of the spleen (nodular infiltration in a patient with chronic lyrnphocytic leukemia).

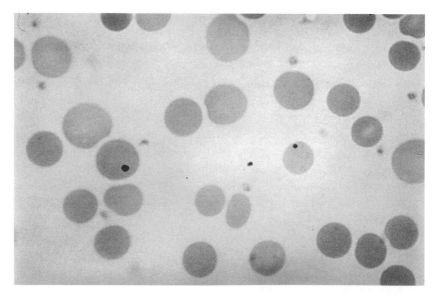

Fig13.3. Howell-Jolly bodies. Cytoplasmic remnant of nucleus, observed after splenectomy.

blood smear. Patients who are splenectomized have a small, but significant, risk of fulminant bacterial infections (overwhelming postsplenectomy infection [OPSI] syndrome). The pathogens seen in OPSI syndrome are pneumococci and meningococci, pathogens that are otherwise phagocytized by an intact spleen. Patients who undergo splenectomy should be vaccinated against pneumococci with a polyvalent vaccine if possible 1 or 2 wk prior to the splenectomy. This vaccination should be repeated every 5 yr. Children should not be splenectomized before the age of 5 yr and should be treated prophylactically with an antibiotic for 1–2 yr or lifelong, depending on the underlying disease. Adults who are splenectomized should receive antibiotic treatment for any febrile infection.

14 Hodgkin's Lymphoma

Erhard Hiller, MD
and Reinhold Munker, MD

CONTENTS

1. INTRODUCTION

Hodgkin's lymphoma (HL) was first described by Thomas Hodgkin in 1832. Carl Sternberg and Dorothy Reed reported on the typical multinuclear giant cells and their relationship to the mononuclear Hodgkin cell. For more than a century, this disease was regarded as a chronic inflammatory disorder, which is reflected by the old term lymphogranulomatosis. However, because aneuploidy and monoclonality were detected in the cells, Hodgkin's disease, or in terms of the World Health Organization (WHO) classification of malignant lymphomas, HL, today is considered a malignant tumor.

HL, together with testicular cancer, has become a prototype for curable neoplasms. Up to 80% of the cases diagnosed in adults and an even higher percentage in children can expect long-term, disease-free survival and cure. The advances in treatment have been brought about by improvements in histopathological diagnosis, by careful staging techniques, and by the combined application of radiation and chemotherapy including stem cell transplantation (SCT).

From: *Contemporary Hematology: Modern Hematology, Second Edition*
Edited by: R. Munker, E. Hiller, J. Glass, and R. Paquette © Humana Press Inc., Totowa, NJ

2. EPIDEMIOLOGY

In the United States, approximately three to four new cases of HL are diagnosed in 100,000 people each year. The age distribution frequency is bimodal, with one peak occurring at 15–30 yr, followed by a second peak in older patients. The incidence of HL has increased in recent years. There is a slight male predominance and, in addition, an increased risk of the disease is associated with higher socioeconomic status.

3. PATHOGENESIS AND ETIOLOGY

HL combines signs of inflammatory reactions as well as signs of a malignant disorder. The etiology of HL remains unknown, and there has been a long debate as to whether the changes seen are of malignant or infectious origin. It has been speculated that a viral infection occurring sometime during young adulthood may trigger the proliferation of premalignant lymphoid cells in certain individuals. A candidate virus is the Epstein-Barr virus (EBV). Indeed, in up to 50% of the cases in North America, this virus has been found to be integrated in the malignant cells. Nevertheless, because not all cases are positive for EBV, EBV is most likely not the only agent or virus implicated in the etiology of HL, but possibly only a co-factor for a yet-unknown agent. The clinical features of patients who are positive for EBV do not differ from those who are not. It has been proposed that EBV promotes genetic instability in susceptible patients. We know today that Hodgkin and the giant Reed-Sternberg cells are pathognomonic for HL, and that these cells are derived from a germinal B-cell in most cases. The cellular progeny of Hodgkin and Reed-Sternberg cells was determined when clonal rearranged immunoglobulin genes were amplified from single Hodgkin and Reed-Sternberg cells that had been micromanipulated from primary HL biopsy specimens. This proved the malignant character of HL by showing the clonality of the pathognomonic Hodgkin and Reed-Sternberg cells. Additionally, the detection of somatic mutations within the rearranged immunoglobulin genes implied a germinal center or postgerminal-center B-cell to be the precursor of Hodgkin and Reed-Sternberg cells, because mutations are introduced into immunoglobulin genes during this particular development stage of the B-cell.

Patients with untreated HL typically have a defect in cellular immunity. The clinical manifestations—for example, B-symptoms and the histological picture—are determined by cytokines secreted in large amounts by Sternberg-Reed cells. Interleukin-1, a cytokine that might explain the fever and night sweats associated with HL, has been demonstrated in HL-derived cell lines. Tumor necrosis factor (TNF)-α and TNF-β; have also been shown to to be produced by such cell lines and like interleukin-1 may cause B symptoms. Recently, transforming growth factor (TGF)-β has been characterized as the major immunosuppressive cytokine in HL.

4. CLINICAL FEATURES

The typical presentation of HL is an indolent enlargement of a lymph node or of several lymph nodes, most often at the neck and less frequently at the axillae. Although any lymphatic region can be affected, inguinal or femoral lymph nodes are involved in less than 10% of the cases as the only disease localization. A typical manifestation of the disease is a mediastinal enlargement that may cause dyspnea or no symptoms, which is only discovered on a routine chest X-ray. Abdominal lymph nodes and the spleen may be enlarged, causing abdominal discomfort, or may be discovered only during staging procedures. Solid organs like the lung or the liver may be involved, generally indicating disseminated disease, but may also be infiltrated by direct extension from a lymphatic mass. This situation has a better prognosis and may still be curable by local treatment. The bone marrow is involved in less than 5% of unselected patients. Involvement of the central nervous system is rare at the time of diagnosis and usually occurs only in late progressive disease. Patients may have B-symptoms, especially in advanced stages (night sweats and unexplained fever, which may be of the Pel-Ebstein type, and weight loss of >10% within 6 mo). An unusual (<2% of cases) but typical symptom is pain in the enlarged lymph nodes or involved tissues felt after the ingestion of alcohol. More often (in about 10% of cases), patients experience nonspecific pruritus. The typical pattern of disease progression is lymphogenous and *per continuitatem*. In its early stages, the disease may progress slowly, and occasionally, enlarged lymph nodes may regress for some time. The lymphatic areas which may become involved by HL and two commonly used radiotherapy fields (mantle field and inverted Y) are shown in Fig. 14.1.

5. DIAGNOSIS AND DIFFERENTIAL DIAGNOSIS, STAGING OF HL

If a suspicious lymph node is larger than 2 cm in diameter or smaller lymph nodes persist for more than 4–6 wk, or if B-symptoms or other signs suggest malignant lymphoma, the lymph node should be biopsied without delay. If no clear diagnosis can be made, the biopsy should be repeated, whenever possible, on a peripheral node. The differential diagnoses are other tumors, the group of non-HLs, and reactive processes, such as toxoplasmosis or pseudolymphomas. If the diagnosis is HL, then the exact stage has to be determined (staging) *(see Table 1)*.

Other staging procedures may also be useful. For example, magnetic resonance tomographies may also detect an enlarged spleen or abdominal lymph nodes. Lymphography is a sensitive, but invasive, method to detect abdominal

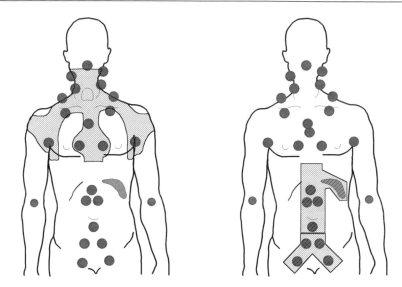

Fig. 14.1. Lymphatic areas and radiotherapy fields (mantle field, left, and inverted Y with spleen, right).

Table 1
Staging Procedures for Hodgkin's Lymphoma

Clinical examination
Complete laboratory status (including lactate dehydrogenase, complete blood count, sedimentation rate, C-reactive protein, alkaline phosphatase)
Chest X-ray
Computed tomography scans of thorax, abdomen, and neck
Ultrasound of abdomen
Positron emission tomography imaging (in selected circumstances)
Bone marrow biopsy
Liver biopsy (if liver involvement is suspected)

lymph nodes and has been abandoned by most centers. In some situations, positron emission tomography (PET) using fluorodeoxyglucose has been found useful for the staging and follow-up of patients with HL. PET is sensitive and, in most instances, specific enough to detect involvement by HL. In untreated patients, a higher stage is found in at least 20% of cases using PET imaging as compared with conventional imaging. However, the clinical relevance of this change in stage is not clear in all instances and must be studied in a prospective trial. PET may also be used in patients with residual tumor masses to discriminate

Table 2
Clinical Stages of Hodgkin's Lymphoma
(Ann Arbor Classification 1971, Cotswold Modification 1990)

I	Involvement of one lymphatic area on one side of the diaphragm or of a single extralymphatic site (I_E)
II	Involvement of two or more lymphatic areas on one side of the diaphragm
III	Lymphatic involvement on both sides of the diaphragm
III_1	1: Lymph nodes in upper abdomen
III_2	2: Para-aortic, mesenteric, or pelvic lymph nodes enlarged
IV	Diffuse involvement of solid organs(s) or bone marrow and/or lymphatic involvement

A or B is indicated for all stages: A, no general symptoms; B, general symptoms (night sweats, fever, weight loss of >10%; E, localized extranodal involvement of a solid organ. X indicates a mass of >10 cm in diameter or a mediastinal mass less than one-third of the thoracic diameter is present.

between active disease and residual fibronecrotic tissue. PET imaging can give further useful information to assess early response to chemotherapy and to prognosticate the outcome of autologous SCT.

The need for staging laparotomies has been controversial for many years. The original observation that up to 40% of patients with HL had a change in their stage of disease led to the introduction of surgical staging; however, as a result of more sensitive imaging techniques, positive staging laparotomies (detecting a change in the stage) have decreased to below 20%. Today, staging laparotomies are no longer performed routinely because of the delay in treatment, late immunological consequences, and the ability of chemotherapy to treat occult abdominal disease.

Table 14.2 describes the clinical stages of HL.

The histopathology of HL is rather distinctive. The Reed-Sternberg cells (large lobulated, multinucleated cells with prominent nucleoli) are generally considered to be a part of the tumor cell population found in the affected tissues along with stroma cells, reactive lymphoid cells, eosinophils, and neutrophils. A section of a lymph node involved by HL is shown in Fig. 14.2 *(see* Color Plate 14). As already mentioned, Reed-Sternberg cells belong in most cases to the B-cell lineage. Marker analysis reveals them to be positive for CD30, frequently positive for CD15 and for CD25, and negative in most cases for CD45 and for CD20. In addition, these cells bear markers of dendritic cells. The reactivity with antibodies against CD30 is typical of Hodgkin's disease, but not specific, as acti-

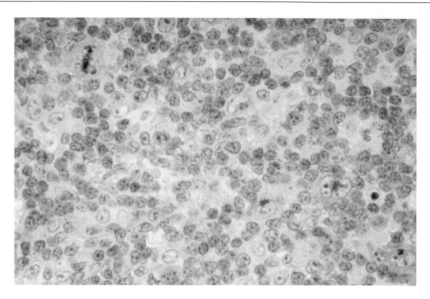

Fig. 14.2. Hodgkin's lymphoma. Lymph node with CD30-positive Hodgkin cells and binucleated Reed-Stemberg cells.

vated lymphoid cells and anaplastic lymphomas are also positive. Nodular lymphocyte-predominant HL has a different immunophenotype, being CD15 and CD30 negative, and CD20 and leukocyte common antigen (LCA)-positive.

The new WHO classification distinguishes only two groups—the nodular lymphocyte-predominant HL and the classical HL. The latter is subdivided in four forms as depicted below.

Nodular lymphocyte-predominant HL	5%
Classical HL:	
1. Lymphocyte-rich HL	5–8%
2. Nodular-sclerosis HL	35–55%
3. Mixed-cellularity HL	20–35%
4. Lymphocytic-depletion HL	3–4%

The frequency of these subtypes differs in different parts of the world. At present, with effective treatments for HL, the subtypes are no longer prognostically relevant. However, some of these types have particular clinical features: nodular sclerosis is more frequent in young women with a large mediastinal mass. The lymphocyte-predominant HL resembles a low-grade, B-cell lymphoma, and can be treated with limited irradiation at least in early stages. Prognostic factors in HL are age, sex, stage, and some serum markers such as sedimentation rate and soluble CD25. Recently, a prognostic score was established for advanced HL. This score, into which seven unfavorable clinical and laboratory parameters enter, predicts treatment failure (low serum albumin, anemia, male sex, age ≥ 45 yr, stage IV, leukocytosis, and lymphocytopenia).

6. TREATMENT OPTIONS AND RESULTS

6.1.Treatment

For the choice of treatment, stage, and systemic B-symptoms are the two major components for stratifying patients with HL. Bulky disease (<10 cm) has emerged as a third prognostic factor in the treatment concept. In the United States, most centers treat patients according to the classifications of early stages (IA–IIA or IIB) and advanced stages (III–IVA or B; I–IIB with bulky disease). In Europe, the European Organisation for Research and Treatment of Cancer (EORTC) and the German Hodgkin's Lymphoma Study Group (GHSG) have defined stage I–II as unfavorable or intermediate if certain adverse factors (large mediastinal mass, age >50 yr, elevated erythrocyte sedimentation rate, >3 involved regions) are present. Most patients who die of HL today present with stage IIIB or IV disease, or are of older age (>60 yr) at the time of diagnosis. Thus, in advanced disease, there is a need for more effective therapy, whereas in early stages, which have an excellent prognosis, a reduction of the treatment-related toxicity is needed. Treatment options for diagnosed HL are radiation, chemotherapy, and the combination of both (combined modality). Because the prognosis of HL is generally good, and because relapses may be salvaged by high-dose chemotherapy, different treatment options may be offered to some patients.

6.1.2. EARLY-STAGE DISEASE (CLINICAL STAGE I AND II)

Until a few years ago, early-stage (favorable) HL was treated in most centers with extended-field radiation without chemotherapy. However, a high incidence of relapse (about 25%) was observed, indicating that rescue therapy was necessary, which led to a very good overall survival of nearly 95% after 10 yr. But extended-field radiation therapy plus rescue therapy administered to about 25% of the patients caused an increased toxicity, such as secondary neoplasm, cardiac toxicity, infertility, and others. For this reason, extended-field radiotherapy has been replaced in favor of combined modality treatment consisting of a short-duration chemotherapy (e.g., two to four cycles of ABVD [Adriamycin® (doxorubicin), bleomycin, vinblastine, and dacarbazine]) followed by involved-field radiotherapy (20–30 Gy). Although a further improvement of overall survival could not to be achieved, the long-term treatment complications could thus be reduced considerably. Whether chemotherapy alone is sufficient to control disease has yet to be determined.

6.1.3. EARLY-STAGE UNFAVORABLE DISEASE

In the past, patients with clinical stage I and II with risk factors who underwent extended-field irradiation had a poor 10-yr relapse-free survival in the 50% range. Therefore, it is generally accepted today that these patients qualify for combined modality therapy. In many institutions, four cycles of ABVD followed by involved-field irradiation has become the standard regimen for unfavorable stage I–II disease. Because 5% of those patients progress and 15% relapse early, more intense regimens are evaluated in clinical studies (Stanford V, BEACOPP [bleomycin, etoposide, Adriamycin (doxorubicin), cyclophosphamide, Oncovin® (vincristine), procarbazine, and prednisone]) in combination with involved-field radiotherapy. For patients not included in clinical studies, at the present time four cycles of ABVD followed by involved-field irradiation can be considered the treatment of choice. Involved-field radiation is sufficient to control occult disease when combined with chemotherapy.

6.1.4. ADVANCED STAGE (CLINICAL STAGES III AND IV)

Advanced-stage HL consists of patients with lymph node involvement above and below the diaphragm, and those in stage IV with additional involvement of extralymphatic manifestations (lung, liver, bone, bone marrow). Until the early 1960s, patients with advanced-stage disease were uncurable. The report of De Vita and colleagues of the effectiveness of MOPP (mechlorethamine, vincristine, procarbazine, and prednisone) with a 50% cure rate remains a landmark in the success story of treatment in HL. Later, it became clear that alternating the regimes MOPP and ABVD was superior to MOPP alone. After 15 yr, the overall survival is around 65%. ABVD alone seems to be as effective as the alternating MOPP/ABVD protocol. The main advantage of ABVD alone is the relatively low incidence of long-term toxic effects as compared with alkylating agents-based regimens.

To address the still considerable rate of treatment failure in advanced disease with conventional regimens, clinical trials with escalation of dose and introduction of etoposide as a novel chemotherapeutic agent were investigated in clinical studies. Stanford V is a seven-drug (mechlorethamine, doxorubicin, vinblastine, vincristine, bleomycin, etoposide, and granulocyte colony-stimulating factor [G-CSF]) regimen that was given weekly for a total of 12 wk in combination with consolidation radiotherapy to sites of initial bulky disease. In a phase-II study of 142 patients, a 5-yr freedom from progression of 89% and an overall survival of 96% at a median of 5.4 yr was achieved. The escalated BEACOPP regimen proposed by a German study group (cyclophosphamide, doxorubicin, etoposide, procarbazine, prednisone, vincristine, and bleomycin; Table 3) administered every 3 wk with G-CSF achieved an 87% freedom from progression and a 91% overall survival after 5 yr. Both schemes are toxic and therefore should only be

Table 3
Chemotherapy Protocols for Treating Hodgkin's Lymphoma

Drugs	Dose (mg/m^2)	Route	Days
MOPP			
Nitrogen mustard	6	i.v.	1, 8
Vincristine	1.4	i.v.	1, 8
Procarbazine	100	Oral	1–14
Prednisone	40	Oral	1–14
ABVD			
Doxorubicin	25	i.v.	1, 15
Bleomycin	10	i.v.	1, 15
Vinblastine	6	i.v.	1, 15
Dacarbazine	375	i.v.	1, 15
Stanford V			
Doxorubicin	25	i.v.	1, 15, 29, 43, 57, 71
Vinblastine	6	i v	1, 15, 29, 43, 57, 71
Nitrogen mustard	6	i.v.	1, 29, 57
Vincristine	1.4	i.v.	8, 22, 36, 50, 64, 78
Bleomycin	5	i.v.	8, 22, 36, 50, 64, 78
Etoposide	60	i.v.	15, 43, 71
Prednisone	40	Oral	for 12 wk
BEACOPP-baseline			
Bleomycin	10	i.v.	8
Etoposide	100	i.v.	1–3
Doxorubicin	25	i.v.	I
Cyclophosphamide	650	i.v.	I
Vincristine	1.4	i.v.	8
Procarbazine	100	p.o.	1–7
Prednisone	40	p.o.	1–14
BEACOPP-escalated			
Bleomycin	10	i.v.	8
Etoposide	200	i.v.	1–3
Doxorubicin	35	i.v.	1
Cyclophosphamide	1200	i.v.	1
Vincristine	1.4	i.v.	1
Procarbazin	100	p.o.	1–8
Prednisone	40	p.o.	1–14

BEACOPP is repeated on day 22.

administered in larger centers with much experience and within clinical trials. The occurrence of nine cases of acute leukemia after increased-dose BEACOPP is a reason for concern; however, this complication must be weighed against the lower rate of early progression and higher rates of failure-free survival and overall survival rates at 5 yr. Outside clinical trials at present, four double cycles of MOPP/ABVD or eight cycles of ABVD may still be considered as a standard treatment.

Through the years, a number of groups have addressed the added benefit of radiotherapy in advanced HL. A number of these studies were underpowered to demonstrate a significant clinical benefit. In a recent multi-center study of the EORTC on 739 patients, involved-field radiotherapy did not improve the outcome in patients with advanced-stage HL who had a complete remission after MOPP/ABV chemotherapy. However, it was concluded that the only patients who benefit from radiotherapy are those in partial remission after chemotherapy.

6.1.5. LYMPHOCYTE-PREDOMINANT HL

Nodular lymphocyte-predominant HL is a rare subtype that accounts for less than 5% of all cases of HL. Mostly peripheral lymph nodes are involved, 75% of the patients have stage IA disease, and organ involvement rarely occurs. The clinical course is indolent with frequent relapses, but responsive to treatment. Patients in stage I–IIA disease should be treated with involved-field radiation (30 Gy). Patients in a higher stage should probably be treated more aggressively by chemotherapy because they show a substantially worse progression-free survival and overall survival than patients with early-stage lymphocyte-predominant disease. Recently, the anti-CD20 antibody rituximab was used for treatment at first diagnosis or relapse. Remission rates of 80% were observed but there are no data as yet for long-term follow-up.

6.2. Prognosis

The prognosis for patients with various stages of HL is as follows:

1. In early stages, 5-yr survival is about 95%. Because of combined modality treatment (i.e., a short-duration chemotherapy prior to involved-field radiotherapy), the freedom from progress comes close to the survival rate after 5 yr.
2. In intermediate stages, the 5-yr survival is 90%, and 75–80% survive without relapse.
3. In advanced stages, the 5-yr survival is decreased to 75–80% and freedom from treatment failure is in the range of 60% with COPP/ABVD (earlier data from GHSG). With the modern dose-intensified chemotherapy regimens (e.g., BEACOPP) the rates of freedom from treatment failure at 5 yr are significantly better and were 76% for the baseline BEACOPP and 87% for the escalated BEACOPP. Beyond 5 yr, relapses are rare and most patients can be considered as cured.

4. The ultimate prognosis for patients depends not only on relapse-free survival and early treatment complications, but also on long-term complications and comorbid conditions. In patients with early-stage HL, it was shown that after 13 yr, deaths from other conditions (i.e., late treatment-related conditions) exceeded death from relapsed HL.

7. TREATING RELAPSED HL

The clinical diagnosis of a relapse must be established with a biopsy. Generally, a relapse of HL is prognostically unfavorable and justifies aggressive treatment. The therapeutic options for recurrences within 1 yr or progressive disease include high-dose chemotherapy followed by autologous SCT. High-dose chemotherapy is generally given following four cycles of salvage chemotherapy with protocols such as ESHAP (etoposide, solu-medrol, high-dose ara-C, and cis-platinum), ICE (ifosfamide, carboplatin, and etoposide), or DHAP (dexamethasone, high-dose cytarabine, and cisplatin). Negative prognostic factors for an autologous transplant are: B-symptoms at relapse, duration of complete remission of less than 1 yr, extranodal disease at relapse, and persistent PET positivity. A different approach exists if a localized relapse occurs after radiotherapy alone, in which case conventional dose chemotherapy (plus additional irradiation if necessary) may still be curative. Similarly, if a localized nodal relapse occurs after chemotherapy alone, radiotherapy (plus further chemotherapy) may result in a durable remission in some situations. The current treatment of choice for HL relapsing, however, is high-dose chemotherapy. If possible, an adjuvant irradiation following high-dose therapy should be considered. The results of allogeneic transplantation for relapsed HL compared unfavorably with autologous transplantation. More recently, promising results were observed with reduced-intensity transplants and might be proposed to young patients with a fully matched donor.

8. LATE EFFECTS OF TREATMENT

Of patients receiving mantle radiotherapy, 20–50% develop some degree of hypothyroidism, which may require substitution by thyroid hormones. These patients are also at a higher risk of developing cardiovascular disease. Shortly after receiving mantle-field irradiation, less than 5% of patients develop a radiation pneumonitis and less than 2% develop pericarditis. Late effects may be lung fibrosis from radiation plus bleomycin. The dose-intensified chemotherapy regimens are associated with a high risk of sterility (80%). A rare (<0.5%) but serious late effect of splenectomy was septicemia caused by pneumococci. This may be prevented to a large extent by immunizing such patients against pneumococci prior to splenectomy. A significant problem emerging in recent years is the appearance of other malignant tumors in patients cured of HL. These second neoplasms have been called the "price of success" and can be observed in about 20% of patients after 20-yr follow-up. Compared with the general population, the risk of second malignancy is about three- to fivefold elevated. The major types of second cancers are acute myelogenous leukemias (increased risk within 3–8 yr), myelodysplastic syndromes, NHLs, and various solid tumors. Some types of second tumors are associated with special treatment features and appear preventable (e.g., the risk of breast cancer is increased only in young women treated with radiation, and smokers have a higher risk of developing second lung cancers). Despite the generally good prognosis, the late complications of treatment mandate a lifelong follow-up of patients treated for HL.

SUGGESTED READING

Aisenberg AC. Problems in Hodgkin's disease management. *Blood* 1999;93:761–779.

Aleman BM, Raemaekers JMM, Tirelli U, et al. Involved-field radiotherapy for advanced Hodgkin's lymphoma. *N Engl J Med* 2003;348:2396–2406.

Diehl V, Franklin J, Pfreundschuh M, et al. Standard and increased-dose BEACOPP chemotherapy compared with COPP-ABVD for advanced Hodgkin´s disease. *N Engl J Med* 2003;348:2386–2395.

Hasenclever D, Diehl V. A prognostic score for advanced Hodgkin's disease. *N Engl J Med* 1998;339:1506–1514.

Horning SJ, Hoppe RT, Breslin S, et al. Stanford V and radiotherapy for locally extensive and advanced Hodgkin's disease: mature results of a prospective clinical trial. *J Clin Oncol* 2002;20:630–637.

Meyer RM, Ambinder RF, Stroobants S. Hodgkin's lymphoma: evolving concepts with implications for practice. *Hematology (Am Soc Hematol Educ Program)* 2004;184–202.

Munker R, Glass J, Griffeth LK, et al. Contribution of PET imaging to the initial staging and prognosis of patients with Hodgkin's disease. *Ann Oncol* 2004;15:1699–1704.

Urba WL, Longo DL. Hodgkin's disease. *N Engl J Med* 1992;326:678–687.

15 The Non-Hodgkin's Lymphomas

Reinhold Munker, MD,
Jay Marion, MD, Gang Ye, MD,
and Martin H. Dreyling, MD

1. INTRODUCTION

Non-Hodgkin's lymphomas (NHLs) are malignant proliferations of the lymphoid tissues that can be distinguished from Hodgkin's lymphoma *(see* Chapter 14) by a variety of clinical and histological features. NHLs are a disease of predominantly elderly persons, with a median age around 50–70 yr, are more heterogeneous in their behavior, and often have an extranodal involvement. The classification of

From: *Contemporary Hematology: Modern Hematology, Second Edition*
Edited by: R. Munker, E. Hiller, J. Glass, and R. Paquette © Humana Press Inc., Totowa, NJ

NHLs continues to evolve. Recently, a new World Health Organization (WHO) classification scheme was introduced, which is based on the revised European American Lymphoma (REAL) classification and incorporates some of the progress in immunology and molecular biology (*see* "Classification"). Considerations that enter into these classifications are the lymphocyte lineage (B- vs T-cell type), and maturation status (precursor vs mature cell type), additional immunophenotypic markers, and characteristic molecular alterations. Based on these criteria, the clinical course and biology of each distinct lymphoma subtype may be more accurately predicted. About 90% of the NHLs are derived from a malignant B-cell, the remaining cases from T-cells, natural killer (NK) cells, or undifferentiated cells. In recent years, the incidence of NHL has steadily increased. NHLs are more frequent than Hodgkin's lymphoma and have an annual incidence of about 15–20 new cases per 100,000 people.

2. ETIOLOGY OF NHLs

The etiology of NHLs cannot be determined in most cases. There is some evidence that chronic antigenic stimulation by viral or bacterial infections increases the likelihood of NHLs. This is true for patients infected with HIV who have a high risk of developing NHLs (most of aggressive histology), as well as for children in Central Africa who develop Burkitt's lymphomas. The genome of the Epstein-Barr virus (EBV) is integrated into the tumor cells of classic Burkitt's lymphomas. As with normal B-lymphocytes transformed by EBV, a number of transformation-associated genes are expressed in the tumor cells. Serologically, patients with Burkitt's lymphoma show an immune response against viral capsid antigens of EBV. Lymphomas in Europe and North America with similar histology (Burkitt's-like lymphomas) do not have a clear correlation with EBV; therefore, other factors play a role in these lymphomas. An increased risk for NHL exists in cases of congenital immunodeficiency syndromes (e.g., ataxia telangiectasia). A human retrovirus (HTLV-1) that is endemic in Japan and in the Caribbean is associated with the development of acute T-cell leukemias or lymphomas. HTLV-1 is found to be clonally integrated into the tumor cells; however, as only a small fraction of the infected individuals develops lymphoma, this retrovirus is considered to be only a co-factor in lymphomagenesis. Another important example is the association between infection of the stomach by *Helicobacter pylori* and mucosa-associated lymphoid tissue (MALT)-type gastric lymphomas. The eradication of the bacterial infection with antibiotics in an early stage results in the regression of the lymphoma. More recently, it was shown that a new human herpesvirus (HHV8) is associated with a rare type of undifferentiated lymphoma (primary effusion lymphomas). Chronic infection with the hepatitis C virus has been associated with the development of NHL predominantly of the marginal zone type. Infections with *Borrelia burgdorferi*,

Table 1
Cytogenetic and Molecular Markers in Non-Hodgkin's Lymphomas

Follicular lymphoma	t(14;18)\Bcl-2
Mantle cell lymphoma	t(11;14)
	Bcl-1/cyclin D1
B-cell chronic lymphocytic leukemia	Trisomy 12, other markers
Burkitt's lymphoma	t(8;14)(q24;q32), c-myc
	t(2;8)(p12;q24)
	t(8;22)(q24;q11)
Anaplastic large-cell lymphoma	t(2;5)
	Alk

the etiological agent of Lyme disease, are associated with some forms of cutaneous lymphomas.

The distinct lymphoma subtypes are reflected by characteristic chromosomal translocations detectable in the majority of cases. Several types of lymphomas have such cytogenetic markers. An example is the translocation t(14;18)(q32;q21) in 80–90% of follicular lymphomas. Translocation t(14;18) leads to an over expression of the *bcl-2* gene thereby immortalizing the tumor cells by suppression of the programmed cell death (apoptosis). However, this translocation can also be found in the peripheral blood of some normal individuals. Thus, the expression of certain oncogenes or antiapoptotic genes is only one factor in the multi-step pathogenesis of lymphomas. Accordingly, *bcl-2*-transgenic mice also do not regularly develop follicular lymphomas. Another example is the translocation t(8;14)(q24;q32) or related translocations, which are present in virtually all cases of Burkitt's lymphoma and lead to an activation of the *Myc* oncogene. Table 1 lists important cytogenetic and molecular changes in NHL.

3. CLASSIFICATION

As mentioned previously, the current WHO classification is accepted worldwide and takes into account clinical, immunological, and molecular observations. Compared with the previous Working Formulation, several additional entities with distinct features are now included (e.g., mantle cell lymphomas, MALT lymphomas, and mediastinal B-cell lymphomas). In the clinical section of this chapter, the clinical features and treatment of the major and some rare categories are discussed. A simplified version of the WHO classification is listed in Table 2. The WHO classification also incorporated some chronic leukemias (chronic lymphocytic leukemias [CLL], hairy cell leukemia [HCL]). Likewise, Hodgkin's lymphoma and multiple myeloma are included in the WHO classification of lymphoid neoplasms, but in this book are described in separate chapters.

Table 2
World Health Organization Lymphoma Classification

B-Cell neoplasms

Precursor B-cell neoplasms
Precursor B-lymphoblastic leukemia/lymphoma

Peripheral B-Cell neoplasms

Small lymphocytic lymphoma (B-Cell chronic lymphocytic leukemia)
Prolymphocytic leukemia
Lymphoplasmacytic lymphoma/immunocytoma (including M. Waldenström)
Hairy cell leukemia

Follicular lymphoma
Marginal zone B-cell lymphoma (extranodal, MALT-type, nodal, splenic marginal zone)

Mantle cell lymphoma
(grade I–III)

Diffuse large B-cell lymphoma
Subtype: Primary mediastinal (thymic) B-cell lymphoma

Burkitt's lymphoma

T-Cell neoplasms

Precursor T-cell neoplasms
Precursor T-lymphoblastic leukemia/lymphoma

Peripheral T-Cell and natural killer (NK)-cell neoplasms
T-Cell chronic lymphocytic leukemia
T-Cell Prolymphocytic leukemia
Large granular lymphocytic leukemia
Mycosis fungoides
Sezary syndrome
Anaplastic large cell lymphoma, CD30 positive, T- and null-cell types
Peripheral T-cell lymphomas (not otherwise specified): Extranodal NK-/T-cell
    lymphoma (nasal type
Angioimmunoblastic T-cell lymphoma Enteropathy-type T-cell lymphoma
Hepatosplenic T-cell lymphoma
Subcutaneous panniculitis-like T-cell lymphoma
Adult T-cell lymphoma/leukemia

4. CLINICAL FEATURES AND DIAGNOSTIC STRATEGIES

Patients with lymphoma present most frequently with lymph node swelling (lymphadenopathy) that may be either peripheral (e.g., axillary, cervical, inguinal) or involve central locations (e.g., mediastinal tumor, abdominal lymph nodes). In most cases, the enlarged lymph nodes are painless. The lymph nodes may enlarge very slowly, as is the case in most low-grade or indolent lymphomas, or show an aggressive growth pattern. Abdominal lymph nodes may sometimes enlarge considerably before clinical symptoms occur. Especially marginal zone lymphoma, but also other lymphoma subtypes, may have an extranodal spread: the gastrointestinal tract or solid organs such as the liver; rarely, the CNS can be involved. In such cases, the clinical symptoms may be different. For example, the first symptoms of gastric lymphoma may be dyspepsia or discomfort in the upper abdomen. When the bone marrow is involved, the patient may present with anemia, leukopenia, or thrombocytopenia. Similarly to patients with Hodgkin's lymphoma, patients with NHL may also have systemic or B-symptoms (fever, night sweats, or weight loss).

The clinical staging of NHL is based on the Ann Arbor classification, which recognizes four clinical stages (I–IV), the presence or absence of systemic symptoms, and/or the presence of extranodal localized disease. The Ann Arbor classification was originally developed for Hodgkin's lymphoma and is described in Chapter 14, Table 2.

If a malignant lymphoma is suspected, a lymph node biopsy should be performed without delay. Biopsies should also be performed on other tissues (e.g., gastric mucosa, solid organs) if clinical or radiological evidence suggests that these systems are involved. A lymph node aspiration may yield some diagnostic information, but is usually insufficient to make the proper classification of malignant lymphoma. The diagnosis of malignant lymphoma is generally made on fixed, paraffin-embedded tissue. For some immunochemical and molecular studies, unfixed tissue is necessary. An accurate diagnosis of malignant lymphomas is important, as the prognosis and the treatment of the different categories of NHL differ considerably.

The diagnostic strategies for NHL are described in Table 3.

The different categories of NHL can be divided into two major groups:

1. Low-grade (indolent) NHL: these lymphomas have an indolent course, do not always need treatment, but cannot be cured by most present approaches. Examples are the follicular lymphomas and CLL.
2. High-grade (aggressive) NHL: these lymphomas have an aggressive clinical course and, if untreated, are rapidly fatal. In a fraction of these NHL, cure is achieved with chemotherapy. Examples are Burkitt's lymphomas and diffuse large B-cell lymphomas (DLBCLs).

Table 3
Diagnostic Strategies for the Non-Hodgkin's Lymphomas

History and clinical examination	Ask for B symptoms and palpate all lymph nodes, liver, and spleen
Lymph node biopsy	Biopsy, if possible, a peripheral lymph node, obtain immunohistochemistry and molecular studies (bcl-2, myc, cyclin-D1, others)
Laboratory studies	Obtain complete laboratory status, including blood counts, sedimentation rate, white cell differential, clotting tests, lactate dehydrogenase, β_2-microglobulin, total protein, serum electrophoresis, quantitative immunoglobulins, immunoelectrophoresis if a monoclonal protein is suspected, creatinine, urea, uric acid, GOT, GPT, γ-GT, alkaline phosphatase; if hemolysis is suspected: haptoglobin, Coombs' test; if risk category: HIV serology
Chest radiograph (in two planes)	**CT scan of the thorax**
CT scans of the abdomen	**Ultrasound of the abdomen and the neck**
FDG-PET scan	
Bone marrow biopsy	**Bone marrow aspiration** (with immunophenotyping to detect lymphoma infiltration) (if leukemic presentation, immunophenotyping can be done from blood)
EKG, cardiac ultrasound, or MUGA scan	
Further studies (dependent on clinical situation and type of lymphoma)	ENT examination, endoscopy, liver biopsy, skeletal X-rays, bone scan, magnetic resonance imaging, lumbar puncture

GOT, glutamic-oxaloacetic transaminase; GPT, glutamic-pyruvic transaminase; γ-GT, γ-glutamyl transpeptidase; CT, computed tomography; FDG-PET, fluorodeoxyglucose-positron emission tomography; MUGA, multiple-gated acquisition; ENT, ear–nose–throat.

The major categories of NHL are described in the following seven sections, based on the WHO classification. Some special forms or presentations of NHLs are described in "Special Forms of NHL."

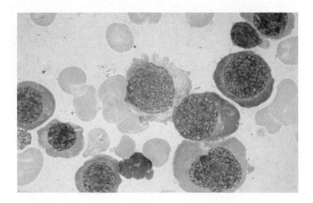

Color Plate 1, Fig. 5.2. Megaloblastic Erythroblasts. (*See* full caption in Ch. 5 on p. 94.)

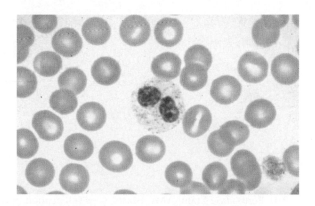

Color Plate 2, Fig. 7.1. Granulocytes. (*See* full caption in Ch. 7 on p. 129.)

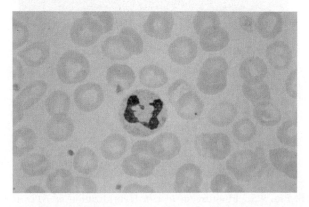

Color Plate 3, Fig. 7.2. Döhle Bodies. (*See* full caption in Ch. 7 on p. 129.)

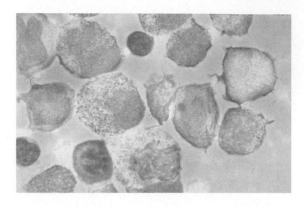

Color Plate 4, Fig. 9.3. APL, Myeloid Blasts. (*See* full caption in Ch. 9 on p. 162.)

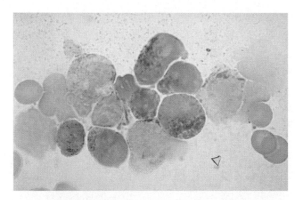

Color Plate 5, Fig. 9.4. Peroxidase Stain, AML Blasts. (*See* full caption in Ch. 9 on p. 162.)

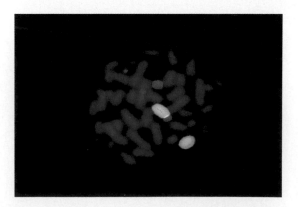

Color Plate 6, Fig. 9.5. Fluorescent *in situ* Hybridization in APL. (*See* full caption in Ch. 9 on p. 163.)

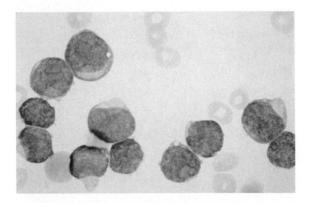

Color Plate 7, Fig. 10.2. ALL Lymphoblast. (*See* full caption in Ch. 10 on p. 179.)

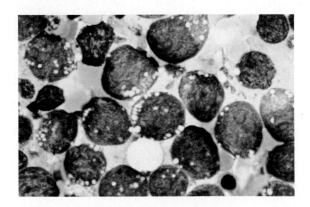

Color Plate 8, Fig. 10.3. Blasts of B-ALL. (*See* full caption in Ch. 10 on p. 179.)

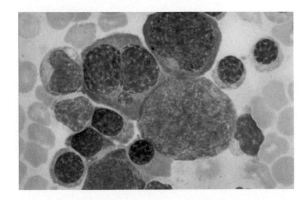

Color Plate 9, Fig. 11.1. Dysplastic Changes in Erythropoiesis (*See* full caption in Ch. 11 on p. 199.)

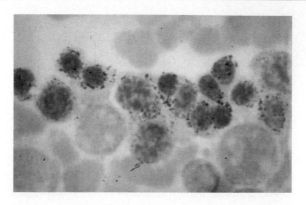

Color Plate 10, Fig. 11.2. Ringed Sideroblasts, MDS. (*See* full caption in Ch. 11 on p. 200.)

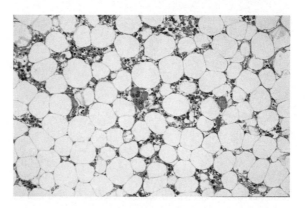

Color Plate 11, Fig. 12.1. Aplastic Anemia, Histology. (*See* full caption in Ch. 12 on p. 212.)

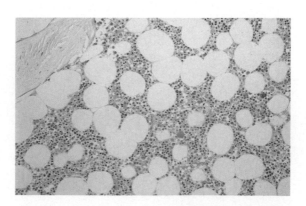

Color Plate 12, Fig. 12.2. Normal Bone Marrow, Histology. (*See* full caption in Ch. 12 on p. 212.)

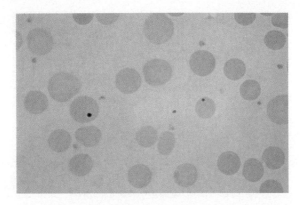

Color Plate 13, Fig. 13.3. Howell Jolly Bodies. (*See* full caption in Ch. 13 on p. 222.)

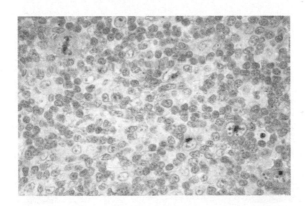

Color Plate 14, Fig. 14.2. Lymph Node, Hodgkin's. (*See* full caption in Ch. 14 on p. 230.)

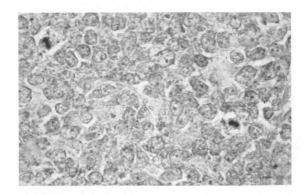

Color Plate 15, Fig. 15.1. Lymph Node, Non-Hodgkin's. (*See* full caption in Ch. 15 on p. 243.)

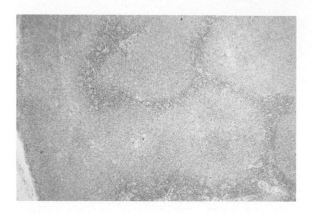

Color Plate 16, Fig. 15.2. Follicle Center Lymphoma. (*See* full caption in Ch. 15 on p. 249.)

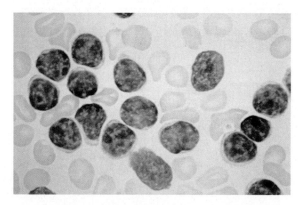

Color Plate 17, Fig. 15.3. CLL Morphology. (*See* full caption in Ch. 15 on p. 254.)

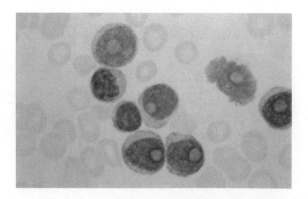

Color Plate 18, Fig. 15.4. PLL Morphology. (*See* full caption in Ch. 15 on p. 257.)

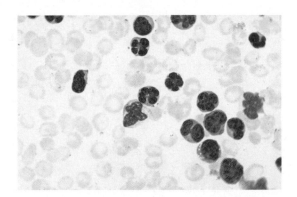

Color Plate 19, Fig. 15.5. Adult T-Cell Leukemia, Lymphoma. (*See* full caption in Ch. 15 on p. 258.)

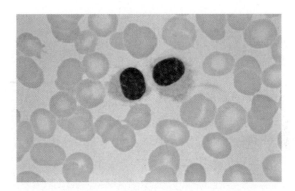

Color Plate 20, Fig. 15.6. Hairy Cell Leukemia. (*See* full caption in Ch. 15 on p. 262.)

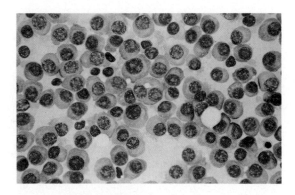

Color Plate 21, Fig. 16.2. Multiple Myeloma, Dense Infiltrate of Neoplastic Plasma Cells. (*See* full caption in Ch. 14 on p. 280.)

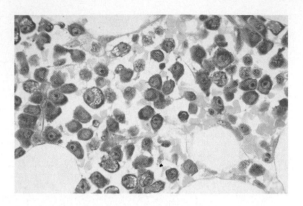

Color Plate 22, Fig. 16.3. Multiple Myeloma, Bone Marrow. (*See* full caption in Ch. 16 on p. 280.)

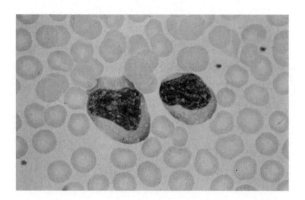

Color Plate 23, Fig. 18.1. Infectious Mononucleosis. (*See* full caption in Ch. 18 on p. 317.)

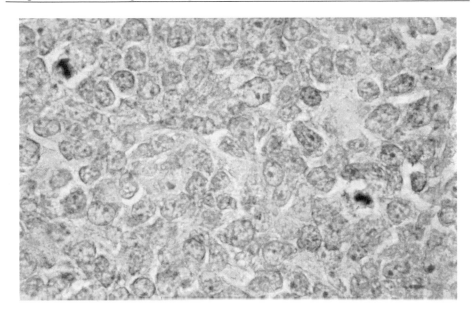

Fig. 15.1. Diffuse large B-cell lymphoma. Lymph node structure destroyed by large neoplastic lymphatic cells, numerous mitoses, Giemsa stain, high-power magnification.

5. DIFFUSE LARGE B-CELL LYMPHOMA

This is the most frequently occurring NHL. It includes lymphomas predominantly classified in the former Working Formulation as diffuse large-cell, diffuse mixed-cell, or immunoblastic, and lymphomas classified as diffuse centroblastic, diffuse centroblastic/centrocytic, and immunoblastic in the Kiel classification.

Histopathologically, a diffuse proliferation of large, transformed lymphoid cells is found. The nuclei have a vesicular chromatin, prominent nucleoli, basophilic cytoplasm, and a moderate to high proliferation fraction. Figure 15.1 is an example of an involved lymph node at high magnification (*see* Color Plate 15). Cytogenetically, about 50% of patients with diffuse large-cell lymphomas have abnormalities of the chromosome region 3q27–29. These abnormalities correlate with the presence of a rearrangement of the *Bcl-6* oncogene. Other oncogenes or antiapoptotic genes like *bcl-2* are also involved in some diffuse large-cell lymphomas. Cases that overexpress *Bcl-2* have a worse prognosis. By marker analysis, most diffuse large-cell lymphomas are positive for B-cell antigens like CD19, CD20, and CD22.

Table 4
International Index for Aggressive Non-Hodgkin's Lymphomas

Risk group	Number of risk factors	Rate of complete remissions	5-yr Survival	
			Relapse-free	Total
Low	0–1	87%	61%	73%
Low-intermediate	2	67%	34%	51%
High-intermediate	3	55%	27%	43%
High	4–5	44%	18%	26%

5.1. Prognostic Factors in High-Grade NHL

The prognosis in NHL is more heterogeneous than in Hodgkin's lymphoma and the Ann Arbor stage is not a good prognostic indicator for all cases. Recently, an International Index was described and was found to permit a better estimation of remission rate and survival. Factors (each contributing one point) that enter into this International Index are age greater than 60 yr, reduced performance status, clinical stage III or IV, increased lactate dehydrogenase (LDH), and extranodal manifestation in two or more locations.

Based on these criteria, four categories are defined (Table 4).

Additional adverse prognostic factors for response to treatment and survival of patients with aggressive lymphomas include the presence of *p53* mutations, lack of class II antigens, some karyotypic abnormalities, deletion of the tumor suppressor genes *p15* and *p16,* and *bcl-6* rearrangements.

5.2. Gene Expression Profiling in Diffuse Large B-Cell Lymphoma

Using clinical prognostic models such as the International Prognostic Index alone cannot identify the molecular basis of clinical heterogeneity of diffuse large B-cell lymphoma. Recent development of DNA microarrays has allowed scientists to take a genome-wide approach towards furthering insights into the disease, predicting the treatment outcomes, and developing novel targeted treatments. Several studies have demonstrated that there are at least two subtypes of diffuse large B-cell lymphoma: germinal center B-cell type and activated B-cell type (*see* Table 5). The gene-based predictor is independent from the international prognostic index. More recently, these findings were confirmed by tissue microarray. This suggests that the findings from gene expression profiling can be translated into clinical application at the level of routine immunohistochemistry. The molecular classification based on gene expression profiling not only shows distinct clinical features in the two subtypes, but also suggests different lymphomagenic mechanisms. Activated B-cell lymphoma cells cannot survive without constitutive activation of nuclear factor (NF)-κB, which may give a potential target for treatment.

Table 5
Gene Expression Profile in Diffuse Large B-Cell Lymphoma

	Germinal center B-cell-type	Activated B-cell-type
Frequency	50%	30%
Genes expressed	CD10, BCL-6, LMO2	PKCb1, CND2, MUM1, CD44
Oncogenic events	BCL-2 translocation REL amplification	Nuclear factor-κB activation
5-yr survival	60%	35%
Median survival	10 yr	2 yr

Primary mediastinal large B-cell lymphoma, a subtype of diffuse large B-cell lymphoma by the WHO classification, serves as another example of the power of this new technology. Gene expression profiling studies have shown that this specific subtype of lymphoma does not belong to either germinal B-cell type or activated B-cell type. Rather, it shares many clinical and molecular features with classical Hodgkin's lymphoma.

5.3. Treatment

The treatment of large-cell lymphomas depends on the stage of disease. Patients with disseminated disease (generally stages III and IV) are given six to eight cycles of CHOP (cyclophosphamide, hydroxydaunomycin, Oncovin® [vincristine], and prednisone) or a comparable regimen (see Table 6). In patients with a B-lineage phenotype, the chimeric monoclonal antibody rituximab should be added to CHOP. With this approach, about 60–70% of the patients obtain a complete remission and approx 35% are cured. The advantage of adding rituximab to CHOP chemotherapy has mainly been demonstrated in older patients, but promising results indicate that both overall survival and relapse-free survival are improved in younger patients when treated with a combined approach. Patients with localized disease (stages I or II) are treated with a shorter course of chemotherapy (three to four cycles) and involved-field radiation. Again, the prognosis seems to be improved when immunotherapy with rituximab is added to chemotherapy. At present, the 5-yr freedom from progression is around 70–85% and the overall survival around 80–85%. High-dose therapy with stem cell or bone marrow support is indicated for certain high-risk patients with large-cell lymphomas. In a French study, four cycles of standard chemotherapy were given followed by either high-dose therapy or further conventional treatment. The total group of patients did not benefit from high-dose therapy, but patients who had more than one risk factor in the International Index had a longer sur-

Table 6
Chemotherapy Protocols for the Treatment of Non-Hodgkin's Lymphomas

1. CHOP protocol (repeat on day 21)

Cyclophosphamide	750 mg/m^2 i.v., day 1
Adriamycin	50 mg/m^2 i.v., day 1
Vincristine	Vincristine 2 mg, day 1
Prednisone	100 mg p.o., days 1—5

2. CHOP Rituximab Protocol (repeat on day 21)

(Same as 1, addition of Rituximab 375 mg/m^2 i.v. on day1)

3. CVP protocol (repeat on day 21)

Cyclophosphamide	400 mg/m^2, intravenous, days 1–5 (modified at some centers)
Vincristine	Vincristine 1.4 mg /m^2 (maximum 2 mg), day 1
Prednisone	100 mg p.o., days 1–5

4. ESHAP protocol (repeat on day 21)

Etoposide	60 mg/m^2 i.v., days 1–4 Methylprednisolone 500 mg i.v., days 1–4
Cytarabine	2 g/m^2 i.v., day 5
Cisplatin	25 mg/m^2 continuous infusion, days 1–4

(continued)

vival. Gene expression profiling may further delineate risk factors and treatment choices. More studies are necessary to define exactly the indications for an initial high-dose treatment. Patients who relapse or who do not achieve a complete response have a poor prognosis. All such patients are candidates for high-dose treatment if the disease is still sensitive to chemotherapy. Common salvage regimens for patients with relapsed diffuse large B-cell NHL are ICE (ifosfamide, carboplatin, and etoposide), which can be combined with rituximab (*see* Table 6), DHAP (dexamethasone, high-dose cytarabine, and cisplatin), or ESHAP (etoposide, solumedrol, high-dose ara-C, and platinol). In an Italian study, 84% of patients with relapsed diffuse large-cell NHL achieved a complete response with high-dose treatment and 46% survived after more than 5 yr vs 44 and 12% in the conventional treatment arm. At present, there is limited experience with allogeneic transplantation for large-cell lymphomas. If a high-dose treatment is not indicated because of age, previous treatment, or co-morbidity, a good palliation may be reached with various protocols including ESHAP and MINE (mitoxantrone, ifosfamide, and etoposide). In selected cases, radiotherapy can

Table 6 (Continued)

5. MINE protocol (repeat on day 21)

Mitoxantrone	8 mg/m^2 i.v., day 1
Ifosfamide	1.33 g/m^2 i.v., days 1—3 (together with Mesna, 1.33 g/m^2)
Etoposide	65 mg/m^2 i.v., days 1-3

6. Rituximab-ICE

Rituximab	375 mg/m^2 i.v. 48 h prior to cycle 1 and on day 1 of cycles 1–3
Etoposide	100 mg/m^2 i.v. days 1–3
Carboplatin	AUC5 (capped at 800 mg i.v. on d 4)
Ifosfamide	5000 mg/m^2 mixed with an equal amount of Mesna (as continuous infusion for 24 h on day 4)

7. Oral chlorambucil

Chlorambucil	0.08 mg/kg p.o. or 2–4 (8) mg absolute dose (continuous treatment, until toxicity is reached or not effective)
	Alternatively 0.4 mg/kg p.o., day 1 (increase dose, if no major toxicity, repeat after 2 wk)

8. Fludarabine protocol (repeat on day 29)

Fludarabine	25 mg/m^2 i.v., days 1–5

9. FCM Protocol (repeat on day 29)

Fludarabine	25 mg/m^2 i.v., days 1–3
Cyclophosphamide	200 mg/m^2 i.v., days 1–3
Mitoxantrone	8 mg/m^2 i.v., day 1

10. FCR Protocol (repeat on day 29/after recovery from toxicity)

Fludarabine	25 mg/m^2 i.v., days 2–4
Cyclophosphamide	250 mg/m^2 i.v., days 2–4
Rituximab	375 mg/m^2 i.v., day 1 (cycles 2+: dose of 500 mg/m^2)

11. Cladribine protocol (in hairy cell leukemia: repeat on day 29, if no complete remission)

Cladribine (2 CdA)	0.1 m/kg i.v., days 1–7

12. CVB protocol (protocol *for autologous transplantation*)

Cyclophosphamide	4.8–7.2 g/m^2 i.v., over 4 d
Etoposide	750–2,400 mg/m^2 i.v., over 4 d
Carmustine (BCNU)	300–600 mg/m^2 i.v., over 4 d
Stem cell infusion	Day 7 (at least 1×10^8 cells/kg for marrow or 2×10^6 CD34+ cells/kg for peripheral blood stem cells)

13. Total body irradiation with cyclophosphamide (protocol *for autologous transplantation*)

Total body irradiation: 12 Gy total dose (days 6–4)
Cyclophosphamide   60 mg/kg (day 3 to -2)
Stem cell infusion: day 0

also give a palliation for refractory lymphomas. Besides autologous stem cell transplantation (SCT), dose-intense therapy is a further way to improve the prognosis of patient with diffuse large-cell lymphoma. Patients with bulky lymphomas (lymph node diameter in excess of 5 or 10 cm) are generally excluded from the approach followed in localized disease and should be treated as for advanced stages.

The subtype of primary mediastinal B-cell lymphoma typically occurs in young adults who have a rapidly enlarging mediastinal mass. As with other B-cell lymphomas, the markers CD19 and CD20 are positive. Histologically, sclerosis and monocytoid lymphoid cells are typical. The recommended treatment at present is an aggressive chemotherapy consolidated by radiotherapy. The prognosis is relatively good.

Primary testicular lymphoma is a rare form of diffuse large B-cell lymphoma (1–2% of all NHL). Despite being initially localized, primary testicular lymphoma commonly relapses in extranodal sites (CNS, lung, pleural, soft tissues).

6. FOLLICULAR LYMPHOMA

The combined group of follicular lymphomas or follicle center lymphomas makes up the second most frequent type of NHL (approx 20–30% of all cases of NHLs). In many countries, an increased incidence of follicular lymphomas has been observed.

Pathologically, the follicular lymphomas have a characteristic picture that resembles normal germinal centers. Centrocytes are mixed with centroblasts and form a neoplastic germinal center. The growth pattern is usually follicular *(see* Fig. 15.2 and Color Plate 16), but may be diffuse in rare cases.

According to number of blasts per high power field, grade I (<5), II (5 to 15 blasts) and III (>15 blasts) may be differentiated. Recently, the latter type was further subclassified in grade IIIa (mixture of centrocytes and blasts) and IIIb (diffuse sheets of blasts). Clinically, grades I–II appear more indolent with a relapsing course whereas grade III lymphomas are more aggressive and should be treated according to the guidelines of diffuse large-cell lymphoma.

At the molecular level, about 90% of patients with follicular lymphomas have the t(14;18) (q32;q21) translocation. Translocation t(14;18) leads to an overexpression of the bcl-2 protein. The immunophenotype of follicular lymphomas (as determined on tissue sections or in cell suspensions) is CD19$^+$, CD20$^+$, CD10$^+$ in most cases, CD3$^-$, and CD5$^-$.

6.1. Clinical Symptoms

The clinical course of follicular lymphomas is indolent in most cases. The median age of patients with follicular lymphomas is around 50–60 yr. The dis-

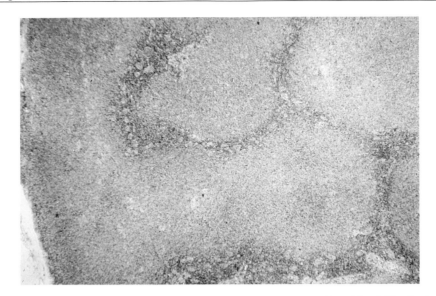

Fig. 15.2. Follicle center lymphoma. Lymph node structure replaced by follicular infiltrate, Giemsa stain, low-power magnification.

ease most often begins with peripheral lymphadenopathy, and the mediastinum is rarely enlarged. Less than one-fifth of the patients have B-symptoms. The bone marrow is involved in about half of the patients, typically showing nodular infiltration. The clinical symptoms are often subtle and caused by the enlarged lymph nodes; para-aortic lymph nodes or an enlarged spleen may cause abdominal fullness or other local symptoms. An extranodal manifestation is observed in about 10% of the patients (gastrointestinal tract, rarely in the skin).

6.2. Prognosis

Generally, newly diagnosed follicular lymphomas respond well to treatment (radiation or chemotherapy). In contrast to high-grade lymphomas, however, follicular lymphomas cannot be cured by the conventional treatment strategies available. A possible exception is the early stages of follicular lymphomas. Taking into account all stages, people with newly diagnosed follicular lymphomas can expect to live an average of 8–10 yr. Risk factors for an adverse prognosis are male sex, older age, systemic symptoms or reduced performance status, a large tumor mass, bone marrow infiltration, and among laboratory criteria, an increased LDH, or increased β_2-microglobulin. The relevance of the International Index established for high-grade lymphomas is limited in low-grade NHL. Recently, a more specific Follicular Lymphoma International Prognostic Index (FLIPI) has been proposed. FLIPI distinguishes three groups of patients according to the number of adverse prognostic factors. In the good prognostic group (0–1 adverse prognostic factors), a 10-yr survival of 70% can be expected. An intermediate group with two adverse prognostic factors has a 10-yr survival of 50%. A poor prognostic group (at least three adverse prognostic factors) has a 10-yr survival of only 35%. Despite the initially good prognosis, up to 40% of follicular lymphomas finally transform into high-grade NHL, which then require more aggressive treatment strategies such as chemotherapy. Gene expression profiling was studied in patients with follicular lymphoma. Interestingly, survival correlates could be established not with genes expressed in tumor cells but with genes expressed in infiltrating immune lymphocytes.

6.3. Treatment

At present, several therapeutic strategies can be considered for the follicular lymphomas: observation, radiation therapy, standard chemotherapy, and high-dose therapy with autologous transplantation.

6.3.1. OBSERVATION (WATCH-AND-WAIT STRATEGY)

Observation is indicated for asymptomatic patients with advanced disease (stage III–IV) who do not have B-symptoms or other complications caused by the lymphoma. Clinical examination, laboratory and ultrasound studies, and, if necessary, computed tomographies should be performed at regular intervals (e.g., quarterly) to estimate the disease activity and behavior. If there is rapidly progressive disease (e.g., B-symptoms, a major increase in the size of the lymph nodes, or if signs of bone marrow failure develop), chemotherapy should be started.

6.3.2. RADIOTHERAPY

Radiotherapy is indicated in stages I and II without bulk (usually as involved- or extended-field radiation with 30–40 Gy). This strategy can induce prolonged remissions and possibly cures especially in stage I whereas in stage II with high tumor load, the majority of patients will finally relapse. The rate of complete remissions is 90–95% after radiotherapy and the survival free from relapse is 60–70% after 5 yr. An initial treatment with combined modality (chemotherapy plus radiation) may induce longer remissions in patients with follicular lymphomas, but the total survival is comparable to that observed with radiotherapy alone. Thus, combined modality treatment cannot be considered as standard treatment in the early stages of follicular lymphomas.

6.3.3. SYSTEMIC CHEMOTHERAPY

Chemotherapy is indicated in all advanced stages if the disease causes symptoms or if the disease progresses after an observation period. Basically, a monotherapy with an alkylating agent (e.g., chlorambucil) is effective but, because of a slow response, is only appropriate for selected patients with contraindications to more aggressive options. Various combination treatments (e.g., CVP [cyclophosphamide, vincristine, and prednisone], CHOP) can achieve a faster (and usually longer) response (see Table 6). Four to six cycles of such protocol should be given and, after a satisfactory response, the patient should be observed again. In recent years, good responses to a treatment with fludarabine combinations (e.g., FCM [fludarabine, cyclophosphamide, mitoxantrone]) have been reported. For treatment of relapses, the same protocol as used initially can be repeated if the remission has lasted several years. If the relapse occurs earlier, a more intensive protocol (e.g., the CHOP or a related protocol) should be used. According to a recent meta-analysis a maintenance treatment with interferon (IFN)-α prolongs the relapse-free survival. However, side effects are more frequently observed.

Younger patients with follicular lymphomas have an unfavorable long-term prognosis, despite the initial good response. Therefore, these patients are candidates for novel treatment strategies, especially if risk factors like B-symptoms or large lymph node masses are present. Such an approach is myeloablative chemoconsolidation with subsequent autologous SCT and results in prolonged progression-free survival (>60% risk of relapse). However, consistent data on overall survival are still lacking, and late side effects (secondary malignancies) represent an inherent risk of this approach. Recent studies attempt to remove malignant cells with immunomagnetic purging or combine high-dose chemotherapy with in vivo purging.

6.3.4. ANTIBODIES/COMBINED IMMUNO-CHEMOTHERAPY

The monoclonal anti-CD20-antibody rituximab destroys lymphoma cells via complement- and antibody-mediated cellular cytotoxicity. Side effects of rituximab are mainly fever and a depletion of normal B-cells; however, no major myelotoxicity has been observed. In a phase II study, a response rate of 50% was observed in patients with relapsed follicular lymphomas, but progression-free survival was rather short (12–18 mo). In recent clinical trials, rituximab given in combination with conventional chemotherapy (R-CHOP, R-CVP, or R-FCM) resulted in a prolonged progression-free survival (up to a median of >7 yr) comparable to the effect of myeloablative consolidation. Currently, different antibody maintenance schedules are being evaluated.

Because of the curative approach with local radiation in early stages of disease, radioactively labeled antibodies represent another promising approach. Recent phase II studies indicate very favorable remission durations especially in patients who are in complete remission.

6.3.5. ALLOGENEIC TRANSPLANTATION

Allogeneic transplantation with either conventional myeloablative or reduced-intensity conditioning remains the only curative treatment approach in advanced stages, but has a substantial treatment-related morbidity and thus remains reserved for relapsed disease.

6.4. Novel Strategies

Molecular approaches (bcl-2 antisense, proteasome inhibitors) and vaccination strategies as well adoptive immunotherapy approaches are currently evaluated in clinical studies.

7. MANTLE CELL LYMPHOMA

7.1. Definition and Incidence

Mantle cell lymphoma accounts for about 5–8% of all cases of NHL and is characterized by an aggressive clinical course despite its apparently "non-blastic" morphological features. As with other forms of NHL, the incidence of mantle cell lymphomas increases with age, the median age being 60–70 yr. There is a striking predominance of males (70%). The mantle cell lymphomas have a specific cytogenetic marker, the t(11;14) translocation, which involves a rearrangement of the *bcl-1* gene with subsequent overexpression of cyclin-D1. Histopathologically, a monomorphic proliferation of small- to medium-sized cells is found mixed with follicular dendritic reticulum cells. The immunological phenotype of mantle cell lymphomas is CD3$^-$, CD5$^+$, CD10$^-$, CD20$^+$, CD23$^-$, and cyclin-D1$^+$.

7.2. Clinical Symptoms

The major symptom of mantle cell lymphomas is the enlargement of lymph nodes. About 80% of patients at diagnosis are already at an advanced stage (III or IV). About 30% of patients have B-symptoms. Almost two-thirds of the patients have an enlarged spleen. The bone marrow is involved in two thirds of the cases, and in some patients a leukemic dissemination can be found already at diagnosis. In about 10% of patients the gastrointestinal tract is involved; for example, as multiple gastrointestinal polyposis.

7.3. Prognosis

Compared with the follicular lymphomas, the mantle cell lymphomas have a rather unfavorable prognosis related to the relative resistance of the neoplastic cells to cytotoxic treatments. The average survival is about 3–4 yr. A high number of mitoses or a blastic transformation in the lymph node section and a leukemic dissemination are unfavorable prognostic signs.

7.4. Treatment

The optimal chemotherapy (CHOP, CVAD [hyper-cyclophosphamide, vincristine, Adriamycin®, and dexamethasone]) has not yet been well established. In recent studies, a combined immuno-chemotherapy (R-CHOP) achieved superior remission rates greater than 90%, but remission duration remained limited, thus effective consolidation strategies are urgently warranted. Myeloablative radiochemotherapy results in a significantly superior progression-free survival and a trend to prolonged overall survival in patients up to 65 yr. Although the majority of patients relapse even after such multi-modal approach, allogeneic transplantation still has to be considered as an experimental approach and remains reserved for relapsed disease. Molecular approaches (especially proteasome inhibitors and rapamycine derivatives) show promising results in current phase I/II studies and may become a part of future treatment strategies. In rare cases with localized disease I/II and low tumor burden, external radiation may achieve long-lasting remissions.

8. CHRONIC LYMPHOCYTIC LEUKEMIA

CLL is typically a leukemia of elderly people and accounts for about 20% of all NHLs. In Western countries, CLL is the most frequent type of leukemia, whereas in Asia, the typical CLL is much rarer. CLL has a clear male predominance and characterized by the monoclonal accumulation of small, mature-appearing lymphoid cells. The morphology of CLL cells is depicted in Fig. 15.3 *(see also Color Plate 17)*. The typical immunophenotype is CD3$^-$, CD5$^+$, CD10$^-$, CD19$^+$, CD20$^+$, and CD23$^+$ (in contrast to mantle cell lymphoma). As in other malignant lymphomas, surface immunoglobulins are light-chain restricted (generally with a weak expressed). The typical CLL belongs to the entity of peripheral B-cell neoplasms, whereas about 5% of all CLLs have a T-cell phenotype. With a sensitive cytogenetic analysis, most cases of CLL have chromosome aberrations. Frequent markers are trisomy 12, aberrations of chromosome 13q, as well as the deletions of chromosomes 11q and 17p (location of the p53 tumor suppressor gene *p53*). Both latter alterations usually predict clinical unresponsiveness. Another important risk factor is the immunoglobulin mutation status, which may be substituted by the fluorescence-activated cell sorting analysis of the closely associated expression of the adhesion molecule zeta chain-associated protein (ZAP)-70. Expression of ZAP-70, as well as unmutated status of the immunoglobulin heavy chain genes confers a poorer prognosis.

8.1. Clinical Features

Most patients present with enlarged lymph nodes. In early stages, the patients are asymptomatic and have a leukocytosis as the only sign of disease. In later stages, anemia, splenomegaly, and hepatomegaly develop. Some patients also have bruising due to thrombocytopenia, and frequent infections due to neutrope-

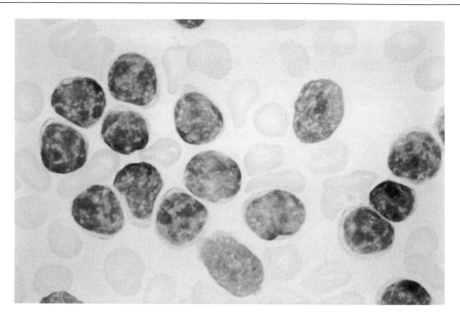

Fig. 15.3. Chronic lymphocytic leukemia. Small, mature-appearing lymphoid cells with a thin cytoplasmic rim.

nia and hypogammaglobulinemia. Some patients develop erythroderma (skin infiltration with CLL cells). Two common classification schemes of CLL based on clinical and laboratory features are shown in Table 7.

8.2. Laboratory Features

A lymphocytosis that may be as low as 5000 or higher than 200,000/µL is constantly found in CLL. In advanced stages, anemia and/or thrombocytopenia are present. The anemia may also be due to autoimmune hemolysis. Bone marrow aspiration shows infiltration of the bone marrow with CLL cells (at least 25% of the aspirate, but in many cases as high as 90%). Bone marrow biopsy shows a nodular, diffuse, or mixed infiltration. The bone marrow trephine biopsy may not be necessary in all cases of CLL, as a nodular infiltration has been not confirmed as independent prognostic factor. In many, and especially in advanced, cases, the serum immunoglobulins are decreased (hypogammaglobulinemia). A monoclonal para-protein is rarely present in CLL. About 5% of patients terminally transform into an aggressive NHL (Richter syndrome).

Lymphocytic lymphomas resemble B-CLL cytomorphologically, but there is no leukemic dissemination or infiltration of the bone marrow. Lymphocytic lymphomas are rare (<2% of all NHL). The treatment is oriented at the principles outlined for other indolent lymphomas.

Table 7
Chronic Lymphocytic Leukemias Classification Schemes

	Rai classification		Binet classification
Stage 0	Lymphocytosis 5000–15000/µL	Stage A	0, 1, or 2 lymphatic areas enlarged
Stage I	Lymphocytosis + lymphadenopathy	Stage B	3, 4, or 5 areas enlarged
Stage II	As 0 + hepato- and/or splenomegaly		Hb >10 g/dL, Platelets > 100000/µL
Stage III	As 0 + anemia (Hb <11 g/dL)	Stage C	Any lymphatic involvement
Stage IV	As 0 + thrombocytopenia (platelets <100000/µL)		Hb <10, and/or platelets <100,000

8.3. Prognosis

The prognosis of B-CLL depends on clinical and molecular laboratory features. In early stages, the survival is more than 12 yr (Binet A); some patients with early CLL (about one third of patients in Binet stage A) do not progress for many years and do not have a reduced life expectancy (smoldering CLL). In contrast, in advanced stages (Binet C, Rai IV) the median survival is less than 2 yr. Mutations of *p53,* deletions of chromosome 11q, and a lymphocyte doubling time of less than 12 mo have a negative impact on prognosis. More recently, it was found that overexpression of the Syk tyrosine kinase ZAP-70 (important in T cell development) confers a poor prognosis in B-CLL.

8.4. Treatment

The conventional treatment of CLL aims at the palliation of symptoms, not at a cure. In the early stages (Rai 0–II or Binet A or B) the disease may be stable for several years; therefore, no treatment is indicated. If the disease progresses rapidly, if B-symptoms develop, or if the disease leads to complications such as frequent infections or an autoimmune hemolytic anemia, treatment with alkylating agents or fludarabine is indicated in later stages. A symptomatic autoimmune hemolytic anemia needs an emergency treatment (high-dose steroids, 1–2 mg/kg prednisone or cyclophosphamide, or both).

Supportive therapy plays a major role in the management of patients with CLL. Infections need prompt treatment. Patients with hypogammaglobulinemia and frequent infections may benefit from prophylactic antibiotics or the administration of polyvalent immunoglobulins in case of life-threatening infections.

8.4.1. Single-Agent Chemotherapy

Chlorambucil is still a commonly used alkylating agent for the first-line treatment of CLL. It can be given as a pulse treatment (18 mg/m^2 on day 1, repeat after 2 or 3 wk, increase dose if no major toxicity is seen) or as a continuous treatment (0.1–0.2 mg/kg for 14 d, then repeat on day 28). The treatment should be continued for 6–12 mo until a maximum response is seen or until the disease is progressive.

8.4.2. Fludarabine

The purine analog fludarabine is the most active single-agent drug in the treatment of CLL. In the second-line treatment, 30–70% of patients obtain partial and complete remissions. Fludarabine is given at the dose of 25 mg/m^2 i.v. for 5 d; this is repeated after 28 d. A side effect of the treatment with fludarabine is a long-lasting immunosuppression and an increase in the incidence of opportunistic infections. Fludarabine must be discontinued if an autoimmune hemolytic anemia develops. Cladribine (another purine analogue) is also active in CLL (about 80% responses in previously untreated patients). Based on the superior remission rates and progression-free survival, purine analogs represent the preferred first-line treatment in younger patients.

8.4.3. Combined Immuno-Chemotherapy

Multi-agent chemotherapy is indicated for patients whose disease progresses after the first- and second-line treatment, or who present with a very aggressive form. For these patients, protocols such as COP (cyclophosphamide, Oncovin, and prednisone), CHOP, or combinations with fludarabine are currently in use. Similarly, first studies suggest a superiority of fludarabine combinations (FC) in comparison to fludarabine alone.

Recently, monoclonal antibodies directed against B- or T-cell antigens (rituximab, alemtuzumab) have been introduced. Rituximab monotherapy has only limited effect as a result of, the low CD20 expression on CLL cells whereas the combination of fludarabine, cyclophosphamide, and rituximab (FCR) has shown considerable activity in relapsed and refractory CLL. FCR is currently tested in newly diagnosed CLL. Especially in refractory cases (frequently associated with p53 deletions), anti-CD52 antibody alemtuzumab (Campath®) shows high efficacy either as consolidation or in combination with chemotherapy (FluCam) but is hampered by its serious immunosuppressive effect on B- and T-cells.

8.4.4. Experimental Strategies

Younger patients with an aggressive clinical course may benefit from an autologous SCT. Patients less than 50 yr of age who have a human leukocyte antigen-identical donor may also be candidates for an allogeneic SCT or bone

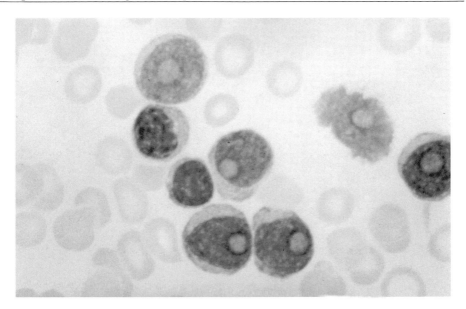

Fig. 15.4. Prolymphocytic leukemia. Large lymphoid cells with a large nucleus and a prominent nucleolus.

marrow transplantation, but such treatments should be performed within controlled clinical trials

For selected patients, splenic irradiation or splenectomy may be indicated (large spleen with hypersplenism).

8.5. Special Forms of CLL

8.5.1. PROLYMPHOCYTIC LEUKEMIA

In prolymphocytic leukemia (PLL), the leukemic cells are larger than in classical CLL, appear to be immature, and have a prominent nucleolus (see Fig. 15.4 and Color Plate 18). Most cases of PLL have a B-phenotype (strong expression of surface immunoglobulin and negative for CD5), but some cases are derived from T-cells. In T-cell prolymphocytic leukemia, alterations of chromosome 11 and the *ATM* gene are frequent. Patients generally present with a huge spleen and a high leukocyte count and do not respond well to the usual treatment for CLL. The median survival of patients with PLL is shorter than for CLL (2–3 yr). For this reason, an intensive chemotherapy (with CHOP-type regimens), or a treatment with purine analogues or monoclonal antibodies should be considered early.

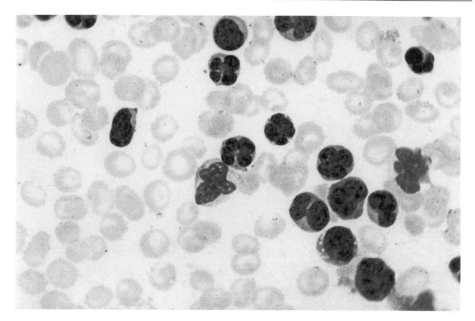

Fig, 15.5. Neoplastic cells of a patient with adult T-cell leukemia/lymphoma (small- to medium-sized lymphoid cells with a highly irregular nucleus, "flower cells").

8.5.2. Smoldering CLL

Some patients with early CLL (about one-third of patients in Binet stage A) do not progress for many years and do not have a reduced life expectancy (smoldering CLL). By definition, the lymphocyte doubling time is longer than 12 mo in such cases.

8.5.3. T-Chronic Lymphocytic Leukemia

A T-cell phenotype is rare in CLL (about 3% of all cases). These patients are younger, often have cutaneous involvement, and respond poorly to therapy. Although these cases are usually derived from CD3$^+$, CD4$^-$, and CD8$^-$ T-cells, an indolent (CD8$^+$) variant is probably derived from immature NK cells.

Some T-cell leukemias and lymphomas are associated with the retrovirus HTLV-1. Figure 15.5 (Color Plate 19; *see also* "Etiology of NHLs") depicts the neoplastic cells of a patient with a HTLV-1-associated lymphoma.

9. LYMPHOPLASMACYTOID/-IC LYMPHOMA/ IMMUNOCYTOMA (INCLUDING WALDENSTRÖM'S DISEASE)

The lymphoplasmacytoid lymphoma or immunocytoma has been grouped as CLL variant in the WHO classification. Lymphplasmocytic immunocytomas also include Waldenström's disease with an immunoglobulin (Ig)M paraprotein and a typical bone marrow morphology.

The clinical signs and symptoms of immunocytomas are comparable to those of other low-grade NHLs. About 80–90% of patients have advanced disease at diagnosis. A special form of immunocytomas involves the eye or the skin; occasionally, an enlarged spleen is the main manifestation of an immunocytoma.

Immunocytoma cells bear the B-lymphoid antigens CD19, CD20, and CD22. In contrast to the typical B-CLL, immunocytoma cells are negative for CD5 and CD23.

The prognosis of immunocytomas is somewhat inferior to that of classical CLL depending on the patient risk profile. The median survival in Waldenström's disease is about 5 yr. As far as the treatment is concerned, radiation is only indicated in the rare localized forms. If immunocytomas are disseminated or leukemic, the treatment is oriented at the principles outlined for CLL or follicular lymphomas.

Waldenström's macroglobulinemia is a special form of immunocytoma with particular features. The bone marrow is involved in virtually all cases, showing a dense infiltrate with small basophilic lymphoid cells and plasma cells. The patients are frequently anemic as a result of bone marrow infiltration. The spleen or lymph nodes are enlarged in about 20–40% of cases. A common feature is an increased number of mast cells. The presence of a typical IgM paraprotein (>30 g/L) can lead to a hyperviscosity syndrome with vertigo, visual disturbances, and mucous membrane bleeding. Further complications are hemolytic anemia with cold agglutinins, peripheral neuropathy, amyloidosis, and renal failure.

If urgent treatment is indicated, a hyperviscosity syndrome can be ameliorated rapidly by plasmapheresis. In general, the treatment indications for Waldenström's macroglobulinemia are similar to those in CLL. Patients who are treated with chlorambucil respond in 50–70% of the cases with a reduction of the paraprotein and the lymphadenopathy. However, fludarabine and other purine analogues represent the preferred treatment option with up to 80% response rate. Whereas only an extended schedule of antibody monotherapy (eight cycles) has some effect, a recent randomized study confirmed the superiority of a combined immuno-chemotherapy. Recent data show a considerable role for autologous SCT in relapsed Waldenström's disease.

10. BURKITT'S LYMPHOMAS, BURKITT-LIKE LYMPHOMAS, AND LYMPHOBLASTIC LYMPHOMAS

In Africa, Burkitt's lymphoma is a disease of children; in Europe and North America, Burkitt-like lymphomas typically occur in young adults. The disease often has an extranodal and abdominal manifestation. Lymphomas of the jaws, kidneys, and retroperitoneum are typical for the African variety (endemic Burkitt's lymphoma).

Histopathologically, a monomorphic infiltration of medium-sized cells with round nuclei containing multiple basophilic nucleoli is typically found. The cytoplasm is deeply basophilic. A starry sky pattern in Burkitt's lymphoma reflects macrophages that have ingested apoptoptic lymphoma cells. The primary genetic abnormality in Burkitt's lymphoma is the translocation t(8;14) or variations thereof, with rearrangements of the *Myc* oncogene. The immunophenotype of Burkitt's lymphomas indicates expression of CD19, CD20, CD22, CD79a, CD10, and CD43 and absence of surface IgM, CD5, CD23, and Bcl-2.

Burkitt's lymphoma is aggressive and urgently requires treatment. Using intensive protocols that include high-dose cyclophosphamide and a prophylaxis for CNS involvement, about 30–50% of patients (especially children) can expect cure. Examples for dose-intense protocols used in Burkitt's lymphomas are the Hyper-CVAD and the CODOX-M (cyclophosphamide, Oncovin, doxorubicin, high-dose methotrexate)/IVAC (ifosfamide, etoposide, and high-dose cytarabine) protocols.

Lymphoblastic lymphomas are rare in adults, but somewhat more frequent in children and adolescents. The WHO classification distinguishes B- and T-precursor lymphoblastic lymphomas. T-lymphoblastic lymphomas often present with a mediastinal mass. If the bone marrow is involved in lymphoblastic lymphoma and more than 25% of lymphoma cells are found, the disease is classified by definition as acute lymphoblastic leukemia (ALL). Most cases of lymphoblastic lymphomas are treated with protocols developed for ALL (including a prophylaxis for CNS involvement).

11. MYCOSIS FUNGOIDES (CUTANEOUS T-CELL LYMPHOMA) AND SÉZARY SYNDROME

Mycosis fungoides is a clonal proliferation of neoplastic helper (CD4$^+$) lymphocytes that manifests in the skin. Mycosis fungoides, or cutaneous T-cell lymphoma, often has a protracted course over many years. The WHO classification includes mycosis fungoides in the group of mature (peripheral) T-cell neoplasms. The tumor cells are atypical lymphocytes with hyperconvoluted cerebriform nuclei. Mycosis fungoides has three clinical stages: premycotic and patch stage, infiltrative and plaque stage, and the tumor stage.

Other staging systems are used for clinical studies, and include the presence or absence of lymph node and visceral manifestations (bone marrow or other organs). The median survival of patients with cutaneous T-cell lymphomas varies between 2 and 15 yr depending on the stage of the disease. In Sézary syndrome, a leukemic dissemination of the neoplastic cells has occurred (about 5% of all patients with mycosis fungoides present with Sézary syndrome) and the patients have a generalized erythroderma.

The treatment of mycosis fungoides is mainly supportive and aims at palliation. Skin care and the treatment of infections are important during all stages.

In the plaque stage, topical alkylating agents (nitrogen mustard or carmustin) are effective in 60–80% of cases. An alternative treatment is photosensitizer with UVA irradiation (PUVA) photochemotherapy. For this treatment, oral methoxypsoralen is combined with UVA irradiation. Remissions last for approx 11–13 mo. PUVA can also be given as an extracorporeal photophoresis, which is especially effective in Sézary syndrome. Retinoids and IFN also have some efficacy in mycosis fungoides. In the tumor stage, an external irradiation with electron beams (30–36 Gy over 8–10 wk) is indicated and controls the disease for several months. A systemic chemotherapy (analogous to high-grade NHL), in some cases also steroids, fludarabine, and other agents such as 2-chloro-deoxyadenosine are also effective for disease control or palliation in the tumor stage and with visceral manifestations. Rarely, cutaneous lymphomas are derived from B-cells, which often have an indolent clinical behavior.

12. SPECIAL FORMS OF NHL

12.1. Hairy Cell Leukemia

HCL is an uncommon B-cell lymphoproliferative disorder that was originally referred to as "leukemic reticuloendotheliosis." Because of the presence of prominent and characteristic thin cytoplasmic projections, its name was changed to hairy cell leukemia several decades ago. It is currently thought of as a low-grade or indolent NHL. If counted among the leukemias, HCL makes up about 2–4% of all leukemias. It is mainly a disease of men, with a male to female ratio of about four to one. The median age of onset is in the mid 50s, with a range of 40–70 yr. The pathogenesis of HCL is not known.

The malignant cells of HCL are B-lymphocytes, which have the previously mentioned fine cytoplasmic projections (see Fig. 15.6 and Color Plate 20). These cells express features that are consistent with late stages of B-cell development. They are often characterized by:

- Tartrate-resistant acid phosphatase (TRAP) positivity.
- The expression of B-cell surface antigen markers (CD19, CD20, CD22) and an early plasma cell marker (PCA-1).
- The expression of surface antigen markers that are not routinely identified on B-cells such as CD11c, CD103, and CD25. The presence of CD103, in the presence of other pan-B-cell markers, is highly suggestive of HCL.

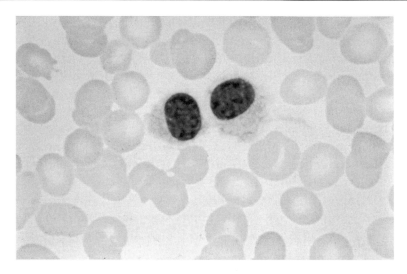

Fig. 15.6. Hairy cell leukemia. Peripheral blood smear with two hairy cells (lymphoid cells with cytoplasmic protrusions).

- No consistent or specific chromosomal mutations (although a partial loss of 7q as well as other abnormalities have been reported).
- The expression of clonal immunoglobulin light- and heavy-chain gene rearrangement as well as monoclonal surface immunoglobulins.
- The production of cytokines like tumor necrosis factor (TNF)-α, fibroblast growth factors (bFGF, FGF-2) and interleukin (IL)-1. In untreated patients, increased serum levels of soluble IL-2 receptors are found. Some of these cytokines may be etiological in the marrow inhibition and fibrosis sometimes seen in HCL.

Clinically, the spleen is enlarged in most patients and is responsible for the presenting symptom of abdominal fullness or discomfort in many. Others may present with constitutional symptoms such as fatigue, malaise, and weight loss. Night sweats are not common, although some will present with fevers due to frequent infections. These infections may be life-threatening as a result of disease-related neutropenia and monocytopenia. Similarly, some patients will present with excessive bleeding and bruising due to disease-related thrombocytopenia. Enlarged lymph nodes and other clinical manifestations are rather infrequent, and approx 25% of patients will be asymptomatic at the time of diagnosis. The diagnosis of HCL in these patients is frequently made during the evaluation of incidentally noted splenomegaly or mild cytopenias.

The typical blood picture most commonly reveals pancytopenia. The majority of patients will present with anemia, neutropenia, monocytopenia, and thrombocytopenia. Despite being called a "leukemia," only about 20% of patients will present with a leukocytosis greater than 10,000/μL.

Most patients have a "dry tap" when the bone marrow is aspirated. Staining of the marrow core for reticulin frequently reveals a moderate to marked increase in reticulin fibrosis. The peripheral blood should be analyzed by flow cytometry and the blood and bone marrow subjected to TRAP staining. Histological investigation of the bone marrow shows a dense infiltration of the bone marrow with hairy cells in virtually all patients and some degree of fibrosis is also typically found. In addition, many patients also have circulating hairy cells. In about 20% of the patients, a frank leukemic blood picture develops. Rarely however is there an extreme leukocytosis.

12.1.1. TREATMENT

Treatment of the patient with HCL is most often indicated in the setting of symptomatic splenomegaly and/or worsening cytopenias. Recurrent infections or leukocytosis (>20,000/μL) are often indications for treatment as well. Some patients with HCL are asymptomatic and can be observed for months or even years without treatment. Once a decision to treat has been made, the patient with symptomatic HCL may have several options. These include purine analog-based chemotherapy, IFN, and splenectomy.

Prior to the early 1980s, splenectomy was the treatment of choice for symptomatic patients. It did relieve symptoms that were directly related to splenomegaly and often resulted in improvement of the cytopenias. It did not affect the underlying disease, however, and is now reserved for the rare patient who has disease that is refractory to pharmacological therapy.

IFN-α has also been very effective in HCL. There is an overall response rate of approx 80%, but complete responses are rare. The majority of patients achieve only partial remissions (defined as normalization of all peripheral blood counts.) Even if IFN does not induce a complete remission, the number of hairy cells in the blood and bone marrow are reduced and the cytopenias are improved. IFN-α is generally given at a dosage of $2-3 \times 10^6$ units three times a week subcutaneously. In order to achieve a maximal response, IFN-α must be given for 12 to 18 mo. The side effects of IFN-α are described elsewhere in this volume.

The therapeutic arsenal has much improved since the introduction of the purine analogs 2-deoxycoformycin (DCF, pentostatin) and 2-chloro-deoxy-adenosine (2-CDA, cladribine). Both drugs induce long-term remission in HCL. After one cycle of 2-CDA, 85% of patients reach a complete remission, which increases to 95% after two treatment cycles. These remissions last for many years. Acute side effects of 2-CDA are fever, a transient bone marrow suppression, fatigue, headache, and some nausea (*see* Table 5 for dose of cladribine). Pentostatin is also very effective in the treatment of HCL (rate of 80–90% complete remissions), but more patients suffer relapses. Pentostatin is also given as monotherapy. Generally three to five cycles are needed to reach a complete response, that is, the disappearance of all hairy cells from blood and bone marrow. The acute side effects of pentostatin are comparable with those of cladribine. Both drugs also induce a long-lasting depression of cellular immunity. In patients with relapsed or refractory HCL, interesting clinical activity was found for the monoclonal antibody rituximab and the immunotoxin BL-22 (a CD22 antibody fused to pseudomonas exotoxin).

12.2. Gastric and MALT Lymphomas

Lymphoma deriving from the MALT was first described as a distinct pathological entity in 1983. Under the current WHO classification, it is classified as extranodal marginal zone lymphoma MALT type, and comprises 8% of all NHL. MALT lymphoma has characteristic features such as homing in epithelial tissue, lymphoepithelial destruction, and an indolent clinical course. They arise in epithelial tissues normally devoid of lymphatic cells, where the lymphatic tissue was acquired after, for instance, a chronic infection. The best example here is the association of gastric MALT lymphoma and the infection of the stomach with *H. pylori*. Gastric MALT lymphoma also exemplifies the translation of biological knowledge of a disease towards improved clinical practice. Rarely, MALT lymphomas arise in tissues other than the stomach (salivary glands, where they are associated with Sjogren's syndrome or lungs). MALT lymphomas of the ileum are also rare and have a less favorable prognosis.

12.2.1. ASSOCIATION WITH *H. PYLORI* AND PATHOGENESIS

Multiple lines of evidence indicate a causative role of *H. pylori* infection in the gastric MALT lymphoma. MALT of the stomach is always a sequela of *H. pylori* infection. Acquired MALT is the precondition for the potential development of a MALT lymphoma. Prior *H. pylori* infection is therefore a pre-MALT lymphoma condition. In more than 90% of cases, MALT lymphoma is associated with *H. pylori* infection. In animal experiments MALT lymphomas can be induced by *H. pylori* infection. *H. pylori* eradication alone can lead to complete remission of the MALT lymphoma. Besides the classical association with gastric MALT lymphomas, there have been reports in which an association between *H. pylori* and DLBCL has been observed as well. Consequently, cure of *H. pylori* infection resulted in remission induction not only in gastric MALT lymphomas, but also in some patients with limited stages of DLBCL of the stomach.

In addition to the association with *H. pylori*, progress has been made with regard to MALT lymphoma biology. Three translocations, t(11;18)(q21;q21), t(1;14)(p22;q32), and t(14;18)(q32;q21) are specifically associated with MALT lymphoma and the genes involved have been identified. t(11;18) results in a chimeric fusion between the *API2* and *MALT1* genes and is specifically associated with gastric MALT lymphomas that do not respond to eradication of *H. pylori*. t(1;14) and t(14;18) deregulate *BCL10* and *MALT1* expression, respectively. These seemingly irrelevant chromosomal translocations share common oncogenic properties by targeting the same NF-κB oncogenic pathway. These genetic events seem specific in that they have been observed only in MALT lymphomas. Once present, at least the more frequently observed translocation t(11;18) renders cells resistant to cure of *H. pylori* infection. The result is *H. pylori*-independent growth and a unique clinical picture characterized by a more advanced presentation and unresponsiveness to *H. pylori* eradication therapy. Although more likely to require cytotoxic therapy, this subtype is paradoxically less likely to undergo large-cell transformation.

12.2.2. CLINICAL FEATURES AND STAGING

The median age of the presentation is 63 yr, with a similar proportion of male and female patients. The majority of patients have insidious onset of disease and a very indolent course. The most common presenting symptoms are nonspecific dyspepsia and epigastric discomfort. Classical B-symptoms are extremely rare. The most common gastric location is the antrum, although multi-focal disease is seen in approximately one-third of cases. At endoscopy, erythema, erosions, or ulcerations are commonly seen whereas masses are rare. MALT lymphomas have characteristic histopathological features. Reactive B-cell follicles surrounded by tumor cells (centrocyte-like cells) are found. The centrocyte-like cells are small- to medium-sized lymphoid cells with an irregular nuclear shape, which selectively penetrate epithelial structures and form lymphoepithelial lesions. The immunophenotyping is that of typical marginal zone B-cells with CD20$^+$, CD21$^+$, CD5$^-$, CD10$^-$, IgM$^+$, IgD$^-$, and cyclin D$^-$. In light of their significance in biology and clinical characteristics, the chromosome translocations, especially t(11;18) should be searched for, and can be done by either fluorescent *in situ* hybridization or reverse-transcription polymerase chain reaction. For staging, either the Ann Arbor system or the Lugano system for gastrointestinal lymphoma (Table 8) can be used.

12.2.3. TREATMENT

Optimal treatment for gastric MALT lymphoma depends upon *H. pylori* status, disease stage, the presence of translocation like t(11;18), and evidence of large cell transformation. *H. pylori* eradication therapy is a worthy goal in all cases, and is probably the only therapy required in a majority (75–80%). A common protocol for the eradication of *H. pylori* is the combination of omeprazole (20 mg twice a day [bid]), clarithromycin (500 mg bid), and amoxicillin (1 g bid) for 10–14 d. For patients who are allergic to penicillin,

Table 8
Lugano Staging of Gastrointestinal Lymphomas

Stage I	Tumor confined to the gastrointestinal tract
Stage II	Tumor extending into the abdomen from the primary site
	II$_1$: Local node involvement (perigastric or perimesenteric)
	II2: Para-aortic or paracaval node involvement
	IIE: Penetration of serosa to involve adjacent organs or tissue
Stage IV	Disseminated disease or supradiaphragmatic lymph node involvement

No stage III defined.

metronidazole (500 mg bid) can be used instead of amoxicillin. Eradication can be achieved in 85% of patients with both regimens. If the lymphoma does not regress after the eradication of *H. pylori,* a local irradiation (of 30 Gy) can lead to prolonged remissions. Patients with advanced stages of disease should be treated like other indolent lymphoma. Options include watchful waiting, chemotherapy, and antibody-based (e.g., rituximab) approaches. The discovery that these cases have constitutive activation of NF-κB suggests a role of novel targeted therapy such as proteasome inhibition.

12.3. Angioimmunoblastic T-Cell Lymphoma

The angioimmunoblastic lymphoma (previously angioimmunoblastic lymphadenopathy) is a rare clonal proliferation of T-cells. Patients present with enlarged lymph nodes, fever, a rash, and an enlarged spleen. The disease is almost always disseminated and shows multiple biochemical abnormalities. There is no standard treatment, but most patients respond well to steroids and alkylating agents. Remissions are usually incomplete and of short duration. High-dose chemotherapy with SCT should be considered as a therapeutic option.

12.4. Anaplastic Large-Cell Lymphoma

About 2–8% of all NHL fit into the category of anaplastic large-cell lymphomas (ALCL). ALCL are characterized by a proliferation of pleomorphic large lymphoid cells that are strongly CD30$^+$ and typically spread into the lymphoid sinuses. Previously, ALCL were diagnosed as malignant histiocytoses or other entities. Clinically, patients with ALCL are younger than patients with other forms of NHL, frequently male and often present with B-symptoms. ALCL have a cytogenetic marker, t(2;5), which is rarely found in other lymphomas. The molecular product of t(2;5) is the fusion gene *NPM-ALK,* which has transforming properties in vitro. Most cases of ALCL have a CD8-positive phenotype, some express no distinct markers (null phenotype). In the WHO classification, ALCL belong to the mature (peripheral) T-cell neoplasms. Of all patients with high-grade lymphomas, those with ALCL generally respond best to treatment, 70% achieving a 5-yr survival.

12.5. Lymphomas in Children

The clinical presentation of NHL in children is aggressive, and in 90% of the cases they have a high-grade histology (large cell, lymphoblastic, Burkitt type). Despite these unfavorable features, children with NHL respond well if treatment is started without delay. At present, 70% of children with NHL can expect cure. The treatment protocols for pediatric NHL are tailored to the type of lymphoma and the individual risk situation. In children with large abdominal masses, the risk of a tumor lysis syndrome has to be considered. In pediatric Burkitt's lymphomas risk-adapted treatments are given, which incorporate high-dose methotrexate and high-dose cytosine arabinoside in addition to vincristine, doxorubicine, prednisone, and cyclophosphamide.

12.6. Lymphomas in HIV-Infected Individuals

NHLs are an AIDS-defining illness in HIV-infected individuals. Of all patients with AIDS, 3–8% have NHL as the first manifestation of their disease. The incidence of AIDS-related lymphomas has recently decreased since the introduction of high-active antiretroviral therapy. These lymphomas most often have an aggressive presentation, intermediate- to high-grade histology and frequently have an extranodal spread (e.g., gastrointestinal tract, CNS). The prognosis of AIDS-associated NHL (mostly B-cell NHLs) is unfavorable but has recently improved (see also Chapter 17, Table 5). Cerebral lymphomas generally arise in the context of advanced immunosuppression with low CD4 counts. All patients with AIDS-related lymphomas, especially if they have CD counts less than 200/µL and B-symptoms, should be investigated for opportunistic infections like cytomegalovirus, toxoplasmosis, and cryptococcosis. EBV is integrated into the genome of lymphoma cells of HIV-infected individuals in about half of the cases of AIDS-related lymphomas. In AIDS-related CNS lymphomas, EBV is found in approx 100% of cases. Patients with a good performance status should be treated with full-dose CHOP-type chemotherapy. Most studies show that antiretroviral therapy can safely be combined with chemotherapy and actually restores the immune competence. The addition of the monoclonal antibody rituximab to chemotherapy has not improved the response to chemotherapy and may even worsen the prognosis of AIDS-related lymphomas. In advanced cases or an extranodal presentation of AIDS-related lymphomas, a CNS prophylaxis is indicated. In selected cases of relapsed AIDS-related lymphomas, autologous SCT was performed successfully.

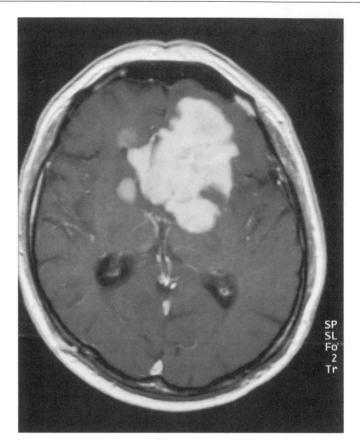

Fig. 15.7. High-grade brain lymphoma (magnetic resonance image with contrast enhancement).

12.7. Cerebral Lymphomas

Most primary cerebral lymphomas are of high-grade histology. The symptoms relate to the location and are comparable with those of a brain tumor. CNS lymphomas have increased in incidence and currently represent 4% of all CNS malignancies. Disturbances of motor and sensory function, intellectual alterations, and other symptoms are found. The diagnosis of cerebral lymphoma can be suspected if computed tomography and nuclear magnetic resonance imaging shows typical findings (see Fig. 15.7). If a meningeal dissemination has occurred, lymphoma cells and an increased protein content are found in the cerebrospinal fluid. If a primary CNS lymphoma is suspected, a histological diagnosis should be obtained by stereotactic (or open) biopsy. Classically, primary cerebral lymphomas were treated with corticosteroids and irradiation with 40 Gy.

This treatment induced remissions for 12–18 mo and less than 5% of patients survived more than 5 yr. More recently, multi-modal concepts were introduced for CNS lymphomas (e.g., intrathecal chemotherapy, irradiation, and systemic chemotherapy including high-dose methotrexate). In a study published by de Angelis and colleagues, five cycles of systemic methotrexate were combined with vincristine and procarbazine. Most patients subsequently received whole-brain radiotherapy and high-dose cytarabine. Of all patients, 94% responded and approx 50% reached a complete remission. In the entire group, the median survival was 3 yr. The major adverse side effect was neurotoxicity (due to the whole-brain radiation).

12.8. Splenic Marginal Zone Lymphoma

This rare entity is the most indolent of the low-grade lymphomas. A large spleen may or may not be associated with villous lymphocytes in the peripheral blood. Following splenectomy, prolonged remissions have been observed. Alternatively, fludarabine and/or antibody may be administered.

SUGGESTED READING

Alizadeh AA, Eisen MB, Davis RE, et al. Distinct types of diffuse large B-cell lymphoma identified by gene expression profiling. *Nature* 2000;403:503–511.

Ardeshna KM, Smith P, Norton A, et al. Long-term effect of a watch and wait policy versus immediate systemic treatment for asymptomatic advanced-stage non-Hodgkin lymphoma: a randomised controlled trial. *Lancet* 2003;362(9383):516–522.

Armitage JO, Weisenburger DD. New approach to classifying non-Hodgkin's lymphomas: clinical features of the major histologic subtypes. *J Clin Oncol* 1998;16:2780–2795.

Canellos GP, Lister TA, Young B, eds. *The Lymphomas*, Second Edition. Philadelphia: W.B. Saunders, 2006.

Cartron G, Watier H, Golay J, et al. From the bench to the bedside: ways to improve rituximab efficacy. *Blood* 2004;104:2635–2642.

Chiu BC, Weissenburger DD. An update of the epidemiology of non-Hodgkin's lymphoma. *Clin Lymphoma* 2003;4:161–168.

Dreyling M, Lenz G, Hoster E, et al. Early consolidation by myeloablative radiochemotherapy followed by autologous stem cell transplantation in first remission significantly prolongs progression-free survival in mantle cell lymphoma - results of a prospective randomized trial of the European MCL Network. *Blood* 2005;105:2677–2684.

Fisher RI. Treatment of advanced stage diffuse large B cell lymphoma. In: *Hematology 2004: American Society of Hematology Education Program Book*. Washington, DC: American Society of Hematology, 2004:pp. 223–225.

Hans CP, Weisenburger DD, Greiner TC, et al. Confirmation of the molecular classification of diffuse large B-cell lymphoma by immunohistochemistry using a tissue microarray. *Blood* 2004;103:275–282.

Isaacson PG. Update on MALT lymphomas. *Best Pract Res Clin Haematol* 2005;18:57–68.

Jaffe ES. Common threads of MALT lymphoma pathogenesis: from infection to translocation. *J Nat Cancer Inst* 2004;96:571–573.

Jaffe ES, Harris NL, Stein H, Vardiman J. *World Health Organisation Classification of Tumours: Tumours of the Haemopoietic and Lymphoid Tissues.* Lyon, France: IARC Press, 2001.

Kahl BS. Update: gastric MALT lymphoma. *Curr Opinion Oncol* 2003;15:347–352.

Lenz G, Dreyling M, Schiegnitz E, et al.: Myeloablative radiochemotherapy followed by autologous stem cell transplantation in first remission prolongs progression-free survival in follicular lymphoma: results of a prospective, randomized trial of the German Low-Grade Lymphoma Study Group. *Blood* 2004,104:2667–2674.

Lorincz AL. Cutaneous T-cell lymphoma (mycosis fungoides) *Lancet* 1996;347:871–876.

Lyons SF, Liebowitz DN. The role of human viruses in the pathogenesis of lymphoma. *Semin Oncol* 1998;25:461–475.

Rohatiner AZ, Gregory WM, Peterson B, et al. Meta-analysis to evaluate the role of interferon in follicular lymphoma. *J Clin Oncol* 2005;23:2215–2223.

Rosenwald A, Wright G, Chan WC, et al. The use of molecular profiling to predict survival after chemotherapy for diffuse large B cell lymphoma. *New Eng J Med* 2002;346:1937–1947.

Rosenwald A, Wright G, Leroy Y, et al. Molecular diagnosis of primary mediastinal B cell lymphoma identifies a clinically favorable subgroup of diffuse large B cell lymphoma related to Hodgkin lymphoma. *J Exp Med* 2003;198:851–862.

Schouten HC, Qian W, Kvaloy S, et al. High-dose therapy improves progression-free survival and survival in relapsed follicular non-Hodgkin's lymphoma: results from the randomized European CUP trial. *J Clin Oncol* 2003;21:3918–3927.

Shipp MA, Ross KN, Tamayo P, et al. Diffuse large B-cell lymphoma outcome prediction by gene-expression profiling and supervised machine learning. *Nat Med* 2002;8:68–74.

Solal-Celigny P, Roy P, Colombat P, et al. Follicular lymphoma international prognostic index. *Blood* 2004;104:1258–1265.

Van Besien K, Loberiza FR, Bajorunaite R, et al. Comparison of autologous and allogeneic hematopoietic stem cell transplantation for follicular lymphoma. *Blood* 2003;102:3521–3529.

Witzig TE, Gordon LI, Cabanillas F, et al. Randomized controlled trial of yttrium-90-labeled ibritumomab tiuxetan radioimmunotherapy versus rituximab immunotherapy for patients with relapsed or refractory low-grade, follicular, or transformed B-cell non-Hodgkin's lymphoma. *J Clin Oncol* 2002;20:2453–2463.

Wundisch T, Kim TD, Tiede C, et al. Etiology and therapy of *Helicobacter pylori*-associated gastric lymphoma. *Ann Hematol* 2003;82:535–545.

16 Multiple Myeloma and Related Paraproteinemias

Jonathan Glass, MD
and Reinhold Munker, MD

1. INTRODUCTION

Multiple myeloma (MM) is a complex clonal malignancy of plasma cells in which the malignant cell has synergistic and complex interactions with the stroma. The first description of the disease was in the 1840s. The patient, Thomas Alexander McBean, was a carpenter born in 1800. He went to his family physician Dr. Thomas Watson in 1844 with sternal pain, which was treated with a plaster cast. The pain recurred 1 yr later and was treated with cupping and then steel and quinine. With relapse in August 1845, the patient was referred to William MacIntyre, a Harley Street physician, who personally examined both the urine and the patient. He noted that with boiling, the urine became opaque, and

From: *Contemporary Hematology: Modern Hematology, Second Edition*
Edited by: R. Munker, E. Hiller, J. Glass, and R. Paquette © Humana Press Inc., Totowa, NJ

that on cooling, a precipitate formed that clarified on reheating. Henry Bence Jones, physician at St. George's Hospital, confirmed the finding and, by chemical analysis, determined the substance to be a protein different from albumin. Mr. Bean died on New Year's Day 1846. John Dalrymple performed the autopsy and, noting bony abnormalities, coined the term "mollities and fragilitas ossium." Subsequently, Bence Jones presented a paper "On a new substance occurring in the urine of a patient with 'mollities ossium'," and 2 years later, MacIntyre described the patient in a paper "Case of mollities and fragilitas ossium accompanied with urine strongly charged with animal matter."

Other early historic landmarks include the description in 1873 by Rustizky, who performed an autopsy on a patient with eight separate tumors of the marrow and designated them MMs. In 1889, Kahler rediscovered Bence Jones' protein and described the clinical problems of loss of stature and kyphosis from osteoporosis in MM. In 1900, Wright made the connection between plasma cell proliferation, MM, and Bence Jones protein in the urine.

2. EPIDEMIOLOG Y OF MM

The incidence of MM in the United States is about 4 cases per 100,000 of the population. In 2004, there were an estimated 15,000 new cases of MM in the United States. The nearly 12,000 deaths from MM in 2004 accounted for about 2% of cancer deaths, with the death-to-new-case ratio of 3:4 being among the worst for all new malignancies. Although the disease is usually characterized as a disease of the elderly, the mean age at diagnosis in men is 62 yr, with 35% of the cases occurring in men under 60 yr of age. In women, the mean age at diagnosis is 61 yr, with 41% of the cases diagnosed in women under 60 yr of age. The incidence is twofold higher in African-Americans and in males in all populations. A map of mortality rates from myeloma shows a several-fold difference across the United States, with a trend toward higher mortality rates in the northern tier of states.

3. PLASMA CELL DYSCRASIAS

The gamut of plasma cell disorders run from the malignant precursor condition monoclonal gammopathy of undetermined significance (MGUS), to a variety of malignant monoclonal gammopathies. MGUS occurs in about 1% of adults and in nearly 10% of the population over 90 yr old. The malignant entities encompass variants of MM and other plasma cell malignancies as noted in Table 1.

The median time for progression of smoldering myeloma to symptomatic myeloma is about 2–3 yr. Currently, patients with MM have a median survival of about 33 mo. Plasma cell leukemia is an uncommon event and can occur either as a primary entity or a secondary event during the progression of myeloma. In

Table 1
Types of Multiple Myeloma and Other Plasma Cell Dyscrasias

Multiple myeloma
    Smoldering multiple myeloma
    Symptomatic multiple myeloma
    Plasma cell leukemia
        Primary
        Secondary
    Nonsecretory myeloma
    Osteosclerotic myeloma (POEMS)
Plasmacytoma
    Solitary plasmacytoma of bone
    Extramedullary plasmacytoma
Waldenström's macroglobulinemia
Heavy chain diseases
Primary amyloidosis
Monoclonal gammopathy of unknown significance (MGUS)

either case, the prognosis is poor, with a mean survival of several months. Although most patients with myeloma have an M-component demonstrable in serum or urine, about 1% of patients will have a nonsecretory disease without synthesis of any portion of a clonal immunoglobulin (Ig). Osteosclerotic myeloma is a rare form of myeloma with an interesting complex of signs and symptoms known as POEMS syndrome: polyneuropathy, osteosclerosis, endocrinopathy, myeloma, and skin lesions. MM can present as solitary growths or plasmacytomas involving the bone or as extramedulary plasmacytomas. Plasmacytomas of the bone have a high frequency of converting to a systemic MM, whereas extramedullary plasmacytomas, especially those that occur in the upper respiratory tract, have a greater tendency to remain localized.

The diagnostic criteria for MGUS are: the concentration of the monoclonal serum protein is below 30 g/L; the levels of the normal (polyclonal) Igs are not decreased; the bone marrow aspirate contains less than 10% plasma cells; a Bence Jones protein cannot be detected; and other malignancies (e.g., malignant lymphoma, MM, solid tumors) have been excluded. Patients with MGUS are generally asymptomatic.

Waldenström's macroglobulinemia is a distinct plasmalymphocytic monoclonal proliferation of B-lymphocytes and plasma cells that produce an IgM monoclonal protein. The morphology of the malignant cells and the clinical progression of Waldenström's macroglobulinemia (described in detail in Chapter 15) are distinct from myeloma. Macroglobulinemia can also occur in other proliferative lymphocytic disorders including MGUS, chronic lymphocytic leukemia (CLL), lymphomas, and primary amyloidosis.

Heavy chain disease (HCD) refers to monoclonal lymphocytic proliferations with the elaboration of only an Ig heavy chain. These entities have distinct clinical-pathological correlates. For example, alpha HCD, which is also known as immunoproliferative small intestinal disease (IPSID), Mediterranean lymphoma, or diffuse small intestinal lymphoma, is a subtype of the indolent mucosa-associated lymphoid tissue (MALT) lymphomas. α-HCD occurs primarily in the Middle East and is characterized by the synthesis of an alpha heavy chain paraprotein and constitutes a form of small intestinal lymphoma called IPSID. In μ-HCD, a monoclonal band is found in the minority of cases and hypogammaglobulinemia is a prominent feature.

Primary amyloidosis is also uncommon. The light chain synthesized by the malignant plasma cell clone diffuses into numerous tissues and stimulates production of amyloid protein. Often, the light chain is so potent in the incitement of amyloid that the amyloid depositions are detected well before it is possible to detect the presence of myeloma.

4. BIOLOGY OF MM

MM is a clonal B-cell malignancy with the myeloma cells derived from postgerminal center bone marrow plasmablasts. In the progression to plasma cells, the B-cells undergo a variety of DNA breaks necessary for variable diversity joining recombinations, somatic mutations, and isotype switching. It is assumed that this inherent genetic instability makes the plasma cell more prone to malignant transformation. Conventional karyotyping reveals abnormalities in only about 20% of patients presenting with stage I disease, increasing to 60% in stage III. By interphase fluorescence *in situ* hybridization (FISH), at least one chromosomal abnormality can be demonstrated in about 90% of cases of myeloma and 40–50% of cases of MGUS. The disparity of karyotyping and FISH analysis may be explained by the low labeling index in the malignant plasma cells and, hence, the difficulty in obtaining metaphases for analysis. FISH analysis demonstrates genetic abnormalities involving the Ig heavy-chain (*IGH*) gene at 14q32 occurring in about 75% of cases. The more common of the translocation partners include 11q13 (*CCND1*), 4p16.3 (*FGFR-3* and *MMSET*), 6p21 (*CCND3*), 16q23 (*c-Maf*), and 20q11 (*mafB*). In addition, deletions of chromosome 13 occur in nearly 50% of patients and, during the evolution and course of the disease, mutations affecting *nRAS*, *kRAS*, *cMyc*, and *p53* are frequently seen.

The traditional hypothesis for the evolution of myeloma is that somatic mutations involving *IGH* at 14q32 lead to MGUS, which has an approx 1% per year conversion rate to myeloma or related B-cell malignancies. Subsequent translocations of 14q32 lead to progression to myeloma either as smoldering myeloma or solitary plasmacytomas. Additional mutations of *N-RAS*, *K-RAS*, *P53*, and/or 13q14 deletions allow for progression to clinically significant myeloma. At odds with this hypothesis for progression is that the mean age at diagnosis of MGUS is far greater than that of myeloma.

Most of the translocations that involve the five recurrent translocation partners seem to be primary event translocations that occur from errors in IgH switch recombination during B-cell development in germinal centers. However, some other translocations may take place as a secondary event after the development of MGUS or MM. For example, *c-myc* translocations appear to be late secondary events that do not involve B-cell–specific recombination mechanisms. The prevalence of occurrence of c-myc translocations increase as the disease advances to late stages. In addition, *p16* methylation occurs both as early change and sometimes later in progression. Activating mutations of *N-* and *K-RAS* appear to mark, if not cause, the MGUS to MM transition in some tumors, but can also occur as later progression events. Other late oncogenic changes include inactivation of *p18* and *p53*.

Altered gene expression in MM has also been analyzed by the use of gene array. Several studies have now demonstrated distinct differences between gene expression in plasma cells from bone marrow of patients with MM versus MGUS and nonmalignant plasma cells. As it is not yet practical to assay gene expression by array analysis for every patient, studies have tried to select genes whose expression best correlates with outcome. For example, after adjusting for the presence of chromosome 13 deletions detected by FISH and for the presence of other chromosomal abnormalities three genes—*RAN*, *ZHX-2*, and *CHC1L*—have correlated with early relapse. *RAN*, which maps to 6p21, is a member of the Ras family of GTPase proteins and has a number of functions including transport into and out of the nucleus, regulation of chromosome condensation, and cell-cycle progression. The *CHC1L* gene (*CH*romosome *C*ondensation *1*-Like), maps to 13q14.3, a region that has been suspected of harboring a tumor suppressor gene for myeloma. *ZHX-2* is a negative regulator of the transcription factor, nuclear factor (NF)-κB, which is a transcriptional regulator of many genes involved in cell cycle control. Increased expression of *RAN* predicted a high probability of early relapse, especially with decreased expression of either *ZHX-2* or *CHC1L*, whereas increased expression of *ZHX-2* and *CHC1L* predicted longer event-free survivals. Recently, high-resolution genomic profiles were established for subgroups of multiple myeloma patients. In this analysis, 87 discrete minimal common regions were defined within recurrent and focal copy number alterations.

The chromosomal abnormalities in MM may have an impact on prognosis and may predict response to therapy. An unfavorable outcome of MM has been associated with increased plasma cell labeling index, hypodiploid cytogenetics compared with hyperdiploid states, monosomy and deletions of chromosome 13, monosomy of chromosome 17, and altered cyclin D1 expression. Activating mutations of K-Ras (but not N-Ras) also represent an adverse prognostic factor. Specific IgH translocations also have a profound prognostic significance, with shortened survival being seen with t(4;14) and with t(14;16) translocations regardless of standard or high-dose therapy. On the other hand, patients with MM who have a t(11;14) translocation appear to have a marginally better survival following conventional chemotherapy and to have a markedly better survival following intense therapy. Deletions of 13 q correlate with an increase of proliferation and stage. Plasma cells in patients with 13q14 have increased expression of Ki67. At least 70% of patients with Stage III myeloma have 13q14 deletions compared with approx 50% of patients with Stage II, and have a lower likelihood of being chemotherapy responsive (41% vs 78%) and a shortened median survival (24 mo vs >60 mo).

Cyclins D1, D2, or D3 interact with cdk4 and/or cdk6 to regulate phosphorylation of retinoblastoma (Rb), facilitating the G1/S cell cycle transition. Recent studies using gene array analysis of plasma cells from patients with myeloma demonstrate that a substantial fraction of of cases of MM express increased *CCND1* in the absence of a t(11;14) translocation and that about 40% of MM tumors bi-allelically express *CCND1* mRNA. Therefore, a novel mechanism that bi-allelically dysregulates *CCND1* is a frequent oncogenic event in MM. Cyclin D1 is expressed in most proliferating tissues, but with little or no expression of *CCND1* in lymphoid tissues or tumors. Presumably, biallelic expression of *CCND1* must be controlled by trans-acting factors, but the candidate factors that increase cyclin D1 expression have not been identified. The expression levels of cyclin D1, cyclin D2, or cyclin D3 mRNA in MM and MGUS cells are distinctly higher than in normal plasma cells. The occurrence of Ig translocations that dysregulate cyclin D1 or cyclin D3 contributes to about 20% of MM tumors. Cyclin D1 is overexpressed in almost all tumors with t(11;14) translocation. Additionally, cyclin D1 is overexpressed in nearly 40% of tumors lacking a t(11;14) translocation, whereas cyclin D2 levels are overexpressed in most of the remaining tumors. Therefore, it seems apparent that almost all MM tumors dysregulate at least one of the cyclin D genes.

The dysregulation of one of the three cyclin D genes may render the cells more susceptible to proliferative stimuli, resulting in selective expansion owing to interaction with bone marrow stromal cells (BMSCs) that produce interleukin (IL)-6 and other cytokines. In addition to the dysregulation of a cyclin D gene, which appears to be a nearly universal event in early pathogenesis, there is evidence that the Rb pathway is further disrupted by *p16INK4a* methylation and inactivation in a substantial fraction of MGUS and MM tumors. Further disruption of the Rb pathway by inactivation of Rb or *p18INK4c* can also occur at a lower frequency and mostly as a late progression event. The frequency and timing of other events, such as inactivation of phosphatase and tensin homolog (*PTEN*), remain to be determined.

Genetic and growth-factor driven events that lead to myeloma occur not only in the malignant plasma cell but also affect the bone marrow microenvironment. During the evolution of myeloma, there is a subtle interaction of malignant plasma cells with stroma, with various paracrine factors being generated by the stroma that affect plasma cell function and various factors generated by the plasma cells that affect the stroma. For example, under the influence of the malignant clone of plasma cells, in particular the secretion of vascular endothelial growth factor (VEGF), BMSCs secrete IL-6, insulin-like growth factor (IGF)1, IL-1β, transforming growth factor (TGF)-β, and tumor necrosis factor (TNF)-α. The secretion of IL-6 in turn increases release of VEGF by MM cells. IL-6 is a major growth and survival factor for myeloma cells. IL-6 triggers signal transduction through the mitogen-activated protein kinase cascade. IL-6 also promotes survival of myeloma cells by upregulation of antiapoptotic molecules such as BCL-x and c-Myc. Finally, IL-6 induction of VEGF has an adverse affect on dendritic cell function and leads to the generalized decrease of Igs, which characterizes myeloma and puts patients at risk for infection. The generalized osteolytic activity that is observed in myeloma derives from the activation by osteoblasts of the receptor activator of NF-κB ligand (RANKL) with a reduction of the decoy receptor osteoprotegerin. As a consequence of the increased ratio of RANKL to osteoprotegerin, osteoclast activity is increased and bone reabsorption occurs. In addition, IGF-1 is elaborated by stromal cells in response to VEGF and other factors from the myeloma cells, and IGF-1 acts on the myeloma cells through activation of Ras, stimulation of the PI3K and Akt pathways, and inhibition of apoptosis by affecting phosphorylation of BCL2 family members.

5. DIAGNOSIS AND STAGING OF MM

The diagnosis of myeloma requires that the clinician be attuned to the presenting symptoms and signs of bone pain, anemia, infections, renal failure, and/or hypercalcemia. The laboratory should be attuned to certain abnormalities on the peripheral smear, namely rouleaux formation and the presence of a "bluish" precipitate on the background staining of a blood smear. The radiologist should be attuned to the classic "punched out" lesions in the skull (Fig. 16.1) and long bones or diffuse osteoporosis that afflicts many patients with myeloma.

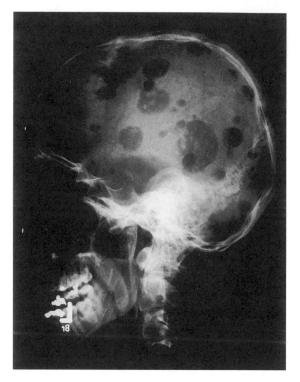

Fig. 16.1. Multiple myeloma with osteolytic bone lesions (lateral radiograph of the skull).

The workup of a person suspected of having MM is summarized in Table 2. This table also indicates parameters that are useful in following response to therapy and/or relapse.

The bone marrow aspiration and biopsy is usually diagnostic with sheets or syncitia of plasma cells (*see* Figs. 16.2 and 16.3). However, as the disease may present with multiple plasmacytomas, the aspiration or biopsy of the marrow between plasmacytomas may, on occasion, allow the marrow to appear normal. Immunohistochemistry often is helpful with the identification of CD38- and 138-positive cells that may be difficult to see on routine Wright stain. In addition, in some patients, it may be of diagnostic importance to obtain flow cytometry, examining for CD38 and 138 (syndecan) and plasma cell labeling index in particular. Other markers that are helpful in diagnosis include CD10, which is expressed in a subset of patients, in contrast to CD19 and CD20, which are rarely expressed. CD28 and CD86 often occur with progressive disease. CD34 is not expressed and CD56 (N-CAM) is expressed in MGUS and plasma cell leukemia but not in all cases of MM.

Table 2
Workup of Suspected Multiple Myeloma

Parameter	Rationale
History and physical examination	Diagnosis, stage, determination of performance status
CBC, differential count, platelelets	Diagnosis, monitoring
BUN/creatinine, electrolytes including Ca^{++} and uric acid	Diagnosis, monitoring
SPEP and immunofixation	Diagnosis, monitoring
Quantitative immunoglobulins	Diagnosis, monitoring
24-h urine PEP and immunofixation	Diagnosis, monitoring
Radiological skeletal survey	Indicates possible need for local intervention
MRI	Possible need for local intervention
PET imaging	Staging, extent of disease (experimental)
Bone marrow aspirate and biopsy (unilateral)	Diagnostic evaluation
Cytogenetics including FISH	Prognostic significance
β_2-Microglobulin	Parameter of response
C-reactive protein	Parameter of response
LDH	Parameter of response
Serum viscosity	Parameter of response

CBC, complete blood count; BUN, blood urea nitrogen; SPEP, serum protein electrophoresis; PEP, protein electrophoresis; MRI, magnetic resonance imaging; PET, positron emission tomography; FISH, fluorescence *in situ* hybridization; LDH, lactate dehydrogenase.

The characteristic finding in patients with MM is a monoclonal protein in the serum and/or urine, which in most (but not all) cases results in a spike in the conventional serum electrophoresis (*see* Fig. 16.4). A clue to the presence of a monoclonal gammopathy is an elevated total protein.

The clinician at all times must contemplate areas of possible complications of the disease and the signs that these complications may cause. For example, hypercalcemia may appear both at the time of diagnosis or as a sign of failure to respond to therapy. The patient with hypercalcemia may present with polyuria, polydypsia, and constipation; also, the sensorium may be muddled in these patients, and end-organ failure, especially of renal function, may occur. Multiple causes of renal failure occur in myeloma and are often present at the time of diagnosis. The precipitants of renal failure include hypercalcemia, hyperuricemia, infiltration of the kidneys with myeloma, precipitation of Igs in the renal tubules, tubular dysfunction from light chain production, and amyloidosis.

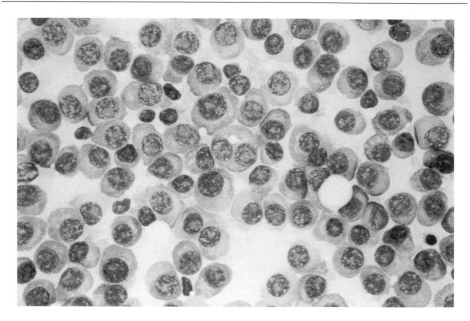

Fig. 16.2. Multiple myeloma. Dense infiltrate of neoplastic plasma cells.

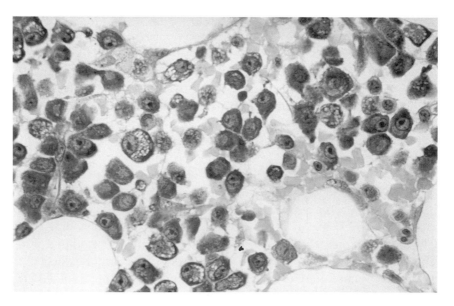

Fig. 16.3. Multiple myeloma. Histological section of the bone marrow.

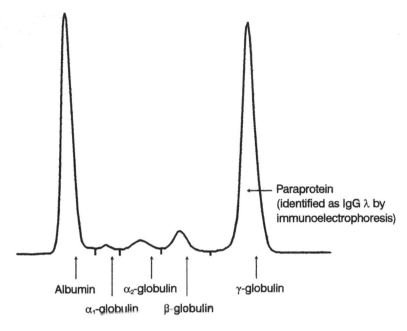

Fig. 16.4. Multiple myeloma. Serum electrophoresis showing a monoclonal peak (paraprotein).

Additionally, in some patients it may necessary to obtain an MRI for suspected cord lesions or to identify a solitary plasmacytoma of the bone. MRI is more sensitive than classic radiography to detect bone involvement of MM. An example of an MRI of the thoracic spine involved with MM is shown in Fig. 16.5. Recently, positron emission tomography (PET) imaging has been introduced into clinical medicine for the staging of tumors. In MM, only a few cases have been imaged by fluorodeoxyglucose (FDG)-PET, but it appears this imaging technique is especially sensitive for highly proliferative myelomas. Hyperviscosity is usually seen with Waldenström's macroglobulinemia; however, patients with high levels of IgG can present with symptoms of hyperviscosity (altered state of consciousness, headaches, visual disturbances) and may respond to vigorous plasmapheresis.

In assessing the workup of the patient with suspected myeloma, it is necessary to distinguish between smoldering (asymptomatic) myeloma and symptomatic myeloma. Smoldering myeloma is usually considered if the monoclonal protein in the serum is greater than or equal to 3.0 g/dL and/or the bone marrow demonstrates clonal plasma cells greater than or equal to 10% with no symptoms and no related organ damage including absence of bone lesions.

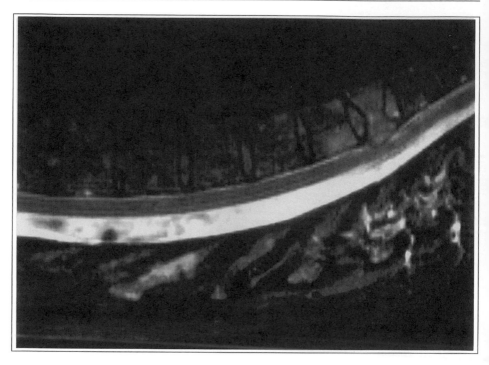

Fig. 16.5. Multiple myeloma. Magnetic resonance imaging (STIR) showing infiltration of the upper thoracic spine.

The criteria generally used for diagnosis of symptomatic myeloma are noted in Table 3.

Many years ago, Durie and Salmon determined three stages of MM based on radiographic and clinical chemistry findings (*see* Table 4). This staging system makes an estimate of the total body plasma cell mass and is widely used. Because this classification relies on conventional bone radiographs which may be insensitive for major bone disease and may not detect aggressive early disease, recently an international study group proposed a new International Staging System. A simple, three-stage classification was developed based on serum β_2-microglobulin (Sβ2m) and serum albumin (SA). Stage I is defined as Sβ_2m less than 3.5 mg/L and SA greater than or equal to 3.5 g/dL. Stage III is defined as Sβ_2m greater than or equal to 5.5 mg/L. The intermediate stage II applies to all patients who are neither stage I or III. In the international survey of more than 10,000 newly diagnosed patients, the median survival in stage I was 62 mo, in stage II 44 mo, and stage III 29 mo.

Table 3
Diagnostic Criteria for Multiple Myeloma

Major criteria	1) Plasmacytomas
	2) Bone marrow >30% plasma cells
	3) Monoclonal Ig (IgG > 3.5 g/L or IgA > 2 g/L)
	or κ or λ > 1 g/d in urine/24 h
Minor criteria	1) 10–30% plasmacytosis
	2) monoclonal Ig spike less than above
	3) lytic bone lesions
	4) normal IgM < 50 mg/dL, IgA < 100 mg/dL, or IgG < 600 mg/dL
Diagnosis	Any two major criteria
	Major criterion 1 plus minor 2, 3, or 4
	Major criterion 3 plus minor criterion 1 or 3
	Minor criteria 1, 2, and 3 or 1, 2, and 4

Table 4
Staging of Multiple Myeloma (According to Durie and Salmon)

Stage	Criteria	Tumor cell burden $(\times 10^{12}/m^2)$
I	All of the following:	<0.6 (low)
	Hgb >10 g/dL	
	Normal Ca^{++}	
	Radiologically normal or only osteolytic lesions	
	Low concentrations of monoclonal protein	
	IgG < 5g/dL	
	IgA < 3 g/dL	
	Light chains in urine < 4 g/24 h	
II	Neither stage I or III	0.6–1.2 (intermediate)
III	At least one of the following:	>1.2 (high)
	Hgb < 8.5 g/dL	
	Elevated Ca^{++}	
	Advanced osteolytic bone lesions	
	High monoclonal protein levels	
	IgG > 7 g/dL	
	IgA > 5 g/dL	
	Light chains > 12 g/24 h	

All stages are appended by A (renal function normal or slightly impaired) or B (renal function impaired, creatinine > 2 mg/ dL). Hgb, hemoglobin.

Table 5
Transplantation Eligibility Criteria

Age	<65 yr
Performance status	0–2
Concomitant diseases	Normal cardiac and pulmonary function

6. THERAPY OF MM

6.1. Stem Cell Transplantation

The decision to treat patients is based on the accuracy of the diagnosis, the staging of the patient, and the presence of complications of the disease. There is no evidence that treatment of asymptomatic smoldering myeloma is beneficial. The median time to progression from smoldering to symptomatic myeloma is about 2–3 yr. However, as there is a wide range as to when the disease will require treatment, each patient requires an individual approach that involves monitoring various laboratory parameters as well as patient symptoms. Because of the proven efficacy of high-dose chemotherapy with subsequent autologous stem cell transplantation (SCT), the approach to treatment can be divided between those patients who are eligible for transplantation and those who are not (*see* Table 5 for transplantation eligibility criteria).

High-dose therapy (HDT) with autologous SCT represents a significant improvement in the treatment of myeloma. The mortality rate for autologous SCT is about 1–2%, with the most widely used preparative regimen being melphalan at a dose of 200 mg/m^2. Most studies demonstrate a survival advantage in individuals who undergo intensive therapy with rescue with autologous SCT compared with those who undergo chemotherapy alone. Tandem (double) autologous SCT allows for a second planned transplantation after recovery from the first. Long-term event-free survival (EFS) is about 40% increased for those who underwent a second transplantation compared with patients who underwent a single procedure. The role of allogeneic transplantation in myeloma remains experimental. Considering the age of patients on presentation, the availability of human leukocyte antigen (HLA)-matched siblings, and end-organ failure, only a minority of patients are candidates for allogeneic transplantation. The graft-vs-myeloma effect of allogeneic transplantation was established without doubt, for example in patients who relapsed with myeloma after a reduced-intensity transplant and then were treated with donor lymphocyte infusions. Currently, protocols incorporating a full-intensity autologous and a reduced-intensity allotransplant are under development. Another interesting idea is to immunize healthy donors with the isotype of the myeloma and then stimulate the immune system further after an allogeneic transplant done in remission.

If patients with myeloma are eligible for (autologous) transplantation, a now commonly used approach is to treat with thalidomide and dexamethasone before stem cell harvesting (induction). The underlying assumption in this approach is that stem cell function is not adversely affected and that the rate of response is sufficient to allow most patients to undergo intense chemotherapy with stem cell rescue. This approach spares potential damage to the stem cell. Four cycles of treatment are usually given with doses of thalidomide 200 mg/d and 40 mg dexamethasone per day on days 1–4, 9–12, and 17–20 on odd cycles and days 1–4 on even cycles. Stem cells are harvested after the fourth cycle. With this program, major responses (prior to high-dose chemotherapy and SCT, defined as greater than or equal to 50% reduction in serum and urine M-protein) of over 60% have been reported. The most common grade 3/4 toxicities include deep vein thrombosis, constipation, rash, and infections.

The outcome of HDT has been evaluated in several ways. Complete remission (CR) has been defined as true CR by negative immunofixation and as near CR by the less-sensitive negative electrophoresis. In most series, CRs are significantly more frequent after HDT than after chemotherapy (17–44% vs 5–15%). The median EFS are always longer with HDT compared with chemotherapy (25–42 mo vs 16–34 mo). It is more difficult to evaluate the effect of HDT on overall survival (OS), as OS will be influenced by salvage therapies. However, significantly increased OSs have been demonstrated in several trials, including the British Medical Research Council (MRC) trial in which the OS was 54 mo after HDT compared with 42 mo after chemotherapy alone. In all HDT studies, the mortality rates were less than 5% and not significantly different from chemotherapy. The data strongly suggest that HDT is now the standard of care of patients up to the age of 65 yr with newly diagnosed MM.

There are several prognostic variables that the clinician should keep in mind when planning HDT. With both HDT and chemotherapy, standard biological markers are important predictors of outcome. These include high levels of β_2m, C-reactive protein, or lactate dehydrogenase (LDH) and low levels of albumin, all of which are associated with poorer outcome. Genetic abnormalities, as evaluated either by conventional cytogenetics or by molecular biology techniques, are also prognostic markers. Hypodiploid states, chromosome 13 deletions, and 14q32 translocations are all poor prognostic markers, with short EFS and OS.

6.2. Cytotoxic Drugs and Other Therapies

For patients who are not candidates for HDT or as alternative treatment programs to thalidomide and dexamethasone, a variety of chemotherapeutic regi-

Table 6
Treatment Regimens for Multiple Myeloma

Regimen	Doses
Melphalan and prednisone	Every 6 wk, Melphalan 8–10 mg p.o. d 1–7 Prednisone 60 mg d 1–7
VBMCP	Every 5 wk Vincristine Carmustine Melphalan Cyclophosphamide Prednisone
VAD	Every 4 wk Vincristine Doxorubicin Dexamethasone
Second-line therapy	
Bortezomib	1.3 mg/m^2 on d 1, 4, 8, 11 every 21 d
Thalidomide	100–200 mg p.o. for maintenance 300–400 mg p.o. for refractory or relapsed myeloma (if tolerated)

mens are available including VAD chemotherapy (vincristine, Adriamycin®
[doxorubicin], and dexamethasone) or melphalan and prednisone. Numerous
other treatment programs have been proposed. It is possible that no chemotherapy regimen is superior to melphalan and prednisone if SCT cannot be accomplished. In stage IIIB disease and with more aggressive-appearing myeloma, VAD
and VBMCP (Vincristine, BCNU [carmustine], melphalan, cyclophosphamide,
prednisone) are often used. Newer programs have also incorporated liposomal
doxorubicin (Doxil®), as this drug may have a lower incidence of myocardial
toxicity. The more common therapies are listed in Table 6.

Patients need to be carefully monitored for toxicity and efficacy of the chemotherapy and for evidence of complications of the myeloma. At a minimum the
monitoring must include the parameters of response listed in Table 2. If there is
no response to therapy when these parameters are reviewed every two cycles it
may be worth considering an alternate therapeutic intervention, bearing in mind
that the number of approaches is relatively limited. The treatment plan may have
to be changed because of drug toxicities. For example, severe neuropathy may
dictate modification of the dose of vincristine whereas psychiatric symptoms or
the appearance of difficult-to-control diabetes may dictate that dexamethasone
is eliminated. The clinician must be astute to the clinical manifestations of

hypercalcemia (hyperdypsia, polyuria, and constipation) and treat hypercalcemia aggressively with bisphosphonates such as zoledronic acid. However, as in most patients, zoledronic acid is used prophylactically (*see* "Bone Diseases and Bone Pain") to prevent bone fractures and pain, and the occurrence of hypercalcemia is not as frequent as previously seen. The major cause of death in myeloma is infection (*see* below) and all febrile episodes must be investigated and appropriately treated.

A number of agents for the treatment of myeloma are now available that are not typical chemotherapeutic drugs. These novel therapies include thalidomide (Thal) and more potent analogs, the proteasome inhibitor bortezomib (Velcade®), and arsenic trioxide (As_2O_3). Thal was proposed as a potential therapy for myeloma because of its known antiangiogenic activity and the demonstration of increased angiogenesis in the involved bone marrow of patients with myeloma. Thal and its analogs such as lenalidomide have other actions including the induction of G1 growth arrest of myeloma cells, the prevention of adhesion of myeloma cells to BMSCs, and the enhancement of natural killer (NK) cell number and activity against myeloma cells. The net result of these actions is decreased production by the bone marrow stroma of IL-6 and VEGF with a resulting decreased stimulation of myeloma cells and of neo-angiogenesis. Hence, Thal acts in part as an immunomodulator and in part as an anticytokine and has been observed to generate a significant response rate either as first-line or second-line therapy. Analogs of Thal, such as lenalidomide, are far more potent stimulators of NK cell and T-cell co-stimulatory activity as well as stimulators of IL-2 and interferon (IFN) production, and may prove to be more efficacious than Thal. Thal is being explored in combination with other agents such as melphalan and preliminary studies in elderly patients suggest a high level of activity. Thal has activity in advanced and refractory myeloma. In a recent randomized, long-term study, Thal was added to high-dose therapy. The frequency of complete responses was increased and the event-free survival was extended, but the overall survival was not improved. In addition, more than 20% of patients on Thal had adverse events such as thrombosis or neuropathy.

Bortezomib (Velcade®) is a proteasome inhibitor and represents a novel class of therapeutic agents that also target the myeloma–BMSC interaction. NF-κB is a transcription factor whose activity is important in stimulating IL-6 production both in the myeloma cell and in the bone marrow stroma. IL-6 production stimulates the growth and survival of myeloma cells. Cellular levels of NF-κB are controlled by the binding of inhibiting factor (IF)- κB, the levels of which are in turn controlled by catabolism via the proteosome. By inhibiting the proteasome, IF-κB remains bound to NF-κB and NF-κB remains inactive. Bortezomib has been shown to induce apoptosis of myeloma cells resistant to known conventional therapies and is synergistic in the antimyeloma effects of dexamethasone.

The net effects of bortezomib are to prevent the binding of myeloma cells to the BMSCs, inhibit the expression of IL-6 that is triggered by myeloma–stromal interactions, and reduce angiogenesis. These clinically relevant actions result from downregulation of growth/survival signaling pathways and upregulation of apoptotic pathways as well as upregulation of the proteasome pathway. The efficacy of bortezomib as a single agent was shown in heavily pretreated patients with myeloma, with about 10% achieving CR and an OS of 35%. Based on preclinical studies, dexamethasone was added, with considerable additional benefit. Responding patients were noted to have improved hemoglobin levels and renal function, decreased blood transfusion requirements, and an increase in the levels of the uninvolved Igs. The major toxicities of bortezomib are significant thrombocytopenia and neuropathy. A number of trials are being conducted with bortezomib in newly diagnosed myeloma patients or using bortezomib as a second-line agent either alone or in combination with other agents, such as pegylated liposomal doxorubicin, melphalan, and Thal.

As_2O_3 also targets the myeloma cell–bone marrow stroma interaction. As_2O_3 induces apoptosis, adds to the efficacy of dexamethasone, and inhibits the antiapoptotic actions of IL-6. In addition, As_2O_3 decreases binding of myeloma cells to the bone marrow stroma and inhibits the secretion of IL-6 and VEGF induced by the adhesion of myeloma cells.

6.3. Maintenance Therapy

The decision to initiate maintenance therapy depends in part on how long induction therapy is continued. With melphalan and prednisone, therapy is continued until there is a plateau of the monoclonal protein that is being monitored. In general, this means that patients are treated from 6 to 12 mo. For the more aggressive therapies such as VAD, assessment of response should be done after two cycles. There are few data to support the use of VAD beyond four cycles. It is extremely important to monitor responses, and if minimal headway is made either in symptoms (e.g., bone pain), signs (e.g., anemia, neutropenia, and/or thrombocytopenia), or in the monoclonal protein, then therapy must be reassessed and changed. There is an insufficient database from which to gauge the appropriate length of treatment with new agents such as bortezomib, Thal, or As_2O_3. In trials with bortezomib, the drug was used for a total of 29 wk. Thal has been used continuously, with the drug stopped for toxicity or disease relapse.

Although a plateau phase can be achieved with chemotherapy, this apparent quiescent state is unlike that of MGUS or smoldering MM in that virtually all patients with MM will relapse. There is no evidence that continued chemotherapy is of benefit in preventing relapse. There are data suggesting that continued exposure to chemotherapy will increase resistance and may lead to the development of myelodysplasia and/or acute leukemia.

There have been trials of IFN-α and prednisone for maintenance therapy. A meta-analysis of trials comparing IFN with no maintenance treatment demonstrated delay of time to progression of 6 mo, with an estimated overall increase in median survival of approx 4 mo. This efficacy must be balanced by the considerable toxicity of the IFN, which is used at an initial dose of five million units subcutaneously three times per week, with the dose reduced for side effects. Over 50% of patients reduce the dose because of toxicity.

The efficacy of prednisone for maintenance therapy has been evaluated in a randomized trial of patients who received and responded to induction therapy with VAD. Maintenance treatment with 50 mg of prednisone p.o. every other day compared with 10 mg p.o. every other day resulted in beneficial effects both in progression-free survival (14 vs 5 mo) and OS (37 vs 26 mo) for the higher-dose regimen. As all of the patients responded to a regimen containing a glucocorticoid, it is not known if responders to other chemotherapies would also benefit from prednisone maintenance.

7. COMPLICATIONS OF MM

7.1. Renal Failure

There are two major categories of causes of renal failure: one related to the metabolic consequences of myeloma and the other directly related to the Ig products of the myeloma cells. The metabolic causes of renal failure include hypercalcemia and hyperuricemia. It is not unusual for patients to present with elevated serum calcium or for elevated calcium to be an early sign of disease progression. Hence, serum calcium must be part of the initial workup and included in the routine surveillance of patients. As the serum albumin will decrease with an increase in tumor load, patients who present with high-stage myeloma or who have relapsed will be hypoalbuminemic, and the serum calcium levels will have to be adjusted. Hypercalcemia leads to renal failure by producing renal vasoconstriction and by direct intratubular calcium deposition. Elevated filtered calcium may also potentiate the toxicity of filtered light chains. The clinician must also be cognizant of symptoms caused by hypercalcium (namely, polyuria and polydypsia, which result from nephrogenic diabetes insipidus), constipation, and an altered sensorium. The renal failure induced by hypercalcemia is generally reversible. Immediate treatment is directed at lowering the serum calcium, and should include isotonic saline with a loop diuretic and bisphosphonates. The underlying disease must also be treated. If renal failue is severe, placing the patient in a poor performance status, the patient can be treated with high-dose decadron and more definitive therapy instituted as the performance status improves. The cell turnover in myeloma, especially with high-stage disease, can lead to production of large amounts of uric acid and result in the deposition of urate crystals in the kidney.

Renal failure may also be the result of direct infiltration of the kidney with myeloma cells. But far more commonly, renal disease in MM results from the toxicity of the Igs being synthesized by the myeloma cells, especially the over-production of monoclonal Ig light chains, which can lead to cast nephropathy, primary amyloidosis, and light chain deposition disease (LCDD). Detection of light chains in the urine is an essential part of the initial workup of a patient suspected of having a plasma cell dyscrasia. Light chains cannot be detected by the common urinary dipsticks, which detect albumin, but should be quantitated with immunoelectrophoresis and immunofixation techniques. The kidney has a large capacity for catabolism of light chains. However, some light chains have properties that make them nephrotoxic. In vitro, light chains from patients with renal failure aggregate to form high-molecular-weight complexes, and it is hypothesized that these aggregates lead to tubule cast formation. Other prop-erties of light chains are important. Most patients with primary amyloidosis have λ light chains, whereas individuals with LCDD usually have κ light chains. Light chains filtered into the tubules can produce renal failure either by intratubular cast formation or direct tubular toxicity. Precipitated light chains lead to intratubular cast formation with obstruction, especially in the distal and collect-ing tubules. The cast formation may be accelerated by the binding of the light chains to the Tamm-Horsfall mucoprotein, a protein excreted by the tubules, and which is commonly found in the casts of patients with myeloma kidney. In other patients, light chains are absorbed by the renal tubule cells and are not catabo-lized by lysozymes, but instead crystallize in the tubule cell, causing tubular dysfunction and renal failure. Renal failure can also occur either from LCDD or, less commonly, from heavy chain deposition disease (HCDD). In these cases, light chains or, occasionally, fragments of heavy chains are deposited on the basement membrane of the tubules, Bowman's capsule, and glomeruli.

7.2. Bone Disease and Bone Pain

Patients with MM commonly present with bone pain in association with ane-mia. The interaction of the myeloma cells with the bone marrow stroma results in the activation of osteoclasts and the inhibition of osteoblasts by many mecha-nisms. The net result of the increased osteoclastic activity is that most patients have significant osteoporosis. Skeletal surveys done at the time of diagnosis demonstrate that osteoporosis is present in nearly 80% of patients and that focal lytic lesions can be found in about half of the patients, with pathological frac-tures, including compression fractures of the spine, in about one-fith of the cases. The increase in bone resorption is the result of an increase in the number and activity of osteoclasts combined with inhibition of osteoblastic activity. A number of factors are involved in these processes, including IL-1, TNF-α, IL-6,

IL-1β, lymphotoxin, TNF, IL-3, vascular cell adhesion molecule-1, receptor activator of NF-κB (RANK), and RANKL (also known as osteoclast differentiation factor and osteoprotegerin ligand). In addition to diffuse osteoporosis, at the site of plasmacytomas within the bone marrow the presumed high concentration of these factors locally gives rise to the classic "punched out" or lytic lesions of myeloma. The interactions between myeloma cell and stroma that result in increased bone resorption also provide a microenvironment that is conducive to the proliferation and survival of myeloma cells. For example, the IL-6 and osteopontin as well as the other factors will promote myeloma cell growth.

The result of these processes is that patients are at risk for small cortical fractures from the diffuse osteoporosis and significant fractures from the larger osteolytic lesions. The approach to the treatment of the ensuing pain from either type of lesion has been to first insure that a critical bone, for example a femoral head, is not imminently going to fracture, in which case prophylactic treatment must be instituted. Patients should be started on primary therapy for the myeloma, and one measure of response will be a decrease in the degree of pain. Simultaneously, appropriate analgesia should be instituted, and a decrease in dose with time serves as another good measure of the efficacy of primary therapy. If pain persists or if a lesion seems to pose the threat of imminent fracture, then radiation therapy should be instituted. It is imperative that the painful areas be well circumscribed so that the radiation ports are delimited. Such an approach will limit radiation to bone marrow-bearing sites and prevent bone marrow compromise, which could lead to a limited tolerance for future chemotherapy. It is wise to consult with the orthopedic surgeon at this point to determine whether concurrent stabilization of the bone is required.

A marked change in the handling of bone disease has occurred with the use of bisphosphonates for the treatment and prevention of osteoporosis in MM as well as other malignancies, such as breast cancer and prostate cancer, in which bone disease plays a major role in morbidity. The use of bisphosphonates prevents skeletal complications and is extremely useful both in breast cancer and prostate cancer in the prevention of treatment-related bone loss, and possibly in delaying skeletal progression. Randomized controlled trials have demonstrated that oral clodronate and intravenous pamidronate and zoledronic acid are superior to placebo in reducing skeletal complications, with a reduction also seen in vertebral fractures. The mechanism of action of the bisphosphonates in myeloma is not clear. Pamidronate has been shown to decrease bone resorption, and this effect correlates with improvement in pain. The American Society of Clinical Oncology has published guidelines on the use of bisphosphonates. The recommendation is to use intravenous pamidronate or zoledronic acid, as these two agents have been demonstrated to delay the time to first skeletal event, and as clodronate is not available in the United States. The choice between pamidronate or zoledronic acid is made based on convenience (pamidronate has a 90-min infusion time vs 15 min for zoledronic acid) and cost (pamidronate is less expensive).

7.3. Infectious Complications

Patients with myeloma are highly susceptible to bacterial infections, which are a leading cause of morbidity and mortality in this disease. The most common sites of infections are the lungs and kidneys, with the most common pathogens being *Streptococcus pneumoniae*, *Staphylococcus aureus*, and *Klebsiella pneumoniae* in the lungs and *Escherichia coli* and other Gram-negative organisms in the urinary tract. The etiology of the increase in infections is multifold. First, all patients with myeloma have a progressive decrease of normal Igs and, hence, decreased titers of opsonins. Interestingly, with treatment with nonclassical drugs such as thalidomide, restoration of normal Igs may be seen. In addition, patients may be neutropenic because of the myelophthisic effect of the myeloma in the marrow, suppressing normal myeloid differentiation. Finally, patients may be neutropenic from chemotherapy. A reasonable approach in newly diagnosed patients or after patients have had one infectious episode is to vaccinate patients with pneumococcal and influenza vaccines. Prophylactic antibiotics may also be used. Certainly, after a single or recurrent pneumococcal infection, daily oral penicillin would be of benefit. Prophylactic use of thrice-weekly oral trimethoprim/sulfamethoxazole may also be helpful. Intravenous Ig (IVIg) may be given if IgG levels minus the monoclonal protein are less than 500 mg/dL, with the intent of infusing IVIg often enough to maintain the IgG levels at more than 500 mg/dL. γ-Globulins may be beneficial for patients with recurrent infections, but the administration is inconvenient and expensive.

7.4. Anemia

Anemia is commonly observed in myeloma and has several causes. Clearly, marrow infiltration will decrease erythropoiesis. In addition, cytotoxic drugs will further impede marrow function and renal failure will decrease erythropoietin production. Several studies have demonstrated the efficacy of administering erythropoietin, both in its ability to increase the hemoglobin and also in the resultant improvement in the quality of life. The patient should be evaluated to determine other possible causes of anemia, including iron levels. A common approach is to use erythropoietin 40,000 units weekly, escalating the dose if no response is seen. If iron stores appear low, then oral iron supplementation or ferrous gluconate can be given intravenously. The clinician should aim to maintain a hemoglobin level of about 10–12 g/dL.

8. AMYLOIDOSIS

Amyloidosis is a multisystem disorder that frequently involves the heart, kidneys, liver, skin, subcutaneous tissues, nerves, and other organs. Amyloidosis is characterized by the deposition of amyloid fibrils. All forms of amyloid are derived from a particular folding of a protein, have green birefringence under polarized light, and stain positive with Congo red. The most common form, amyloid L (AL) or light chain amyloidosis, is derived from the deposition of monoclonal light chains. Less common is secondary amyloidosis (or amyloid A amyloidosis), which is observed in chronic infectious or inflammatory disorders. Light chain amyloidosis is associated in only about 10% of cases with frank MM. Rare forms of amyloidosis are heredofamilial forms of amyloidosis, localized amyloidosis, and amyloidosis associated with certain neurodegenerative disorders. Systemic amyloidosis should be suspected in nephrotic range proteinuria, unexplained heart failure, peripheral neuropathy in patients without diabetes, unclear hepatomegaly, or a combination of these findings. If AL amyloidosis is a possible diagnosis, the serum and urine should be screened for monoclonal light chains by immunofixation and free lights should be measured by the free light chain assay. Interestingly, λ light chains are a more frequent cause of AL amyloidosis than κ light chains. A tissue biopsy for amyloid can be obtained from many organs, but a bone marrow biopsy and a biopsy of subcutaneous fat are recommended, as these have both a low risk and a high diagnostic yield. The clinical manifestations of amyloidosis are multiple and protean. Most patients suffer from fatigue. Kidney disease, often with massive proteinuria, is present in most patients. Many patients develop congestive heart failure. Echocardiography shows a biventricular thickening and hypokinesia. A typical finding in advanced cases is "granular sparkling" of the interventricular septum. Other clinical findings are hepatomegaly, orthostatic hypotension, macroglossia, peripheral neuropathy, thickening of muscles ("shoulder pad" sign), and malabsorption. The prognosis of AL amyloidosis was poor in most cases until now. Heart failure especially is a sign of poor prognosis (median survival 6 mo or less). Serum troponin and brain natriuretic peptide are serum markers of cardiac failure and portend a poor prognosis if elevated. More recently, it was shown that high-dose, melphalan-based chemotherapy with stem cell rescue improves the prognosis of patients with early amyloidosis. Major complications, including death from transplantation, occurred mainly in older patients and in patients with advanced heart failure or the involvement of multiple organs. In good- to average-risk patients, a transplant-related mortality of 10–15% was observed. At least 50% of patients had a clonal response to high-dose chemotherapy, including complete responses.

All patients with amyloidosis need symptomatic treatment of heart failure, kidney failure, and gastrointestinal complications. Patients with progressive renal failure need dialysis. Selected patients with end-stage renal disease may benefit from kidney transplantation. An alternative to high-dose therapy may be dexamethasone pulses. Patients in poor performance status may stabilize when treated with melphalan-prednisone pulses. Experimental therapies for amyloidosis include proteasome inhibitors, thalidomide analogs, and inhibitors of TNF-α.

SUGGESTED READING

Barlogie, B, Tricot G, Anaissie E, et al. Thalidomide and hematopoietic stem cell transplantation for multiple myeloma. *N Engl J Med* 2006;354:1021–1030.

Bruno B, Rotta M, Giaccone L, et al. New drugs for treatment of multiple myeloma. *Lancet Oncol* 2004;5:430–442.

Carrasco DR, Tonon G, Huang Y, et al. High-resolution genomic profiles define distinct clinico-pathogenetic subgroups of multiple myeloma patients. *Cancer Cell* 2006;9:313–325.

Gertz MA, Merlini G, Treon SP. Amyloidosis and Waldenström's macroglobulinemia. *Hematology (Am Soc Hematol Educ Program)* 2004;8:257–282.

Harousseau JL, Shaugnessy J Jr, Richardson P. Multiple myeloma. *Hematology (Am Soc Hematol Educ Program)* 2004;8:237–256.

Hideshima T, Bergsagel PL, Kuehl WM, et al. Advances in biology of multiple myeloma: clinical applications. *Blood* 2004;104:607–618.

Sirohi B, Powles R. Multiple myeloma. *Lancet* 2004;363:875–887.

17 Congenital and Acquired Immunodeficiencies

Vishwas Sakhalkar, MD
and Reinhold Munker, MD

CONTENTS

1. INTRODUCTION

The development of the immune system and its function are outlined in Chapter 1. Congenital immunodeficiencies are rare; more details can be found in pediatric textbooks. Here, only the most important entities are discussed. Acquired immunodeficiencies are observed in many lymphoproliferative disorders and during treatment with steroids or chemotherapy with cytostatic drugs. The deficiency of cellular immunity induced by HIV infection is a common problem in many countries. In this chapter, we describe only some hematological consequences of HIV infection.

The following are common tests of immune defense or immune status of an organism. These tests are indicated if a patient has frequent infections—bacterial, fungal, viral, or protozoan. Which tests are used depends on the clinical situation and the type of particular immune defect suspected.

1. **Blood count with white cell differential count, flow cytometry:** this permits exclusion of morphological abnormalities (e.g., a granulation defect of granulocytes). Full blood counts of lymphocyte, neutrophil, and eosinophil numbers are helpful. The mononuclear cell populations can be further differentiated and

From: *Contemporary Hematology: Modern Hematology, Second Edition*
Edited by: R. Munker, E. Hiller, J. Glass, and R. Paquette © Humana Press Inc., Totowa, NJ

analyzed with monoclonal antibodies (*see* Appendix 2, "CD Nomenclature").
This can be done both with flow cytometry or immunocytochemistry.

2. **Functional studies of granulocytes and monocytes:** chemotaxis (Boyden chamber), phagocytosis, bactericidal capacity, nitroblue of tetrazolium reduction, myeloperoxidase activity, CD18 expression.

3. **Studies of humoral immunity:** serum immunoglobulins (Igs) (IgG, IgA, IgM, IgE, IgG, subclasses), isohemagglutinins (not helpful in blood type AB patients), complement levels, components of the complement cascade, levels of specific antibodies, e.g., IgG antivaccine levels: pneumococcus, tetanus, and diphtheria (depends on immunization history). In vivo studies can be done by immunizing with specific antigens (e.g., tetanus toxoid). Ig synthesis is tested in vitro by incubating B-lymphocytes with certain mitogens.

4. **Studies of cellular immunity** (lymphocyte subpopulations, *see* Item 1).
   – *In vitro:* stimulation of lymphocytes with mitogens and antigens, production of cytokines such as interleukin (IL)-2 or granulocyte-macrophage colony-stimulating factor, cytotoxic activity of T-cells, activity of natural killer (NK) cells, antibody-dependent cellular cytotoxicity activity. Measurements of T-cell effector cytokine production.
   – *In vivo:* skin tests (purified protein derivative [PPD], tetanus, streptokinase, *Candida*, and other antigens). Sensitization with dinitrochlorobenzol.

5. **Further studies:** sedimentation rate, total serum protein, serum electrophoresis, complement factors (total complement, CH50), classical and alternate pathway, global tests of complement (if complement defect is suspected).

2. CONGENITAL IMMUNODEFICIENCIES

Congenital immunodeficiencies are subdivided into the following:
- Defects of the phagocytic system (*see* Table 1).
- Defects of combined immunodeficiencies (*see* Table 2).
- Defects of humoral immunity (Ig synthesis) (*see* Table 3).
- Defects of cellular immunity (*see* Table 4).
- Defects of complement components (*see* Table 5).

Most congenital immunodeficiencies manifest themselves within the first 2 months of life. A defect of humoral immunity often becomes apparent several months later when Igs transferred via the placenta disappear. Tables 1–4 also indicate the clinical features and the treatment of these immunodeficiency states. The group of complement deficiencies (C1–C9) has autosomal-recessive inheritance and, in some cases, is associated with frequent infections. Some patients with complement defects suffer from autoimmune disorders. The majority of the congenital immunodeficiencies have autosomal- or X-linked-recessive inheritance. Only four congenital immunodeficiencies appear to have dominant inheritance: isolated congenital asplenia, hyper-IgE syndrome, isolated chronic

Table 1

Congenital Defects of the Phagocytic System

Disease	Defect	Symptoms	Treatment
Chronic granulomatous disease	Defect of bactericidal capacity (oxidative metabolism)	Abscess forming infections	Symptomatic, interferon γ
Defect of myeloperoxidase	Enzyme defect	Asymptomatic or frequent infections with *Candida*	No treatment or antimycotic
Defect of adhesion molecules	Chemotaxis, phagocytosis	Frequent bacterial infections, sepsis	Symptomatic
Chediak–Higashi syndrome	Giant granules in neutrophils, functional defect	Severe bacterial infections	Symptomatic or bone marrow transplant (BMT)
Hyper-IgE syndrome (multisystem disorder)	Chemotaxis	Cutaneous infections, candidiasis	Symptomatic
Reticular dysgenesis	Defect of hematopoietic stem cell	Lethal within first 3 mo	BMT (?)

Table 2
Congenital Defects of the B- and T-Cell Systems (Combined Immunodeficiency)

Disease	Defect	Symptoms	Treatment
Severe combined immunodeficiency	B- and T-cells	Severe intestinal and pulmonary infections	BMT, infusions of ADA (gene therapy; *see also* Chapter 2)
Hyper-IgM syndrome	CD40-ligand defective	Pyogenic infections, lymphoproliferative syndrome	Symptomatic
Defect of major histocompatibility complex expression	Transcription	Severe infections	BMT
Ataxia telangiectasia	Cellular immunity (IgA, IgE deficiency) (defective *ATM* gene, cell cycle regulation, and DNA repair defective)	Neurological disturbances, lymphatic malignancies	Symptomatic

BMT, bone marrow transplantation; ADA, adenosine deaminase; Ig, immunoglobulin.

Table 3
Congenital Defects of Humoral Immunity

Disease	Defect	Symptoms	Treatment
X-linked agammaglobulinemia (type Bruton)	No mature B-cells present, T-cell defect	Relapsing infections of sinuses and bronchi, diarrhea	Immunoglobulins (Igs)
Common variable immunodeficiencies (manifestation often after puberty)	Heterogeneous, usually in B-cells	Pyogenic infections, autoimmune disorders, malignancies	Igs
Transient immunoglobulin deficiency of newborns	Delayed synthesis	Infections	Symptomatic
IgA deficiency	IgA synthesis defective	Gastrointestinal disturbances, anaphylactic reactions to transfusions	Symptomatic

Table 4
Congenital Defects of Cellular Immunity (T-Cell System)

Disease	Defect	Symptoms	Treatment
Di George syndrome (thymic hypoplasia, cardiac malformations, impaired development	Cellular immunity	Abscess forming infections, hypocalcemia, malignancies	Transplantation of fetal thymus, bone marrow transplant (BMT)
Purine nucleoside phosphorylase deficiency	Cellular immunity	Variable, infections (symptoms start between 3 and 18 mo)	BMT, enzyme replacement
Wiskott–Aldrich syndrome	Cellular immunity	Infections, thrombocytopenia, eczema, low immunoglobulin M	BMT

Table 5
Congenital Defects of Complement Components

Disease	Inheritance/Defect	Presentation	Laboratory findings
C1 deficiency	Autosomal recessive, nonfunctional, or absent protein/1p36.3, 12p13	Pyogenic (neisserial) infections, SLE-like syndromes	Abnormal total hemolytic complement
C1 inhibitor deficiency	Autosomal dominant/11q11	Physical trauma-induced hereditary angioedema	Nonfunctional or diminished C1 inhibitor levels
Factor I, H, D, properdin deficiency	Autosomal recessive (properdin is X-linked)/ factor I-4q25, H-1q32, D-?, Properdin-Xp11.4	Pyogenic (neisserial infections, urticaria, immune complex disease; H: hemolytic uremic syndrome)	Abnormal TH50, AH50, properdin levels
C2 deficiency	6p21.3	50% asymptomatic; pyogenic infections, vasculitides (SLE, HSP)	
C3 deficiency	Autosomal recessive/ 19p13.3	Pyogenic (neisserial infections, urticaria, immune complex disease)	Low C3 levels
C4 deficiency	Autosomal recessive/ 6p21.3	SLE, CVID, IgA deficiency, auto-immune disease	Low C4 levels

SLE, systemic lupus erythematosus; HSP, Henoch-Schonlein purpura; CVID, common variable immunodeficiency; IgA, immunoglobulin A.

mucocutaneous candidiasis, and Di George syndrome (DGS; which is associated with deletions on chromosome 22q11.2 and may involve several genes). Several newly described immunodeficiency syndromes have autosomal-dominant inheritance. The pathogenesis of these and other syndromes was elucidated recently. Isolated congenital asplenia is often asymptomatic in early childhood and manifests itself by sudden overwhelming infections. The diagnosis of asplenia can be made by ultrasound showing the absence of a spleen and peripheral blood smears showing Howell-Jolly bodies. In the WHIM syndrome (warts, hypo-gamma-globulinemia, infections, and myelokathexis), patients have an abnormality of the chemokine receptor CXCR4. Patients with WHIM syndrome suffer from common bacterial infections and display a defect in the maintenance of memory B-cells. Both in the partial interferon gamma receptor 1 (IFNγR1) deficiency and in the partial signal transducer and activator (STAT)1 deficiency, patients suffer from infections by mycobacteria and *Salmonella*. Deletions or missense mutations of the respective genes lead to abnormal signal transduction. Anhydrotic ectodermal dysplasia with immunodeficiency has X-linked inheritance in most cases. Patients with this condition suffer from severe infections with Gram-positive bacteria. Recently, the responsible gene was identified as NEMO/IKKγ, which leads to impaired NF-κB activation in response to various receptors. As described in Table 3, in Bruton's agammaglobulinemia, no mature B-cells are present. Bruton's agammaglobulinemia is caused by mutations in the gene encoding Bruton tyrosine kinase.

2.1. Severe Combined Immunodeficiencies

Patients with severe combined immunodeficiencies (SCIDs) exhibit profound disturbance in function of both T- and B-cells (*see* Table 2). They develop recurrent, severe, life-threatening infections (bacterial, viral, fungal), intractable diarrhea, and failure to thrive in early infancy. Opportunistic infections are common. Approximately 20 defective genes have now been identified as associated with SCIDs, classified according to the specific mutation present, the associated lymphocyte phenotype, and type of inheritance. Early diagnosis and immune reconstitution by stem cell transplant (SCT) is critical.

X-linked form (termed X-linked SCID or XSCID), which is due to a mutation in the *IL2RG* gene, is the most common form of SCID. It is present in 44–50% of cases in the United States. This mutation leads to an abnormality in the "common" gamma chain (γ_c) receptor shared by several cytokine receptors (including interleukin [IL]-2, IL-4, IL-7, IL-9, IL-15, and IL-21). The lack of γ_c leads to early arrest of T-cell and natural killer (NK)-cell development and to the production of immature B-cells. The lymphoid tissue and thymus develop poorly. SCT without myeloablation is indicated because the disease is lethal without therapy.

Gene therapy for XSCID is currently on hold, as a result of leukemia developing in two of these patients (*see* Chapter 2). Patients with an autosomal recessive mutation in the α-chain of the IL-7 receptor also have severe immunodeficiency; however, both NK- and B-cell numbers are normal in these patients. An autosomal recessive mutation in the JAK3 enzyme, a tyrosine kinase associated with γ_c required for signal transduction, lead to a similar phenotype in 8% of patients with SCID.

Adenosine deaminase (ADA) deficiency is the most common form of SCID with autosomal recessive inheritance, seen in approx 15% of patients with SCID (*see* Table 3). This and another milder and very rare disorder, purine nucleoside phosphorylase (PNP) deficiency, are the only disorders of nucleotide synthesis resulting in immunodeficiency. These purine salvage pathway defects lead to increasing lymphopenia due to metabolic self-poisoning of these cells by byproducts (5'-triphosphates) of deoxyadenosine and deoxyguanosine, usually within the first few months of life, and about 15% are symptomatic later in childhood. ADA activity of less than 2% of control or mutations in both alleles of ADA must be present in order to diagnose this condition. Skeletal abnormalities (cupping and flaring of the costochondral junctions) are seen in 50% of patients with ADA deficiency, and there may also be associated hepatic, renal, and neurological abnormalities. Enzyme replacement therapy with percutaneous endoscopic gastrostomy (PEG)–bovine ADA can lead to partial immune reconstitution. Red blood cell (RBC) transfusions help patients with ADA deficiency (and *not* with PNP deficiency), as RBCs are rich in ADA. Gene therapy has been successful.

Defects in the recombinase-activating genes, *RAG1* and *RAG2* leads to an early arrest of lymphocyte development. Thirty percent of SCID patients manifesting *RAG1* or *RAG2* mutations account for the majority of patients with autosomal recessive type T(–)B(–)NK(+) SCID. During the process of Ig and T-cell receptor gene recombination in differentiating lymphocytes, the RAG proteins introduce DNA double-stranded breaks, which are repaired via nonhomologous end joining. Clinical manifestations are similar to those seen in XSCID. Omenn syndrome (OS) is caused by a partial loss of function in RAG1 or RAG2, and has an early onset associated with severe infections, diarrhea, erythroderma, lymphadenopathy, and hepatosplenomegaly. T-cell function is markedly defective in OS; however, increased IgE levels and eosinophilia are characteristic of this syndrome.

2.2. Antibody Deficiencies

2.2.1. Defects of B-Cell Maturation

Abnormalities in B-cell maturation and function result in impaired Ig production and antibody deficiency. This leads to recurrent bacterial infections in the first year of life, including otitis, sinusitis, and pneumonia, and these may manifest soon after the loss of maternal IgG antibodies. The respiratory tract, skin, and gastrointestinal tract are the common sites of infection. Patients with significant defects in B-cell development require Ig replacement and sometimes prophylactic antibiotics.

2.2.2. X-LINKED AGAMMAGLOBULINEMIA

X-linked agammaglobulinemia (XLA) is the most severe of the antibody deficiency syndromes (*see* Table 3) and is due to a mutation in the gene for a cytoplasmic (Bruton's) tyrosine kinase (BTK). It was described in 1993. Mutations of BTK impair B-cell receptor signaling and lead to the maturational arrest of B-cells. More than 400 different mutations in BTK have been described, most resulting in absent BTK protein due to unstable BTK mRNA or protein; 30% of these mutations are sporadic. Most patients with XLA have profoundly decreased peripheral B-cells, virtually undetectable serum Ig, and hypoplastic or absent lymphoid tissue. T-cell numbers and function in XLA are normal, although severe viral infections, such as with enteroviruses, may result in meningoencephalitis. Patients with XLA are exempt from autoantibody-driven autoimmune disease. The median age at presentation for patients with sporadic XLA was 26 mo in a recent study, whereas the age at presentation in patients with familial disease is more variable. Male patients have less than 2% CD19+ B-cells and at least one of the following criteria is required for definitive diagnosis: (1) mutation in the BTK gene; (2) absent BTK mRNA on Northern blot analysis of neutrophils or monocytes; (3) absent BTK protein in monocytes or platelets; (4) maternal cousins, uncles, or nephews with less than 2% CD19+ B-cells.

2.3. B-Cell Defects of Unknown Cause

2.3.1. COMMON VARIABLE IMMUNODEFICIENCY

Common variable immunodeficiency (CVID) is a heterogeneous group of distinctly separate disorders resulting in hypogammaglobulinemia with sporadic inheritance in most cases (*see* Table 3). The prevalence is approx 1 in 30,000 to 50,000 individuals. Diagnosis of CVID requires decreased Ig of at least two isotypes (serum IgG, IgA, and/or IgM reduced by two or more standard deviations from the normal mean) with impaired specific antibody formation. Multiple defects in B-cell maturation and differentiation as well as T-cell abnormalities have been associated with CVID. However, lymphocyte subsets are usually preserved. The mean age at diagnosis is 29 yr for males and 33 yr for females, although symptoms start 5 to 10 yr prior to diagnosis. It is a diagnosis of exclusion. Patients present like XLA, with recurrent bacterial infections, most notably sinopulmonary; 78% experience at least one pneumonia prior to diagnosis. Chronic enteroviral infections are also seen. Autoimmune disease (particularly idiopathic thrombocytopenia and autoimmune hemolytic anemia) and malignancy (most frequently lymphoreticular) are increased, with frequencies of 22 and 8%, respectively. Chronic inflammatory diseases (e.g., chronic lung disease, hepatitis, granulomas, inflammatory bowel disease), malabsorption, and autoimmune syndrome may also occur in a significant percentage of patients.

2.3.2. IgA Deficiency

Isolated IgA deficiency (IGAD) (*see* Table 3) is the most common primary immunodeficiency of humans, with both IgA1 and IgA2 subclasses being equally affected. The rate of prevalence varies from 1:400 to 1:3000 with some studies. Prevalence of 1:700 in whites and 1:18,500 in Japanese in one study suggests population genetics differences. It results from unknown defects causing the failure of B-cells to differentiate into IgA-secreting plasma cells and is defined by a serum IgA of less than 7 mg/dL with normal serum IgG and IgM in a patient older than 4 yr of age. Specific antibody production following immunization is normal. The majority of patients are asymptomatic; however, some have increased susceptibility to sinopulmonary infections. Those with severe infections are more likely to have an associated IgG subclass deficiency (IGGSD), particularly IgG2 and IgG4. Gastrointestinal diseases (especially giardiasis and celiac disease), atopic diseases, and a number of autoimmune diseases occur with increased frequency in patients with IGAD. Unless significant IgG antibody defects are found, Ig replacement is not necessary; prophylactic antibiotics may be helpful.

The specific defects leading to the development of IGGSD, transient hypogammaglobulinemia of infancy (THI), and specific antibody deficiency with normal immunoglobulins (SADNI) remain unknown. These may result in recurrent bacterial infections of the upper and lower respiratory tracts. In IGGSD, especially in IgG2-deficient patients, there is an increased risk of infection from encapsulated bacteria (e.g., *Streptococcus pneumoniae* or *Hemophilus influenzae*). Infants with THI have a delay in the onset of Ig synthesis; however, spontaneous recovery occurs between 18 and 36 mo of age. In SADNI, specific antibody production following immunization with protein vaccines or, more commonly, to unconjugated polysaccharide-based vaccines is impaired even though serum Igs and IgG subclass concentrations are normal. Immunization with newer protein-conjugate vaccines may help in reducing infections in all of these disorders. The use of prophylactic antibiotics and Ig replacement may also be required in IGGSD but more rarely, as a temporary measure, in THI.

2.4. Cellular Deficiencies

2.4.1. T-Cell Activation Defects—Defects of the T-Cell Antigen Receptor

Several mutations have also been associated with defects in signaling through the T-cell antigen receptor (TCR). CD45 is a transmembrane tyrosine phosphatase critical for both T- and B-cell antigen receptor transduction. Deficiency in this surface protein results in a phenotype similar to that of most other patients with SCID. CD3 deficiencies (due to mutations in the γ and ε chains) result in defective expression of the TCR–CD3 complex, and have clinical manifestations that may range from mild to severe. Patients with zeta chain-associated protein (ZAP)-70 (tyrosine kinase) deficiency have profound CD8[+] lymphocytopenia; although CD4[+]/CD8[+]-double positive cells are present in the thymic cortex of these patients, only CD4, and not CD8, single-positive cells appear in the thymic medulla, suggesting a selective block of positive selection of CD8[+] cells. As a consequence of the signaling defect, there are normal or elevated numbers of CD4[+] cells that are defective and fail to differentiate.

2.4.2. CYTOKINE AND SIGNALING DEFECTS LEADING TO MYCOBACTERIAL INFECTIONS

Mutations in five genes (*IFNGR1, IFNGR2, STAT1, IL12B,* and *IL12RB1*) cause Mendelian susceptibility to mycobacterial infection (MSMD), a rare clinical syndrome that leads to increased susceptibility to nontuberculous mycobacteria in the first few years of life. These patients also develop disseminated disease following vaccination with bacillus Calmette–Guerin, and increased rate of infections with nontyphoid *Salmonella*. In familial cases, an autosomal recessive inheritance is observed. All of these defects affect the cytokine pathway involved with IL-12 and IFN-γ production, and granuloma formation appears impaired. Antimycobacterial prophylaxis is required, and in the more severe forms of MSMD, bone marrow transplant (BMT) or SCT may be necessary.

2.5. Field Defects That Lead to T-Cell Dysfunction

2.5.1. DI GEORGE SYNDROME

Deletions in chromosome 22q11.2 are seen in most patients with DGS (deletions of 10p13 reported in some patients); it is associated with abnormal development of the third and fourth pharyngeal pouches during embryogenesis (*see* Table 4). Conotruncal cardiac defects (in 50% of patients with DGS), thymic aplasia (or hypoplasia), and hypoparathyroidism are common. Other clinical features include dysmorphic facies, cleft lip/palate, neurodevelopmental delay, and autoimmunity. Complete aplasia of the thymus is associated with a SCID-like phenotype, although varied severity of hypoplasia of the thymus and parathyroids is more common (partial DGS). Increased susceptibility to viral or opportunistic infections is seen with T-lymphocytopenia, and immune function may often improve in time. Fluorescence *in situ* hybridization (FISH) analysis is used to diagnose DGS. Supportive care is usually adequate enough for those patients with mild immunodeficiency; however, severe cases (complete DGS) have required BMT or thymic transplants.

2.6. Combined Deficiencies

2.6.1. WISKOTT–ALDRICH SYNDROME

The classic triad of eczema, thrombocytopenia, and immunodeficiency manifests in the first year of life with bloody diarrhea as the presenting feature (*see* Table 4). Autoimmunity, vasculitis, and risk of lymphoreticular (Epstein-Barr virus [EBV]-induced) malignancy are significantly increased. The platelets are small and dysfunctional, resultant excessive bleeding can lead to significant morbidity and mortality in Wiskott–Aldrich syndrome (WAS). This X-linked disorder is due to a defect in the WAS protein (WASP). Mutations in WASP have also been found in patients with X-linked thrombocytopenia (XLT) and X-linked neutropenia. Patients with XLT also have thrombocytopenia with small platelets, but they do not share the other clinical findings that are observed in classic WAS. Patients with WAS often have poor specific antibody production and progressive lymphopenia. Hematopoietic SCT is the only cure for classic WAS and is the treatment of choice in presence of a matched sibling donor. Ig replacement and prophylactic antibiotics may suffice in more mild cases. Splenectomy may be required for uncontrollable bleeding and by itself can prolong lifespan from 5 to 25 yr. IL-2 infusions have been helpful in some cases.

2.7. Defects in Pathways of T-Cell Death and Regulation

2.7.1. AUTOIMMUNE LYMPHOPROLIFERATIVE SYNDROME

The autoimmune lymphoproliferative syndrome (ALPS) is due to abnormal survival of lymphocytes leading to massive proliferation of these cells as a result of a defect in the Fas–Fas ligand cell death pathway. There is an autosomal dominant inheritance pattern in most families with mutations found in the Fas-encoding gene (*TNFRSF6*, or tumor necrosis factor receptor superfamily member 6). Altered lymphocyte apoptosis leads to massive lymphadenopathy and splenomegaly in infants and children that may regress over time. Unusual or severe infections are unlikely, but autoimmunity and lymphoreticular malignancies are encountered. Diagnosis of ALPS necessitates all of the following: (1) chronic accumulation of nonmalignant lymphoid cells; (2) defective lymphocyte apoptosis in vitro; and (3) the presence of 1% or more double-negative T-cells in peripheral blood or the presence of double-negative T-cells in lymphoid tissue.

Immunosuppressive treatment is required for autoimmune manifestations in ALPS, and BMT has been successful in patients with severe disease.

2.7.2. X-Linked Lymphoproliferative Disease

XLP was first reported in 1975 in male members of a large kindred who died following primary EBV infection due to an abnormal and uncontrolled immune response. The clinical manifestations that characterize most patients with XLP include fulminant infectious mononucleosis, malignant lymphoma, and dysgammaglobulinemia. In the first two forms, XLP is generally fatal in the first decade of life. Lymphocyte function is generally normal in patients with XLP prior to EBV infection. Aggressive treatment of EBV infection and related complications is necessary, but definitive treatment requires SCT before development of typical XLP manifestations (*see also* Chapter 18).

2.8. Defects of T-Cell Regulation

2.8.1. Autoimmune Polyendocrinopathy–Candidiasis–Ectodermal Dystrophy

Multiple autoimmune endocrinopathies, severe and recurrent chronic mucocutaneous candidiasis, and ectodermal dystrophies occur in this disorder and symptoms often start in early childhood. This disorder is also referred to as autoimmune polyglandular syndrome type 1 (APS-1). Autosomal recessive inheritance is found in autoimmune polyendocrinopathy–candidiasis–ectodermal dystrophy (APECED) with a defect in the autoimmune regulator (*AIRE*) gene. Autoantibody-induced polyendocrinopathy include hypothyroidism, adrenal failure, hypoparathyroidism, insulin-dependent diabetes mellitus, and gonadal failure. Ectodermal dystrophies include alopecia, vitiligo, and keratopathy. Antifungal prophylaxis and management of associated autoimmune complications are important in treatment.

2.9. Defects of DNA Repair

2.9.1. Ataxia Telangiectasia

This autosomal-recessive disorder (*see* Table 2) includes progressive ataxia followed by oculocutaneous telangiectasias, sensitivity of cells to radiation damage being the hallmark of this disease. The ataxia is usually evident in the second year of life after the child begins to walk. Recurrent sinopulmonary infections are seen ultimately leading to early death and a median life span of 20 yr, although in some cases the immunodeficiency may be mild. Patients with ataxia telangiectasia (AT) have an increased incidence (1% per year) of malignancy (85% are lymphoreticular), which is frequently fatal. Additional features of AT are hypogonadism, insulin-resistant diabetes mellitus, and skin abnormalities (atrophy and pigmentary changes). The AT-mutated (*ATM*) gene product was first identified as the cause of this disorder in 1995, and more than 400 mutations have subsequently been identified. This protein is important in the detection of double-stranded breaks in DNA, and the failure to correctly repair breaks in DNA and delayed induction of p53 (a protein that halts cell cycle until DNA damage is repaired) leads to dysregulated recombination, cell division in cells (with unrepaired DNA), and apoptosis. As a result, absence of the *ATM* gene leads to abnormalities in both lymphocyte function and development. Progressive lymphopenia is common (with selective CD4$^+$ lymphopenia), with decreased serum IgA, IgG2, and IgE levels noted in many patients. Serum α-fetoprotein (AFP) levels are also elevated. Supportive care and antibiotic therapy are recommended, as is close monitoring for the development of malignancy. Patients with AT respond poorly to treatment regimens that include ionizing radiation and certain chemotherapies (e.g., topoisomerase inhibitors), so modification of standard protocols is required.

2.9.2. NIJMEGEN BREAKAGE SYNDROME

Similarly to patients with AT, patients with Nijmegen breakage syndrome (NBS) have chromosome fragility. It is transmitted with autosomal-recessive inheritance. Patients with NBS are also immunodeficient and radiosensitive, and have an increased risk of malignancy (particularly lymphoma). This disorder is associated with short stature, microcephaly, and mental retardation, and is more common in eastern Europeans. The immunological and laboratory manifestations of this disorder are also similar to those seen in AT; however, AFP levels are normal in NBS.

2.10. Congenital Defects of Complement Components

The complement system has 20 serum proteins, 5 complement receptors, and has varied distribution among leukocytes and most cell membranes. The manifestations of their defects is briefly discussed in Table 5.

3. ACQUIRED OR SECONDARY IMMUNODEFICIENCIES

Acquired immunodeficiencies are seen not only in HIV infection, but also during many hematological disorders. The Ig synthesis is decreased in low-grade malignant lymphomas, especially in chronic lymphocytic leukemia and in multiple myeloma resulting in hypogammaglobulinemia and frequent infections. In patients with a paraprotein, as, for example, in multiple myeloma, the synthesis of normal polyclonal Igs is inhibited. The normal T- and B-cell immunity is defective or delayed for some time after the transplantation of bone marrow or stem cells. Nonhematological causes of secondary immunodeficiency are malnutrition, protein-losing enteropathy, diabetes, and alcoholism. A disturbance of cellular and humoral immunity is a frequent side effect of the treatment with corticosteroids, immunosuppressive drugs like cyclosporine A, tacrolimus, and a number of cytostatic drugs. The immunity is also transiently defective during radiation therapy and some viral infections.

At present, there are only limited possibilities of stimulating the immune system to fight malignancies or bacterial or viral infections. An exception is the treatment with Ig preparations of patients with hypogammaglobulinemia. Patients with leukemias or lymphomas, or who had SCT or BMT, should not be immunized with live vaccines because of the risk of a disseminated infection. Although it has been shown in healthy persons that the efficacy of inactivated vaccines is decreased, these vaccines should be given to immunosuppressed individuals if the clinical situation makes it necessary.

4. HEMATOLOGICAL ASPECTS OF AIDS

AIDS is caused by HIV, a human retrovirus. Worldwide, at least 60 million people are infected with HIV. Despite public health education, in the United States, currently 40,000 new cases of HIV infection are observed annually. There are two subtypes of HIV: HIV-1 is the most common type, HIV-2 is less common and is observed in some cases in Africa and Europe. The infection with HIV proceeds in three stages (I–III) and categories (A–C): the initial primary infection may be mononucleosis-like; later, the infection is commonly asymptomatic (category A). These patients may also present with lymphadenopathy. In category B, patients have symptoms with AIDS-defining illnesses (*see* Table 5). In category C, AIDS-defining illnesses are observed (a list of 23 such diseases as defined by the Centers for Disease Control and Prevention [CDC] is listed in Table 5). The interval between categories A and C may be months to many years. Because of the effective treatment with antiretroviral drugs, some patients will never progress from category A to B or C. For epidemiological purposes, three stages of HIV infection have been defined. CD4 counts also enter into this definition of stages. HIV is transmitted by homosexual and heterosexual intercourse, by needle-sharing among drug addicts, by occupational exposure (in the case of medical personnel), and perinatally; in the past, the virus was also transmitted by contaminated blood products. Prognosis of the HIV infection has improved in recent years as a result of a combination treatments with inhibitors of reverse transcriptase and proteases.

The HIV virus is a retrovirus, with RNA encoding three groups of structural genes (*gag, pol,* and *env*). HIV infects CD4$^+$ helper lymphocytes through a cell surface receptor. There is a specific interaction of gp120 envelope glycoprotein with the CD4 molecule and members of the chemokine receptor family (usually CCR5 or CXR4). Some cells are lysed on infection, whereas in other cells, the virus remains latent until the cells are activated. The long-term consequence of

Table 6
Clinical Categories and Stages of the HIV Infection[a]

CD4 category (counts/μL)	Clinical category A	Clinical category B	Clinical category C
Laboratory and Clinical Categories			
1. ≥500	A1	B1	C1
2. 200–499	A2	B2	C2
3. <200	A3	B3	C3
Stages			
1. ≥500	Stage I	Stage I	Stage III
2. 200–499	Stage I	Stage II	Stage III
3. <200	Stage II	Stage II	Stage III

[a]According to the 1993 revised classification of the Centers for Disease Control.

Definitions of clinical categories: **A:** Asymptomatic HIV infection, persistent generalized lymphadenopathy, acute (primary) HIV infection with accompanying illness or history of acute HIV infection. **B:** Symptomatic conditions, not included in category C, that are related to HIV infection and a defect in cell-mediated immunity or conditions that are complicated by HIV infection. Examples are bacillary angiomatosis, oropharyngeal candidiasis, persistent vulvovaginal candidiasis, cervical dysplasia or carcinoma *in situ*, constitutional symptoms, oral hairy leukoplakia, *Herpes zoster* in two dermatomes, or relapsed, idiopathic thrombocytopenic purpura, listeriosis, pelvic inflammatory disease, peripheral neuropathy. **C:** *Pneumocystis carinii* pneumonia, toxoplasma encephalitis, candida infection of esophagus, lungs, trachea, chronic *H. simplex* ulcers, bronchitis, pneumonia, esophagitis, cytomegalovirus retinitis, relapsing salmonella septicemias, relapsing pneumonias, extrapulmonary cryptoccocal infections, chronic intestinal cryptosporidiasis, chronic intestinal infection with isospora belli, coccidiomycosis, disseminated or extrapulmonary histoplasmosis, tuberculosis, infections by *Mycobacterium avium* or *M. kansasii* (disseminated or extrapulmonary), Kaposi sarcomas, malignant lymphomas, invasive cervix carcinoma, HIV encephalopathy, progressive multifocal leukencephalopathy, wasting syndrome.

HIV infection is a progressive depletion of CD4$^+$ cells, although other cells, such as antigen-presenting cells, neural cells, and hematopoietic progenitor cells, may also become infected with HIV. During HIV infection, the cellular immune defense is progressively and irreversibly lost. Chronic B-cell stimulation often leads to a polyclonal hyper-gammaglobulinemia. The absolute number of CD4 cells (per μL blood) is an established prognostic factor for the complications and progression of HIV infection. The diagnosis of an HIV infection is made by demonstrating antibodies against HIV antigens. The screening test is done with ELISA techniques.

Positive or unclear results are confirmed by Western blot, which detects specific antibodies against viral proteins (e.g., p24, p41 or p120/160). ELISA results become positive 4–8 wk after the initial infection. Other tests (p24 antigen, polymerase chain reaction, or viral culture) may be positive somewhat earlier or later.

The signs and symptoms of HIV infection according to the category of the disease are described in Table 6. Many patients with HIV infection have hematological manifestations. During the acute infection, a mononucleosis-like syndrome is often found. At this stage, fever, which lasts a few days or weeks, lymph node swelling, anorexia, and lethargy are typical. Other patients have a mild meningoencephalitis or are asymptomatic. An atypical lymphocytosis in the peripheral blood can be seen in about half the patients.

A thrombocytopenia is frequent in HIV-infected patients (3–8% in early stages, 30–50% in AIDS). Pathogenic factors are a decrease in production and an increase in platelet destruction, due in some cases to antiplatelet antibodies. In severe symptomatic cases, steroids or high-dose Ig are as effective as in idiopathic thrombocytopenic purpura without HIV infection. Steroids, however, may further decrease cellular immunity. A splenectomy may be indicated in some refractory cases. Some patients improve with antiviral treatment. A thrombotic-thrombocytopenic purpura developing in some HIV-infected patients can be treated similarly as that diagnosed in non-HIV-infected patients (plasma infusions or plasma exchange).

Many patients with HIV infection are leukopenic (granulocytopenia and/or lymphopenia). This may be due to the infection itself but may also be due to drugs used to treat HIV-infected patients. Examples are zidovudine, cotrimoxazole, gancyclovir, and pentamidine, among others. The leukopenia of HIV-infected patients responds well to colony-stimulating factors, such as granulocyte colony-stimulating factor.

In advanced stages of HIV infection, anemia is frequent. It may be due to disturbed maturation of erythroblasts, but is also caused by drugs like zidovudine. Especially in cases of low serum erythropoietin levels (<500 IU/L), the anemia of patients with AIDS responds well to erythropoietin. Some rare cases have anemia due to a persistent infection with parvovirus B19.

HIV-associated lymphomas are a consequence of the depressed immunity and belong (according to the CDC classification) to the AIDS-defining illnesses. These non-Hodgkin's lymphomas (NHLs) are often extranodal (about 25% with bone marrow involvement) and aggressive. Histologically, most NHLs in patients with AIDS are high-grade (Burkitt's lymphomas, Burkitt-like lymphomas, diffuse-large cell lymphomas) and have a B-cell phenotype. The incidence of NHLs in patients with AIDS has increased (up to 25% of all NHLs in the United States are HIV-related). A reason is the longer life expectancy of HIV-infected patients due to better antiviral treatment and improved treatment of opportunistic infections.

Those lymphoma patients in good general condition should undergo combination chemotherapy while continuing antiretroviral therapy. This approach has dramatically improved the complete remission rate and survival of patients with HIV-related NHLs (*see* Chapter 15). Hodgkin's lymphoma is not mentioned in the original definition of AIDS-related conditions, but is also observed more frequently in HIV-infected patients.

The bone marrow in HIV-infected patients often shows megaloblastic and myelodysplastic features. The cellularity is often increased. Common bone marrow findings are megakaryocyte abnormalities with bare megakaryocyte nuclei, giant metamyelocytes, detached nuclear fragments in granulocytes, and gelatinous degeneration (especially in late stages). In the peripheral blood, the granulocytes often show detached nuclear fragments. These changes are reactive and cannot be considered as preleukemic. In some cases, a fibrosis or polymor phic lymphocellular infiltrates are evident. In other cases, pathogens such as mycobacteria, cryptococci, or histoplasma can be demonstrated. A common finding in bone aspirates is a polyclonal plasmacytosis, which is related to the B-cell hyperactivity in HIV-infected patients.

SUGGESTED READING

Bain BJ. The haematological features of HIV-infection. *Br J Haematol* 1997;99:1–8.

Henry DH, Hoxie JA. Hematologic manifestations of AIDS. In: Hoffmann R, Benz EJ, Shattil SJ, et al., eds. *Hematology Basic Principles and Practice*, 4th ed. Philadelphia: Elsevier Churchill Livingstone, 2005:pp. 2585–2612.

Lawrence T, Puel A, Reichenbach J, et al. Autosomal-dominant primary immunodeficiencies. *Curr Op Hematol* 2005;12:22–30.

Bonilla FA, Geha RS. Primary immunodeficiency diseases. In: Nathan DG, Orkin SH, Ginsberg D, et al., eds. *Hematology of Infancy and Childhood*, 6th ed. Philadelphia: WB Saunders, 2003:pp. 1043–1078.

Riminton DS, Limaye S. Primary immunodeficiency diseases in adulthood. *Int Med J* 2004;34: 348–354.

18   Infections Relevant to Hematology

Reinhold Munker, MD

1. INTRODUCTION

In this chapter, several infections are discussed that occur particularly in hematological patients. It is important to recognize these infections, as some of them elicit special changes in hematological parameters. Some viruses have transforming properties. Other infections belong to the group of opportunistic infections common in immunosuppressed patients. The vast group of infections caused by bacteria and fungi is not discussed here, but is covered in Chapter 3 (supportive therapy).

From: *Contemporary Hematology: Modern Hematology, Second Edition*
Edited by: R. Munker, E. Hiller, J. Glass, and R. Paquette © Humana Press Inc., Totowa, NJ

2. INFECTIOUS MONONUCLEOSIS
AND OTHER EPSTEIN-BARR VIRUS SYNDROMES

Infectious mononucleosis is characterized by fever, lymph node swelling, splenomegaly, and pharyngitis and is caused by the Epstein-Barr virus (EBV). In most parts of the world, more than 80% of the adult population has become infected with EBV: in children, the infection is often subclinical, whereas in young adults, the typical signs and symptoms of "glandular fever" or "kissing fever" appear. EBV is a double-stranded DNA virus belonging to the group of herpesviruses that mainly infects B-lymphocytes and epithelial cells. The receptor for EBV on B-lymphocytes was characterized as complement receptor type 2 and has been assigned CD21 in the CD nomenclature. After an infection, EBV persists indefinitely in a small percentage of B-lymphocytes.

EBV-associated malignomas are Burkitt's lymphoma in the tropics and in HIV-infected patients, nasopharyngeal carcinoma, and some cases of Hodgkin's lymphoma and of T-/natural killer (NK) cell lymphoma. In the last few years, an increasing number of EBV-associated lymphomas have been observed in immunosuppressed patients (patients with AIDS and recipients of organ transplants).

The incubation time of infectious mononucleosis is around 4–8 wk; the transmission commonly occurs through the saliva of persons with a latent infection. After a prodromal stage of several days, the disease manifests itself acutely with a generalized, painful lymph node swelling and an exudative pharyngitis or tonsillitis. About 10% of patients have an exanthema; in about half of the patients, an enlarged spleen can be felt. A hepatomegaly, sometimes associated with jaundice, can also be observed. More severe complications can be expected in 1–5% of adults: an acute obstruction of the upper airways can occur as a complication of tonsillitis; encephalitis, meningoencephalitis, or Guillain-Barré syndrome can occur as complications of the CNS; in addition, hepatitis, myocarditis, and, on rare occasions, splenic rupture are possible complications.

A leukocytosis of 10,000–30,000 white blood cells/μL is a characteristic change in the blood parameters observed after the second week. The differential count shows more than 70% atypical cells with a large nucleus, rough chromatin, and basophilic cytoplasm, sometimes with azure granulations (*see* Fig. 18.1 and Color Plate 23). These cells correspond to a reactive proliferation of CD8 T-lymphocytes and contribute to the elimination of infected B-lymphocytes. Occasionally, these cells are misdiagnosed as blasts of an acute leukemia.

A specific diagnosis is possible with the demonstration of antibodies to EBV. Antibodies against capsid antigens (VCA) become positive within the first disease phase. Immunoglobulin (Ig)M antibodies decrease in titer after 4–6 wk, whereas IgG antibodies remain positive indefinitely. Antibodies against early antigens (EA) and Epstein-Barr nuclear antigens (EBNA) become positive some-

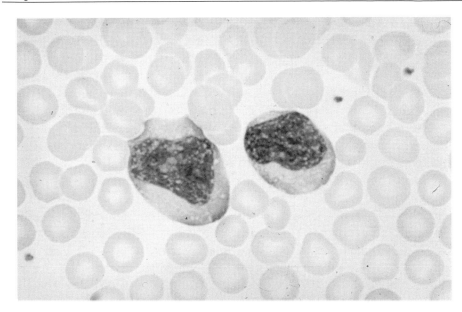

Fig. 18.1. Infectious mononucleosis. Large lymphoid cells with an irregular nucleus and clear cytoplasm.

what later and also remain positive permanently. High-titer antibodies are often produced within a few days in adults, whereas in children the serology becomes positive only after a certain delay. Several fast reactions take advantage of heterophilic antibodies (e.g., directed against horse erythrocytes) that are formed in the context of a nonspecific immune stimulation. Heterophilic antibodies are seen in 80–90% of adults with infectious mononucleosis and are specific in more than 95% of cases. Besides the atypical lymphoid proliferation, a neutropenia or a thrombocytopenia is occasionally observed. A mild hemolysis is only rarely seen in infectious mononucleosis.

Infectious mononucleosis generally heals within 1 or 2 wk after the start of acute symptoms without leaving sequelae. In some cases, weakness persists for a few weeks. In complicated cases, steroids are recommended. The value of a virostatic treatment with acyclovir has not been proven.

The differential diagnosis of the disease caused by EBV includes syndromes resembling infectious mononucleosis, which are caused by other agents such as cytomegalovirus (CMV), HIV, or other viruses and *Toxoplasma gondii*.

Rarely, EBV causes atypical lymphoid proliferation, for example, in children with an X-linked lymphoproliferative syndrome (XLPS). In these children, an uncontrolled proliferation of lymphoid cells develops in the context of immune deficiency and leads to death as a result of multiorgan failure. This condition is generally fatal and happens when male offspring of female carriers of the XLPS mutation are infected with EBV. The underlying defect is the functional absence of the serum alkaline phosphatase (SAP) molecule. In patients with AIDS or in recipients of organ or stem cell transplants, polyclonal and oligoclonal lymphoid proliferation can occur, which are caused by EBV and frequently progress into malignant lymphomas. This condition has also been named EBV-associated B-cell lymphoproliferative disease or posttransplant lymphoproliferative disease. Regression could be achieved by a reduction of the immune suppression. Some complete responses were observed using the monoclonal antibody rituximab. EBV-specific cytotoxic T-lymphocytes from stem cell donors show promise for the treatment of posttransplant lymphoproliferative disease after allogeneic transplants. Anecdotal reports show some activity of acyclovir. A further rare condition is chronic active EBV infection. Vaccines are currently under development for EBV-associated disorders and malignancies. There is a low risk of transmitting EBV by blood transfusion; however, at present, there are insufficient data as to whether this risk can be further reduced by depleting leukocytes from blood products with special filters (*see* Chapter 22).

3. CMV INFECTIONS

CMV belongs to a group of herpesviruses and can cause a clinical picture similar to infectious mononucleosis in immunocompetent patients: lymph node swelling, fever, and changes in the white cell differential count. Serologically, 40–80% of the adult population has antibodies against CMV as a sign of a previous infection. Most infections have a subclinical course, but occasionally immunocompetent persons may develop a pneumonia, myocarditis, or encephalitis caused by CMV. In most cases, the restitution is faster compared with EBV-mononucleosis. When the acute infection has subsided, the virus persists indefinitely in leukocytes. CMV may cause life-threatening complications in immunosuppressed individuals, for example, in patients with AIDS and after organ transplants (especially lung and bone marrow transplants [BMT]). Approximately 20–50% of patients transplanted with allogeneic bone marrow develop a CMV infection or reactivation, which manifests itself in most cases between 30 and 80 d after transplantation. Risk factors are graft-vs-host reactions, total body irradiation, and the transfer of CMV-positive bone marrow, stem cells, or blood products into a CMV-negative recipient. The infection may remain clinically unapparent or manifest itself as gastroenteritis, unclear fever, or hepatitis. Interstitial pneumonias are the most feared complication of CMV infection and still have a lethality of up to 80%.

The presence of a CMV infection can be proved in biopsates by histological, immunological, and molecular methods. A likely diagnosis can be made if serologically the virus titers increase or if the virus can be isolated from urine or from throat washings.

Therapeutically, the virostatic drug gancyclovir (7.5 mg/kg body weight daily) is given for a 14-d treatment course and may be combined with hyperimmune globulins. Major side effects of gancyclovir are leukocytopenia and thrombocytopenia. After a course of gancyclovir, the drug should be continued at a lower dose for several weeks. An alternative drug is foscarnet, which has a different toxicity profile (renal toxicity, hypocalcemia, neuropathy). Cidofovir is a new antiviral drug with a mechanism of action similar to gancyclovir but that does not require viral enzymes for activation. Cidofovir is administered once weekly as an intravenous infusion for two doses (5 mg/kg) and then as maintenance treatment once every 2 wk. Cidofovir may be active against resistant CMV strains. Common side effects are neutropenia and nephrotoxicity. After allogeneic transplantation involving CMV-seropositive donors or recipients, regular monitoring by an antigen assay or molecular monitoring is indicated. If the patient develops antigenemia, a pre-emptive treatment should be given. This strategy has reduced the transplant-related mortality in CMV-positive patients to that observed in CMV-negative patients, at least for matched related allogeneic transplantation. In some patients treated with this strategy, late relapses (beyond day 100 after transplantation) of CMV antigenemia and disease are observed. The transfusion of CMV-specific cytotoxic T-lymphocytes is an elegant strategy for the prophylaxis or treatment of CMV disease. However, this adoptive immunotherapy is not universally available.

For the prophylaxis of CMV infections, the transfusion of CMV-negative blood products is recommended in CMV-negative transplant recipients. If these are not available, leukocyte-depleted blood products might offer some degree of protection. Ganciclovir has also been shown to be active in the prophylaxis of CMV infections.

4. PARVOVIRUS B19 INFECTIONS

Parvovirus B19 was originally discovered serologically by screening healthy blood donors. The majority of the US population is immune to parvovirus. In children, the virus causes erythema infectiosum (fifth disease). In adults, the infection is often unapparent or causes arthralgias. Parvovirus infections may also be a rare cause of hydrops fetalis. The main hematological relevance of parvovirus infections is that hematopoietic (erythroid) precursor cells may become infected thus leading to transient aplastic crises in patients with hemolytic anemias (examples are thalassemias and sickle cell anemias, but also autoimmune hemolytic anemias). The cellular receptor for parvovirus is globoside, a neutral glycolipid. Globoside is also known as the erythrocyte P antigen. Therefore, rare individuals lacking P are not susceptible to an infection with parvovirus B19. A chronically compensated hemolysis decompensates when the patient becomes infected with parvovirus. From time to time, an aplastic crisis due to parvovirus may be the first sign to reveal a chronic hemolytic anemia. Infections with parvovirus B19 manifest themselves particularly in patients with immune defects (among them, BMT recipients and HIV-infected individuals). Occasionally, these infections cause an isolated erythroblastopenic anemia (persistent parvovirus infections). In this situation, antibodies to parvovirus are usually absent; however the virus can be readily detected in the circulation, often at extremely high levels ($>10^{12}$ genome copies per mL).

The genome of parvovirus B19 has approx 5600 nucleotides. The genome encodes only three proteins of known function: the nonstructural protein NS1 and the capsid proteins VP1 and VP2. Folding of the proteins creates α-helical loops that appear on the surface of the assembled capsids, where the host immune system can recognize them.

The diagnosis can be made serologically by demonstrating IgM antibodies (which is unreliable in immunosuppressed patients) or by detecting viral DNA in serum or bone marrow by molecular methods. As far as bone marrow cytomorphology is concerned, giant pronormoblasts are considered as pathognomonic. Occasionally, the infection may also be accompanied by neutropenia and/or thrombocytopenia. DNA assays are required to diagnose persistent infection, because antibody production is absent or minimal. Parvovirus DNA can be found early in the course of an aplastic crisis. DNA direct hybridization is reliable for detecting viral titers of 10^6 copy numbers or higher. DNA amplification techniques are more sensitive but may detect low-level viremia in normal persons without clinical relevance.

The treatment of parvovirus B19 infections with hematological manifestations consists of administering commercially available Ig preparations (a dosage of 0.4 g/kg body weight for 5 successive days has been suggested). Patients who present with an aplastic crisis during hemolytic anemias or who are immunodeficient and develop a persistent anemia with decreased erythroblasts should always be screened for an infection with parvovirus.

5. PROGRESSIVE MULTIFOCAL LEUKOENCEPHALOPATHY

The disease called progressive multifocal leukoencephalopathy (PML) is caused by an infection of the CNS with human polyomavirus JC (JCV). During the course of AIDS up to 3% of patients may develop PML; in patients with hematological diseases, the risk is much lower. Factors that increase the risk are irradiation of the CNS, intrathecal application of methotrexate, and severe immunosuppression. In healthy individuals, the JCV is latent in the organism. When immunosurveillance is lacking, the virus can cause demyelinization, beginning in the deeper structures of the brain and progressing rapidly. This damage can be depicted as an area of high signal density with nuclear magnetic resonance imaging.

The clinical signs and symptoms of PML are fatigue, disorientation, dementia, depression, seizures, hemiparalysis, and other focal neurological signs. An increase in titer of antibodies to the JCV can raise the suspicion of PML; an accurate diagnosis may be made when the virus is demonstrated in brain tissue with immunological or molecular methods. In most cases, the disease has a fatal course within weeks or months. In singular cases, remissions were described following a treatment with cytosine-arabinoside.

6. TOXOPLASMOSIS

Toxoplasmosis can manifest itself in otherwise healthy persons as a lymph node swelling, hepatosplenomegaly, and changes in the white cell differential count, similarly to infectious mononucleosis. Quite often, however, toxoplasmosis remains clinically inapparent. A large segment of the population is immune against *T. gondii*. Transmission occurs by means of insufficiently cooked meat and by contact with domestic animals. Toxoplasmosis may also be transmitted via blood transfusions. If the prime infection occurs during pregnancy, the fetus may become infected via the placenta.

The diagnosis of an acute infection can be made serologically by demonstrating IgM antibodies and an increase in titer of IgG antibodies (by indirect immunofluorescence or complement binding reactions). A histological diagnosis from lymph nodes can be made showing toxoplasma parasites or cysts.

Immunosuppressed patients (especially in cases of AIDS, also after organ transplants, rarely after BMT) can experience a life-threatening disseminated form of toxoplasmosis. Disseminated toxoplasmosis leads to a generalized lymph node enlargement or involves the brain, the eyes, or the myocardium. A cerebral toxoplasmosis shows pleocytosis in the spinal fluid. In computed tomography (CT) scans, focal lesions are visualized, which typically show enhancement after intravenous contrast agents.

Patients with intact immune function generally do not need a specific treatment. In patients with immune deficiency, a combination treatment with pyrimethamine (oral daily dose 25–50 mg) and sulfadiazine (daily dose 100 mg/ kg body weight, orally [p.o.] or intravenously [i.v.]) is recommended. Because pyrimethamine is an antagonist of folate, folinic acid (10 mg daily p.o. i.v.) should be administered. Side effects of the combination treatment are myelodepression, gastrointestinal disturbances, exanthemas, and, in rare cases, seizures. As alternative treatment, clindamycin (daily dose 1.2–2.4 g p.o. or i.v.), often in combination with pyrimethamine, has been recommended.

7. *PNEUMOCYSTIS CARINII* PNEUMONIAS

The pathogen *Pneumocystis carinii* has been classified as protozoan, and most likely persists in the lungs of healthy individuals at a latent stage. During states of immunosuppression, pneumocystis may cause life-threatening interstitial pneumonias. In patients with AIDS, *P. carinii* pneumonias are the most frequent opportunistic infection. In hematological patients not infected with HIV, the risk of contracting pneumocystis pneumonias has been estimated to be between 0.1 and 1%. At risk are recipients of BMT, patients with acute lymphoblastic leukemias, and those treated with high-dose steroids. Untreated, pneumocystis pneumonias lead to a rapidly worsening respiratory failure.The first signs are cough, an increased respiratory rate, fever, and, in the chest X-ray, interstitial infiltrates that may be absent in a radiograph taken during the first hours of worsening respiratory distress. A diagnosis can be made by invasive means, demonstrating the etiological agent in the sediment of bronchial lavage or in a biopsate (staining with methenamine silver or toluidine blue).

The standard treatment of pneumocystis pneumonias consists of high-dose trimethoprim-sulfamethoxazole (TMP/SMX, daily dose 20 mg/kg trimethoprim and 100 mg/kg sulfamethoxazole, given in three to four single doses). The duration of treatment should be 3–4 wk, and during the initial phase the addition of corticosteroids (3×40 mg prednisone equivalent) has been proved to be beneficial. Similarly to patients with AIDS, pentamidine (4 mg/kg i.v. once daily) can be administered. The lethality of pneumocystis infections in patients with hematological disorders is still in the range of up to 40%, especially if the diagnosis is delayed. If bronchoscopy or an open-lung biopsy are considered to be hazardous because of impending respiratory failure, an empiric treatment is justified. Most BMT centers give a prophylactic treatment against pneumocystis until day 100 after transplant. Such a prophylaxis is also recommended in patients who recovered from a pneumocystis pneumonia. A common regime is to administer oral TMP/SMX twice weekly (e.g., Mondays and Thursdays). Possible side effects of TMP/SMX are myelosuppression, renal toxicity, rash, and fever. Another prophylactic regime consists of pentamidine inhalations (once monthly, 300 mg). Recently oral dapsone (50 mg/m^2) was proposed as pneumocystis prophylaxis for persons intolerant to TMP/SMX. Because pneumocystis pneumonias are generally responsive to treatment, the possibility of this opportunistic infection should be considered early in hematological patients with unclear interstitial infiltrates. A prophylaxis is indicated in high-risk cases.

8. INFECTIONS CAUSED BY HUMAN HERPESVIRUS-6

Human herpesvirus (HHV)-6 is a herpesvirus discovered in the 1980s and has two variants. HHV-6 causes exanthema subitum in children. In individuals undergoing stem cell transplantation or BMT, HHV-6 can cause a skin rash, marrow suppression, encephalitis, or pneumonitis and exacerbate graft-vs-host disease. HHV-6 as detected by PCR is found in 50–70% of BMT recipients. Because the virus is ubiquitous in mononuclear cells, it is recommended serum or cerebrospinal fluid be used for diagnostic purposes. Using sensitive techniques, an infection is generally detectable 2–4 wk after transplantation. HHV-6 can also reactivate other herpesviruses. HHV-6 infections are due to exogenous transmission from the donor, an endogenous reactivation, or a transmission from other sources. As to treatment, gancyclovir or foscarnet are recommended.

9. INFECTIONS CAUSED BY HUMAN HERPESVIRUS-8

9.1. Introduction

HHV-8 is a newly discovered herpesvirus associated with Kaposi's sarcoma (KS) and rare lymphoproliferative disorders. Together with non-Hodgkin's lymphomas, KS is the most frequently found neoplasm in patients with AIDS. Patients with AIDS and KS most often come from the high-risk group of male homosexuals. KS tumors not associated with AIDS are rare, although they were observed long before the current AIDS epidemic. An endemic increase has been reported in central Africa and in parts of the Mediterranean countries. In addition, KS is occasionally associated with patients who are immunosuppressed because of organ transplants.

According to the epidemiological evidence, an infectious etiology has been suspected for many years. Finally, a new herpesvirus (HHV-8) was discovered in the tumor tissue of KS by representational display analysis, a new PCR technique.

9.2. Biology of HHV-8

According to sequence homology, HHV-8 (also known as KS-associated herpesvirus [KSHV]), belongs to the subfamily of γ-herpesviruses, similar to EBV and herpesvirus saimiri. The genome of HHV-8 consists of approx 140,000 base pairs and is flanked by several repetitive sequences (size 800 base pairs). HHV-8 has several similarities with EBV:

1. The structure of the genome is very similar.
2. HHV-8 infects B-lymphocytes.
3. HHV-8 is also considered as a possible tumor virus.

Table 1
Diseases and Disorders Associated With HHV-8

Kaposi's sarcomas (all varieties, patients ± HIV infection)
Primary effusion lymphomas
Castleman's disease (especially multicentric variety)
Angioimmunoblastic lymphadenopathy
Mycosis fungoides[a]
Angiosarcoma[a]
Multiple myeloma and Waldenström's disease[a]
Sarcoidosis[a]
Encephalitis in HIV-infected patients[a]

[a]Unconfirmed or controversial. HHV, human herpes virus

Several genes of HIV-8 play a role in its transforming potency. HHV-8 encodes the genes for cytokines and related molecules. The pathogenesis of HHV-8-associated disorders is multifactorial, with HHV-8, immunosuppression, cytokines, and other factors playing a role.

Because of the relationship with EBV, malignant lymphomas were initially screened for HHV-8 sequences. However, most cases turned out to be negative, and only a rare group of malignant lymphomas, primary effusion lymphomas (PEL), was found to be consistently infected with HHV-8. Similar to KS, PEL occur in HIV-infected and noninfected patients.

PEL proliferate as ascites and pleural or pericardial effusions—they do not form tumors; they are often coinfected with EBV; and they have the phenotype of immature B-cell tumors. In addition, HHV-8 can be found in some atypical lymphoproliferative disorders like Castleman's disease or angioimmunoblastic lymphadenopathy. Some cytokines, such as interleukin-6, are involved in the pathogenesis of these diseases as they are in KS. In other disorders, the detection of HHV-8 sequences is not confirmed or universally accepted. The diseases and disorders associated with HHV-8 are summarized in Table 1.

9.3. Diagnosis and Epidemiology of HHV-8 Infections

Initially, it was shown that HHV-8 is specifically detected in KS and rare lymphoproliferative disorders. In patients with KS, HHV-8 could also be detected in CD 19+ cells, which points toward B-lymphocytes as a possible sanctuary of virus. Later, HHV-8 was also found in blood and other tissues of HIV-negative immunosuppressed individuals. HHV-8 sequences have also been found in rare cases in the blood of otherwise healthy normal individuals. In some studies, the detection of HHV-8 in the peripheral blood correlates with disease activity (as far as KS and Castleman's disease are concerned).

Patients with KS and other HHV-8-associated disorders develop antibodies to the virus. In normal persons in Europe and the United States, a low prevalence of HHV-8 is detected serologically. In some regions of Africa, a high prevalence of HHV-8 that correlates with the incidence of KS is observed.

9.4. Treatment of HHV-8-Associated Disorders

Currently, only retrospective data point to some efficacy of antiviral drugs against HHV-8-associated diseases, especially KS. Prospective studies are being undertaken. In established KS, the treatment depends on the stage of the disease and currently ranges from local measures such as surgery or irradiation to systemic treatments such as vinblastine, doxorubicin, or interferon-α. The discovery of HHV-8 may also open perspectives for immunotherapy against KS and related disorders.

SUGGESTED READING

Levy JA. A new human herpesvirus: KSHV or HHV-8? Lancet 1995;346;798,

Macsween KF, Crawford DH. Epstein-Barr virus: recent advances. *Lancet Infect Dis* 2003;3:131–140.

Moore PS, Chang Y. Detection of Herpesvirus-like DNA sequences in Kaposi's sarcoma in patients with and those without HIV infection. *N Engl J Med* 1996;332:1181–1185.

Wang FZ, Dahl H, Linde A, Brytting M, Ehrnst A, Ljungman P. Lymphotropic herpes-viruses in allogeneic bone marrow transplantation. Blood 1996;88:3615–3620.

Winston DJ, Gale RP. Prevention and treatment of cytomegalovirus infection and disease. after bone marrow transplantation in the 1990s. *Bone Marrow Transplant* 1991;8:7–11.

Yoshikawa T. Human herpesvirus 6 infection in haematopoietic stem cell transplant recipients. *Br J Haematol* 2004;124:421–434.

Young NS, Brown KE. Parvovirus B19. *N Engl J Med* 2004;350:586–597.

19   Basic Principles of Hemostasis

Erhard Hiller, MD

1. NORMAL HEMOSTATIC MECHANISMS

The hemostatic system consists of blood vessels, platelets, and the plasma coagulation system including the fibrinolytic factors and their inhibitors. When a blood vessel is injured, three mechanisms operate locally at the site of injury to control bleeding: (1) vessel wall contraction, (2) platelet adhesion and aggregation (platelet plug formation), and (3) plasmatic coagulation to form a fibrin clot. All three mechanisms are essential for normal hemostasis. Abnormal bleeding usually results from defects in one or more of these three mechanisms. For a better understanding of the pathogenesis of pathological bleeding, it is customary to divide hemostasis into two stages (i.e., primary and secondary hemostasis). Primary hemostasis is the term used for the instantaneous plug formation upon injury of the vessel wall, which is achieved by vasoconstriction, platelet adhesion, and aggregation. The fibrin formation is not required for hemostasis at this stage. Primary hemostasis is, however, only temporarily effective. Hemorrhage may start again unless the secondary hemostasis reinforces the platelet

From: *Contemporary Hematology: Modern Hematology, Second Edition*
Edited by: R. Munker, E. Hiller, J. Glass, and R. Paquette © Humana Press Inc., Totowa, NJ

plug by formation of a stable fibrin clot. Finally, mechanisms within the fibrin-olytic system lead to a dissolution of the fibrin clot and to a restoration of normal blood flow.

2. ENDOTHELIUM AND THE VASCULAR SYSTEM

Normal, intact endothelium does not initiate or support platelet adhesion and blood coagulation. Endothelial thromboresistance is caused by a number of antiplatelet and anticoagulant substances produced by the endothelial cells. Important vasodilators and inhibitors of platelet function are prostacyclin (pros-taglandin I_2, PgI_2) and nitrite oxide (NO), formerly called endothelium-derived relaxing factor (EDRF). The thrombin-binding protein thrombomodulin and hep-arin-like glycosaminoglycans exert anticoagulant properties. Thrombomodulin not only binds thrombin, but also activates protein C as a thrombin–thrombomodulin complex. Endothelial cells also synthesize and secrete tissue factor pathway inhibitor (TFPI), which is the inhibitor of the extrinsic pathway of blood coagu-lation. In addition, tissue plasminogen activator (t-PA) and its inhibitor plasmi-nogen activator inhibitor-1 (PAI-1), which modulate fibrinolysis, are secreted by endothelial cells. Endothelial cells also possess some procoagulant properties by synthesizing and secreting von Willebrand factor (VWF) and PAI-1. Following injury, these procoagulant factors and tissue factor (TF) activity are induced. This leads to adhesion and activation of platelets and local thrombin generation. The hemostatic properties of the endothelial cells are modulated by cytokines such as endotoxin, interleukin (IL)-1, and tumor necrosis factor (TNF), resulting in an increased TF activity and downregulated thrombomodulin.

Small blood vessels comprise arterioles, capillaries, and venules. Only arte-rioles have muscular walls, which allow changes of the arteriolar caliber. Upon contraction, arterioles contribute to hemostasis, thus temporarily preventing extravasation of blood. Platelet secretion of thromboxane A_2, serotonin, and epinephrine promotes vasoconstriction during hemostasis.

3. THE ROLE OF PLATELETS

Platelets are anuclear cells released from megakaryocytes in the bone marrow. Their life span in the peripheral blood is approx 9 d. The average platelet count in peripheral blood ranges from 150,000 to 400,000 per microliter. The mecha-nism for their production, release, and aging is described in Chapter 1 under the heading "Megakaryopoiesis." The exterior coat of platelets is comprised of sev-eral glycoproteins, including integrins and leucine-rich glycoproteins. They mediate platelet adhesion and aggregation as receptors for agonists such as adenos-ine diphsophate (ADP), arachidonic acid, and other molecules. Electron micro-scopic examination shows the presence of many cytoplasmatic bodies such as

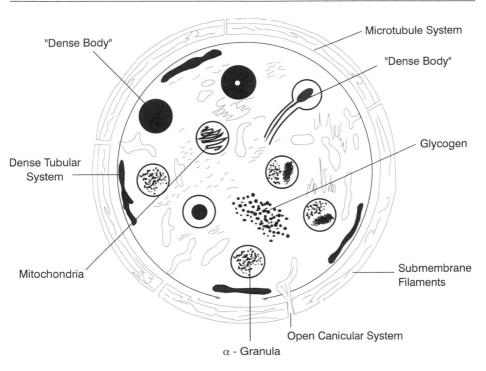

Fig. 19.1. Ultrastructure of a platelet.

α-granules and dense bodies (*see* Fig. 19.1). α-Granules are the storage site of β-thromboglobulin, platelet factor (PF) 4, platelet-derived growth factor (PDGF), VWF, fibrinogen, factor V, PAI-1, and thrombospondin. Dense bodies contain ADP, ATP, calcium, and serotonin. Platelets also contain actin filaments and a circumferential band of microtubules, which are involved in maintaining the shape of the platelets. The open canicular system has its role in the exchange of substances from the plasma to the platelets and vice versa.

Whereas normal platelets circulate in the blood and do not adhere to normal vasculature, activation of platelets causes a number of changes resulting in promotion of hemostasis by two major mechanisms:

1. Formation of the hemostatic plug at the site of injury (primary hemostasis).
2. Provision of phospholipids as a procoagulant surface for plasmatic coagulation.

The formation of the initial platelet plug can be divided into separate steps, which are very closely interrelated in vivo: platelet adhesion, shape change, the release reaction, and platelet aggregation (*see* Fig. 19.2). Within seconds after endothelial injury, platelets attach to adhesive proteins, such as collagen, via specific glycoprotein surface receptors (*platelet adhesion*). In this context, VWF serves as a bridge that first adheres to collagen fibers and then changes its con-

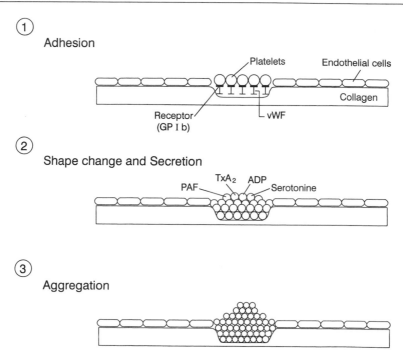

Fig. 19.2. Platelet adhesion, shape change with secretion, and platelet aggregation following activation.

firmation. This is followed by the binding of platelets to VWF via the platelet membrane glycoproteins (GP) Ib and IX (*see* Fig. 19.3).

Two congenital bleeding disorders, von Willebrand disease and Bernard-Soulier syndrome, are characterized by the absence of VWF and GP Ib/IX and thus by defective adhesion, which causes a life-long bleeding tendency. Following adhesion, platelets undergo a *shape change* from a disc shape to a spherical shape and extend pseudopods. Almost simultaneously the *release reaction* occurs by which a number of biologically active compounds stored in the platelet granules are secreted to the outside. These released substances, which include ADP, serotonin, Thromboxane A_2 (TxA_2), βTG, PF4, and VWF, accelerate the reaction of plug formation and also initiate platelet aggregation, i.e., the adhesion of platelets to each other. As a result of *platelet aggregation*, the platelet plug increases in size and a further release of granular contents is initiated in order to induce more platelets to aggregate. The prostaglandins play an additional role in mediating the platelet-release reaction and aggregation. Thromboxane A_2 is a very potent inducer of platelet secretion and aggregation. It is formed from arachidonic acid by the enzyme cyclooxygenase. Arachidonic acid is liberated

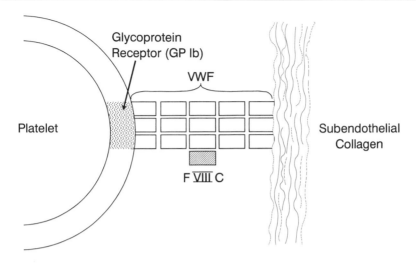

Fig. 19.3. von Willebrand factor as a bridge between the injured vessel wall (collagen fibers) and platelet.

from the platelet membrane by phospholipases following activation of the platelets by collagen and epinephrine. At the end of the aggregation process, the hemostatic plug consists of closely packed degranulated platelets. Fibrinogen is required for platelet aggregation binding to specific glycoprotein receptors (GP IIb/IIIa) (*see* Fig. 19.4). In Glanzmann's thrombasthenia, a disease characterized by the absence of these receptors, the bleeding time is markedly prolonged, platelet aggregation is absent, and clinically a life-long bleeding tendency is present.

4. THE ROLE OF BLOOD COAGULATION

The fibrin clot is the end product of a multiplicity of complex reactions of plasma proteins called coagulation or clotting factors. Most of the clotting factors are zymogens of serine proteases and are converted to active enzymes during the process of blood coagulation. The six serine proteases are the activated forms of the clotting factors II, VII, IX, X, XI, and XII. The letter "a" accompanying a Roman numeral (e.g., factor Xa) indicates that the factor is in its activated form. Factors V and VIII are not enzymes but co-factors, which, after activation, modify the speed of the coagulation reaction. The reactions of the coagulation factors take place on the surface of phospholipids. Following platelet activation, certain phospholipids (i.e., phosphatidyl ethanolamine, phosphatidyl serine, and phophatidyl choline) that were not present on the surface of the resting platelet become exposed on the platelet surface. These newly exposed phospholipids

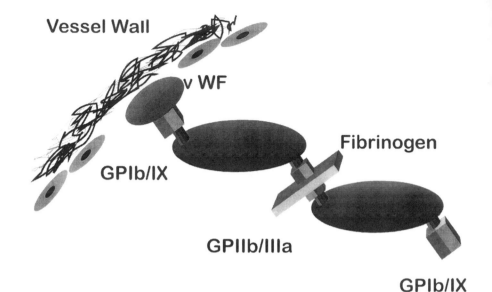

Fig. 19.4. Scheme of platelet adhesion and aggregation. Surface glycoprotein (GP) Ib and IX interact with von Willebrand factor to adhere to subendothelial tissue. Aggregation involves the GP Iib/IIIa receptor and fibrinogen as essential co-factors.

provide the appropriate phopholipid surface upon which reactions of the coagulation factors take place (Fig. 19.5).

The plasmatic coagulation traditionally has been divided into two different pathways—the intrinsic and extrinsic pathway. This understanding of coagulation has been built on studies of clotting in a relatively cell-free plasma system in vitro. However, such a division does not really occur in vivo because factor VIIa-TF complex is a potent activator of factor IX as well as factor X. The principal initiating pathway of in vivo blood coagulation is the extrinsic system. The critical component is TF, an intrinsic membrane component expressed by cells in most extravascular tissues. The nomenclature "extrinsic" continues to be used today, despite being somewhat outdated. TF is not always extrinsic to the circulatory system, but it is expressed also on the surface of the endothelial cells and leukocytes under certain pathological conditions. TF functions as a co-factor of the major plasma component of the extrinsic pathway, factor VII. A complex of these two proteins leads to the activation of factor VII to factor VIIa, which then converts factor X to factor Xa, the identical product as formed by the intrinsic pathway. As mentioned previously, factor VIIa-TF complex also activates factor IX to factor IXa. As factor Xa levels increase, however, factor VIIa-TF complex is subject to inhibition by factor Xa-dependent TFPI.

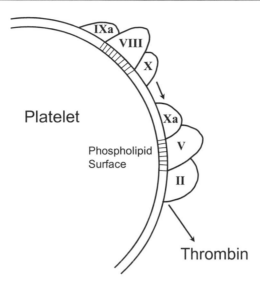

Fig. 19.5. Exposed phospholipids on the surface of platelets providing surface for coagulation reactions.

The early part of the intrinsic pathway is called contact phase. This phase is carried out by factor XII (contact factor), prekallikrein, and high-molecular-weight (HMW) kininogen. In vitro contact phase is initiated by the binding of factor XII to negatively charged surfaces, such as glass or kaolin. This leads to the formation of the enzyme factors XIIa and kallikrein, and the release of brady-kinin from HMW kininogen. Factor XIIa then activates factor XI. The resulting factor XIa converts factor IX to factor IXa, a reaction that requires the presence of calcium. Factor IXa then forms a complex with its co-factor protein factor VIIIa on a negatively charged membrane surface. This enzymatic complex, also referred to as tenase complex, converts factor X to factor Xa.

After both the extrinsic and intrinsic pathways have resulted in the formation of factor Xa, the ensuing reactions of the coagulation pathway are the same and are referred to as the common pathway.

Based on the discovery that the factor VIIa-TF complex also activates factor IX to factor IXa, which appears to be the favored reaction, a new revised concept of coagulation was suggested in which factor VIIa-TF complex is thought to be the main initiator of coagulation, whereas the intrinsic pathway is considered necessary to sustain the coagulation response.

4.1. Formation of Fibrin

Fibrinogen is a large plasma protein with a molecular weight (MW) of 340 kDa. It is synthesized in the liver and its concentration in normal individuals is in the range of 200 to 400 mg/dL. The half-life of fibrinogen is about 4 to 5 d. It is a dimeric protein of extremely low solubility composed of two pairs of three nonidentical polypeptide chains, designated as A-α, B-β, and γ (A-α-2, B-β-2, γ-2). The chains are covalently linked together by disulfide bonds. The conversion of fibrinogen to fibrin proceeds in three stages. In the first step, thrombin cleaves four small peptides—the fibrinopeptides A (FPA) and fibrinopeptides B (FPB)—from the fibrinogen molecule, resulting in the formation of a new molecule called fibrin monomer. The release of these fibrinopeptides exposes sites on the A-α and the B-β chains that seem to be essential for the polymerization of the fibrin. In the second step, polymerization occurs spontaneously by noncovalent end-to-end and side-to-side associations to form fibrin polymers. These polymers are easily dissolved in denaturing agents such as urea or monochloroacetic acid. In the third step, a resistent and stable fibrin molecule is formed by the action of factor XIII (fibrin-stabilizing factor) and calcium ions. Factor XIII must first be activated by thrombin before it becomes a transglutamase capable of crosslinking fibrin polymers by forming covalent bonds (γ-glutamyl/epsilon-lysil). The fibrin gel is now stabilized and insoluble in urea or monochloroacetic acid.

5. INHIBITORS OF THE PLASMATIC COAGULATION SYSTEM

Human plasma contains a number of antiproteases that inhibit the activity of most of the activated coagulation factors and fibrinolytic enzymes. These inhibitors include antithrombin (AT), protein C and S, TFPI, and PAI, among others. All belong to the serine protease inhibitors (SERPINs). Their task is to limit thrombosis on the one side and fibrinolysis on the other side. A defect or decrease of activity of these inhibitors can thus lead to thrombosis or hyperfibrinolysis.

5.1. Antithrombin

This glycoprotein with an MW of 65 kDa is synthesized in the liver, is composed of a single polypeptide chain, and migrates with the α_2-globulins. The normal concentration of AT in plasma is in the range of 18 to 30 mg/dL. It is the major inhibitor of thrombin, but it also inhibits the factors XIIa, XIa, Xa, IXa, VIIa, plasmin, and plasma kallikrein. It inhibits thrombin as the other serine proteases by forming a stable 1:1 complex between an arginine residue of AT and the serine-active site of thrombin or the other clotting factors. The presence of heparin greatly accelerates the reaction by inducing a conformational change in AT, which renders arginine at the reactive site more readily available for the

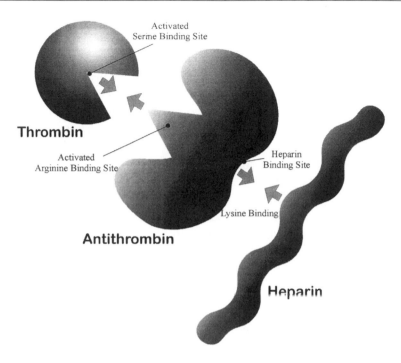

Fig. 19.6. Antithrombin inhibits thrombin and other serine proteases. This reaction is greatly accelerated in the presence of heparin.

binding of thrombin (*see* Fig. 19.6). A congenital deficiency of AT may lead to the occurrence of repeated episodes of venous thrombosis.

5.2. Protein C and Protein S

Protein C is the zymogen of a serine protease with an MW of 56 kDa and a plasma concentration of about 0.4 mg/dL. Protein S (MW 69 kDa) serves as a co-factor for activated Protein C and like protein C is a vitamin K-dependent protein. Its plasma concentration is about 2.5 mg/dL. Protein S exists in plasma either in a free form or bound to the C4b-binding protein, a component of the complement system. Only the free form of protein S can serve as a co-factor for activated protein C. When thrombin escapes the localized area of vascular injury, it must be kept from freely circulating in blood. This is accomplished by the upregulation of thrombomodulin on the cell surface of the vascular endothelium, primarily in the microcirculation. Thrombomodulin binds thrombin, thus switching off the procoagulant activity of thrombin. Thrombin in this bound form changes its substrate specificity from fibrinogen to protein C. The thrombomodulin/thrombin-complex activates protein C. Following activation, activated protein C forms a complex with protein S. This complex degrades factor Va and factor VIIIa by limited proteolysis, dramatically reducing the local generation of thrombin. Activated protein C also increases fibrinolysis by inactivating PAI-1. The downregulation of thrombin generation and the role of protein C and protein S are shown in Fig. 19.7. The physiological significance of the protein C-thrombomodulin pathway in the control of thrombin generation is emphasized by the increased incidence of thrombosis in individuals with hereditary deficiencies of protein C or protein S. Recent studies revealed that in addition to a deficiency state, an inherited poor anticoagulant response to activated protein C also exists in patients with a point mutation in the factor V gene (Factor V Leiden). Because this mutation involves the cleavage site of factor V by activated protein C, the activated factor V in these individuals is resistant to cleavage and thus to the ability of activated protein C to control thrombin generation (*see* Chapter 21).

6. ROLE OF FIBRINOLYSIS

The fibrinolytic system is essential for removal of excess fibrin deposits in order to preserve vascular patency. Figure 19.8 depicts its individual components. The circulating proenzyme plasminogen is a single-chain glycoprotein with an MW of 90 kDa. Cleavage of the Arg_{560}–Val_{561} bond converts plasminogen to an active two-chain plasmin molecule. Plasmin digests a number of plasma proteins including fibrin, fibrinogen, and factors V and VIII . Conversion of plasminogen to plasmin is achieved by a variety of plasminogen activators that include physiological substances such as urokinase and tissue plasminogen activator, as well as streptokinase, a compound derived from streptococcus Lancefield group C. The most important circulating plasminogen activator in humans is t-PA, which is a serine protease existing either in a single-chain or two-chain form. Both t-PA and plasminogen bind to the fibrin gel and are incorporated into the developing thrombus. The stage is set for dissolution of the fibrin clot from its inception. t-PA is not only present in human vascular endothelial cells but is also found in other human tissues and cell lines. The control of plasmin generation is as important as the previously described control of thrombin. The strongest inhibitor of plasmin is α_2-antiplasmin, a single-chain protein that forms a 1:1 complex with plasmin so rapidly that under normal circumstances free plasmin is never detectable. Other inhibitors of minor significance are α_2-macroglobulin and α_1-antitrypsin. The most important inhibitor of t-PA is the PAI-1, which not only inhibits t-PA but also urokinase plasminogen activator (u-PA). PAI-1 circulates in plasma in a free, noncomplexed form of 48 kDa and as a complex with t-PA of 110 kDa. In normal human plasma, most of the t-PA is complexed. Plasma-PAI-1 behaves as an acute-phase reactant, rising in

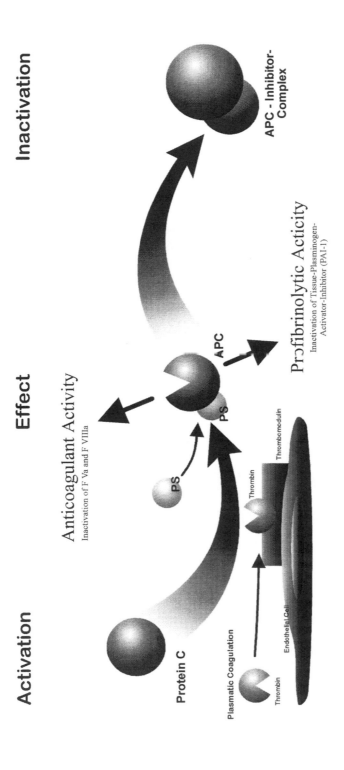

Activation **Effect** **Inactivation**

Anticoagulant Activity
Inactivation of F Va and F VIIIa

APC - Inhibitor-Complex

Profibrinolytic Acticity
Inactivation of Tissue-Plasminogen-
Activator-Inhibitor (PAI-1)

APC

PS

PS

Protein C

PS

Plasmatic Coagulation

Thrombin

Thrombin

Thrombomodulin

Endothelial Cell

Fig. 19.7. Thrombin is inactivated by endothelial thrombomodulin. The thrombin/thrombomodulin complex thereafter activates protein C.

337

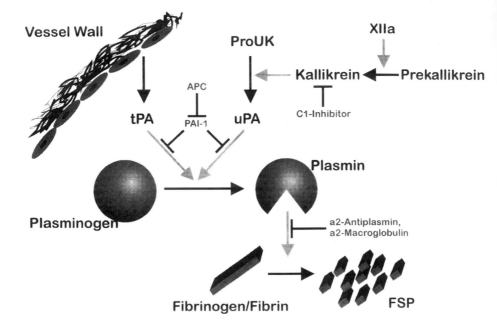

Fig. 19.8. Fibrinolytic system with the components of activation and inhibition.

a variety of pathological conditions and occuring in relatively large quantities in platelets. A second inhibitor, known as PAI-2, has been identified in the placenta and in plasma samples of pregnant women.

7. CLINICAL EVALUATION OF HEMORRHAGIC DISORDERS

7.1. The Bleeding History

The initial evaluation of a patient with hemorrhagic problems involves obtaining a detailed history of bleeding symptoms and inspecting any current lesions. The bleeding history forms the basis of the laboratory tests and therapy. Asking patients if they are bleeders is not always helpful, as patients with mild to moderate bleeding abnormalities may not admit that their bleeding episodes are significant. Questioning must be specific and designed to ascertain whether bleeding occurs in response to mild trauma. The diagnostic value of any single hemorrhagic symptom varies with the different disorders. Valuable information may be obtained if a patient has undergone major surgery; however, if this is not the case, inquiries as to minor surgical procedures, such as dental extractions and tonsillectomy, should be made. It is important to get information on the duration of bleeding, the type of bleeding and what procedure was necessary to stop the bleeding (blood transfusion?).

7.2. *Physical Examination*

The clinical examination of a patient is important to evaluate the nature and extent of any current hemorrhage. Several clinical as well as laboratory features help differentiate clinical disorders associated with qualitative and quantitative platelet defects and abnormalities of the blood vessel wall (diseases of primary hemostasis) from those associated with disorders of the coagulation factors. Diseases of primary hemostasis have also been referred to as "purpuric syndromes." Purpuric syndromes are characterized by capillary hemorrhages occurring chiefly in the skin and mucous membranes. The usual lesions encountered are spontaneous petechiae and ecchymoses, which result from a breakdown of the anatomic and physiological integrity of small vessel walls. Petechiae are pinpoint to small areas of skin bleeding, which characteristically appear as crops of lesions in dependent portions of the microvasculature. Larger accumulations of skin lesions are usually called ecchymoses. It is often difficult to differentiate petechiae secondary to a platelet disorder from purpura caused by a defect of the blood vessel wall. The latter can only be proven by the absence of defects in number and function of platelets. Gastrointestinal and genitourinary bleeding may occur spontaneously with abnormalities of platelets and/or coagulation factors. Deep hematomas, areas of palpable skin or soft tissue bleeding, and hemarthroses are most often associated with coagulation factor deficiencies or abnormalities. It is important to note the relationship of excessive bleeding to antecedent trauma or surgery, such as tooth extraction, tonsillectomy, or circumcision. Recurrent bleeding for several days usually indicates an underlying bleeding disorder. In women, a careful and thorough history of their menstrual bleeding pattern gives valuable information about the nature of their hemostatic mechanism.

8. LABORATORY EVALUATION OF HEMOSTATIC DISORDERS

Understanding of the physiology of primary and secondary hemostasis is important for the interpretation of diagnostic laboratory tests and for the subsequent management of patients with hemostatic disorders. The type of bleeding may be of significant help in designing the program of hemostatic laboratory tests. Patients who have a severe hemostatic defect usually present no problems in either clinical recognition or laboratory diagnosis. Unfortunately, difficult diagnostic problems frequently arise because most patients who present for evaluation show only mild or equivocal bleeding symptoms and the results of the screening tests often turn out to be normal.

Familiarity with a number of laboratory procedures will enable one to place a hemostatic defect in one of several broad categories, i.e., a disorder of the platelets or a disorder of the plasma coagulation factors. More specialized tests are subsequently employed to establish a definite diagnosis. Thus, when evaluating a bleeding disorder, the first task is to establish whether the disorder is attributable to damage to the microvasculature (vasculitis), to an inadequate number or function of platelets, or to impairment of the reactions leading to thrombin generation and fibrin clot formation. This is accomplished by performing a platelet count, a bleeding time, an activated partial thromboplastin time (aPTT) and a prothrombin time (PT), and a thorough review of the patient's peripheral blood smear.

8.1. Screening Tests

The *platelet count* is performed to detect thrombocytopenia, which is defined as a platelet count of less than 150,000/μL. The test is usually performed as part of an automated blood cell profile and can be considered as reliable down to a platelet count of 30,000/μL. The finding of an unexpected thrombocytopenia should be confirmed by a review of the peripheral blood smear. The possibility of the existence of red blood cell fragments or of a pseudothrombocytopenia may provide clues for further evaluation of the patient.

The *bleeding time* is defined as the time between the infliction of a small standard cut and the moment the bleeding stops. Although the test is quite simple, bleeding time has many variables and is difficult to standardize. Bleeding time measures the interactions of the platelets with the vessel wall and the subsequent formation of the primary hemostatic plug. A long bleeding time will be recorded either when the number of platelets is decreased, their function is abnormal, or there is defect of the vessel wall. The bleeding time may also be prolonged when there is a decrease of plasmatic factors, especially the VWF or fibrinogen. The various methods for performing the bleeding time are basically modifications of two techniques: the bleeding time according to Duke, in which a puncture is made in the earlobe, or the bleeding time according to Mielke, in which an incision is made in the forearm while the capillaries are under increased constant pressure from an inflated blood pressure cuff. The depth, width, and position of the skin incision are difficult to standardize and thus the diagnostic usefulness is of limited value as an individual test. Evaluation of the closure time ("in vitro bleeding time") with PFA-100™ (Platelet Function Analyzer) allows a rapid and simple determination of VWF-dependent platelet function. This high shear stress system was demonstrated to be sensitive and reproducible for the screening of von Willebrand disease.

The *prothrombin time (PT)* is performed by adding a crude preparation of TF (usually an extract of brain) to citrate-anticoagulated plasma, recalcification of the plasma, and measurement of the clotting time. Both thromboplastin and $CaCl_2$ are usually added in a single step. The prothrombin time may be prolonged because of a deficiency of a factor(s) of the extrinsic coagulation pathway, i.e, factors II, V, VII, X, and/or fibrinogen. A circulating anticoagulant directed against on or more of these factors may also cause a prolongation of the PT. The assay of coagulation factor deficiencies depends on the type of thromboplastin used because each thromboplastin has a different sensitivity. Therefore, the World Health Organization has proposed that thromboplastins be calibrated against an international reference preparation to derive an international sensivity index (ISI). Once the ISI of the thromboplastin is assigned, the results can be reported as the international normalized ratio (INR). The INR has two major advantages: it allows comparison between results obtained from different laboratories, and it allows investigators to standardize anticoagulant therapy in clinical trials and scientific publications.

The *aPTT* is performed by adding a surface activating agent, such as kaolin or ellagic acid, and phospholipid to citrate-anticoagulated plasma. After a standardized incubation time to allow optimal activation of the contact factors, the plasma is recalcified and the clotting time recorded. In the old "cascade" theory of coagulation, the aPTT involves factors of both the intrinsic and common pathway (*see* Fig. 19.9). The aPTT may be prolonged as a result of a deficiency of one or more of these factors or of the presence of inhibitors that affect the functions of the factor(s) or the phopholipid reagents. A decrease in factor levels to less than 30% of normal are usually required to prolong the aPTT. The aPTT will not detect deficiencies of factors VII and XIII, the factor that crosslinks fibrin. In some instances it may be helpful to perform a *thrombin time (TT)* as part of the screening procedures. The test consists of adding a diluted solution of thrombin to anticoagulated plasma and performing a clotting time. The thrombin time will be prolonged when the levels of plasma fibrinogen are very low, and when fibrinolytic split products, abnormal fibrinogen (dysfibrinogenemia), and/or heparin are present. The presence of an inhibitor is identified when a mixture of patient and normal plasma fails to correct the prolonged clotting time of the test in question.

8.2. Interpretation the Screening Tests of Hemostasis

Discrimination of the majority of the inherited and acquired hemostatic disorders is possible by looking at the results of the three screening tests: aPTT, PT, and TT.

Patients with a prolonged aPTT and normal PT have abnormal activities of factors in the first stage (intrinsic) of the coagulation mechanism (i.e., factors VIII, IX, XI, and XII). Deficiencies of prekallikrein and HMW kininogen are possible. Whereas deficiencies of factor XII, prekallikrein, and HMW kininogen are not associated with bleeding, deficiencies of factors VIII, IX, and XI will cause bleeding. A prolonged PT and a normal aPTT and TT may indicate a factor VII deficiency. Inherited or acquired deficiencies of factors II, V, VII, and X have

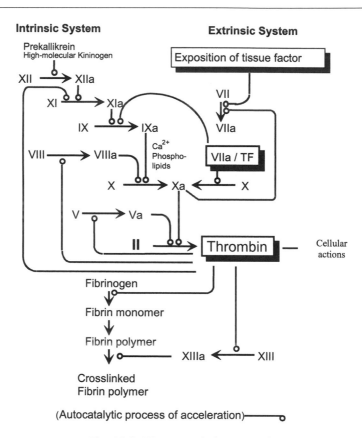

Fig. 19.9. The coagulation cascade.

to be considered if a prolonged PT and aPTT and a normal thrombin time are found. A prolongation of aPTT, PT, and thrombin time may reflect fibrinogen deficiency or dysfibrinogenemia. Most congenital deficiencies are single, whereas acquired abnormalities caused by vitamin K deficiency, liver disease, disseminated intravascular coagulation (DIC), or anticoagulant therapy cause multiple coagulation defects. A prolonged bleeding time in the presence of a normal platelet count usually is a sign of an abnormality of platelet–blood vessel interaction (e.g., von Willebrand disease). The proper interpretation of the screening tests of hemostasis will be time- and cost-effective with regard to determining which coagulation factor assays are necessary to clearly identify the specific factor deficiency and its level in patient plasma.

8.3. Specific Assays of Coagulation

Factors II, V, VII, and X are usually assayed by determining the ability of various dilutions of the patient's plasma to correct the PT of a plasma congenitally deficient in the factor to be assayed. The degree of correction is compared to that produced by equivalent dilutions of normal pooled plasma. Factors VIII, IX, XI, and XII are determined in a similar manner except that the specific factor assays are based on the aPTT.

A number of procedures for the determination of fibrinogen have been devised. In most laboratories, however, the assays are based on the original method of Clauss. This procedure involves an initial (10-fold) dilution of the plasma sample to ensure that fibrinogen is rate limiting for clotting and the subsequent measurement of the clotting time by the addition of an excess of thrombin to the sample. The length of the clotting time is inversely related to the concentration of fibrinogen. The presence of inhibitors of fibrin polymerization, such as degradation products of fibrinogen or fibrin produced by plasmin (DIC, fibrinolytic therapy) may, however result in an underestimation of the actual fibrinogen concentration in this assay.

The screening test for factor XIII is based on the ability of monochloric acid to dissolve a fibrin clot in the presence of a severe factor XIII deficiency. Quantitative assays depend on factor XIII transamidase properties (i.e., the incorporation of monodansylcadaverine into casein). Chromogenic assays are also commercially available.

Although a prolonged bleeding time is the hallmark of von Willebrand disease, this laboratory finding is not specific. Thus, the diagnosis has to be established by additional laboratory tests. These usually include measurements of the amount of von Willebrand antigen present in the plasma, the functional activity of the VWF, and the procoagulant activity of the associated factor VIII molecule. Analysis of the multimeric structure of VWF is useful in some special settings. The VWF protein is quantitated by ELISA. In most patients with von Willebrand disease the antigenic level of the VWF protein will be reduced. The mean VWF antigenic level in individuals with blood group 0 is approx 25% lower than that found in individuals with other blood types. The functional activity of VWF is assessed by measurement of the ristocetin co-factor activity of the patient's plasma. In this assay, the ability of VWF in the plasma to agglutinate a standardized suspension of fixed normal platelets in the presence of ristocetin is determined from either the rate or the extent of platelet agglutination.

Clinical *platelet function tests* measure platelet adhesion (retention) and aggregation, the release reaction, and coagulant activity. These tests must be meticulously performed and are usually available only in specialized laboratories. Platelet aggregation is monitored by the increase in light transmission

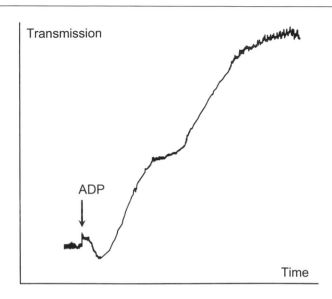

Fig. 19.10. Curve of ADP-induced platelet aggregation. The "second peak" is caused by secretion of platelet granule contents, such as intrinsic ADP.

through a suspension of platelet-rich plasma as aggregation occurs. A sample platelet aggregation curve is depicted in Fig. 19.10. Collagen, ADP, epinephrine, arachidonic acid, and ristocetin are the agonists usually used in the hematological laboratory. Platelet aggregation is affected by many drugs. In recent years flow cytometry of platelets has become a most valuable tool to assess platelet function in the specialized coagulation laboratory. This technique offers a number of advantages, such as the examination of full blood samples, a multiparamter examination (expression of glycoproteins, size of platelets, granularity of platelets), and the chance to identify asymptomatic heterozygotes of rare platelet disorders such as Glanzmann's disease.

8.4. Tests of Hypercoagulability and Fibrinolysis

Failure of the coagulation mechanisms may cause bleeding, but failure of the control mechanisms may give rise to thrombosis. These modulators of coagulation include AT, protein C, and protein S. AT can be measured by immunological and functional techniques. The functional assays that use chromogenic substrates measure AT as a heparin co-factor. Heparin is added to form an AT–heparin complex. This step is followed by adding an excess of thrombin, some of which is neutralized by the AT–heparin complex. A chromogenic substrate is used to measure the excess, uninhibited thrombin, which is inversely proportional to the concentration of AT.

For *protein C*, a number of functional assays exist that are based on the prolongation of the aPTT due to the inactivation of factors V and VIII by activated protein C. Determination of *protein S* is complicated by the existence of a free protein S and a complex of protein S with C4b-binding protein. Only the free protein S serves as cofactor of activated protein C. A functional assay for protein S is available using protein S-deficient plasma and activated protein C. The anticoagulant effect of activated protein C is proportional to the amount of protein S added to the deficient plasma.

In the past, the fibrin/fibrinogen degradation products were measured by a variety of methods. In most laboratories today, only the D-dimer, a cross-linked fragment of fibrin not produced by the digestion of fibrinogen, is measured as a diagnostic parameter for DIC and other thrombotic events. A monoclonal antibody has been produced that can detect the fibrin D-dimer in plasma. The fact that the antibody does not react with fibrinogen allows the test to be performed in plasma.

For the evaluation of hypercoagulability in the scientific laboratory, prothrombin fragment 1 and 2 (F1 +2), thrombin-antithrombincomplex (TAT), β thromboglobulin, and PF 4 can all be measured by ELISA. However, these assays are usually not applied for evaluation of a bleeding patient or a patient with thrombotic disorders.

SUGGESTED READING

Bowie EJW, Owen CA. Clinical and laboratory diagnosis of hemorrhagic disorders. In: Ratnoff OD, Forbes CD, eds. *Disorders of Hemostasis*, 3rd ed. Philadelphia: WB Saunders, 1996:pp. 53–78.

Colman RW, Hirsh J, Marder VJ, Clowes AW, George JN. *Hemostasis and Thrombosis. Basic principles and clinical practice*, 4th ed. Philadelphia: JB Lippincott Williams & Wilkins, 2001.

Michelson AD. Flow cytometry: A clinical test of platelet function. *Blood* 1996;87:4925—4936.

Morrissey JH. Tissue factor and factor VII initiation of coagulation. In: Colman RW, Hirsh J, Marder VJ, Clowes AW, George JN, eds. *Hemostasis and thrombosis. Basic principles and clinical practice,* 4th ed. Philadelphia: JB Lippincott Williams & Wilkins, 2001:pp. 89—102.

Ratnoff OD, Forbes CD. *Disorders of Hemostasis*, 3rd ed. Philadelphia: WB Saunders, 1996.

Reitsma PH. Genetic principles underlying disorders of procoagulant and anticoagulant proteins. In: Colman RW, Hirsh J, Marder VJ, Clowes AW, George JN, eds. *Basic principles and clinical practice*. 4th ed.Philadelphia: JB Lippincott Williams & Wilkins, 2001:pp. 59—88.

Rodgers RPC, Levin J. A critical reappraisal of the bleeding time. *Semin Thromb Hemost* 1990;16:1–20.

Ruggeri ZM. Von Willebrand factor, platelets and endothelial cell interactions. *J Thromb Haemost* 2003;1:1335–1342.

Saito H. Normal hemostatic mechanisms. In: Ratnoff OD, Forbes CD, eds. *Disorders of Hemostasis*, 3rd ed. Philadelphia: WB Saunders, 1996:pp. 23–52.

Verstraete M. The fibrinolytic system: from Petri dishes to genetic engineering. *Thromb Haemost* 1995;74:25–35.

20 Bleeding Disorders

Erhard Hiller

Contents

1. VASCULAR DISORDERS ASSOCIATED WITH BLEEDING

Vascular disorders of bleeding are classified into congenital disorders and acquired disorders. Congenital disorders are caused by either vascular malformations (telangiectasias, hemangiomas) or disorders of connective tissue. Acquired disorders usually present with purpura. The different vascular causes of bleeding are classified in Table 1.

1.1. Hereditary Vascular Malformations

1.1.1. Hereditary Hemorrhagic Telangiectasia (Osler-Weber-Rendu Disease)

Hereditary hemorrhagic telangiectasia (Osler-Weber-Rendu disease) is the most common inherited vascular bleeding disorder, with an autosomal-dominant transmission and a positive family bleeding history in both sexes. Bleeding occurs spontaneously or after minor trauma from teleangiectases (i.e., malformations of dilated small vessels in the skin and mucosa). These abnormal, small vessels have very thin walls lacking smooth muscle. They rupture easily and do not contract effectively, causing prolonged bleeding. The lesions have a diameter of 2–4 mm, appear dark red, and are frequently localized on the face, the lips, the

From: *Contemporary Hematology: Modern Hematology, Second Edition*
Edited by: R. Munker, E. Hiller, J. Glass, and R. Paquette © Humana Press Inc., Totowa, NJ

Table 1
Vascular Causes of Bleeding

Congenital disorders	Hereditary hemorrhagic telangiectasia (Osler)
	Cavernous hemangioma (Kasabach-Merritt)
	Ataxia telangiectasia
	Connective tissue disorders
	Ehlers-Danlos syndrome
	Osteogenesis imperfecta
	Pseudoxanthoma elasticum
	Marfan syndrome
Acquired disorders	Purpura simplex
	Purpura senilis
	Purpura due to infections
	Purpura due to chemicals or drugs
	Henoch-Schönlein purpura (vasculitis)
Miscellaneous	Amyloid
	Excess corticosteroids
	Paraproteinemia
	Vitamin C deficiency (scurvy)
	Cushing syndrome

mucous membranes of the mouth or nose, and the fingertips. Bleeding becomes more common in adulthood as the number of lesions increases. Recurrent epistaxis and gastrointestinal hemorrhage are the most common bleeding patterns, and can lead to iron deficiency anemia. Arteriovenous malformations may develop in the lungs and can cause shunting of blood between the right and left heart.

Coagulation studies are normal. A causative treatment does not exist, and treatment is symptomatic. Acute epistaxis must be treated by local measures (compression, topical hemostatic drugs). In some instances, antifibrinolytic therapy with tranexamic acid may be beneficial. Recurrent gastrointestinal bleeding and recurrent pulmonary bleeding must be treated by surgical means. The other hereditary vascular disorders listed in Table 1 are very rare. They are caused by defects of the connective tissue or elastic fibers. The most important diseases are Ehlers-Danlos syndrome, osteogenesis imperfecta, and pseudoxanthoma elasticum. In all three diseases, the inborn defects of connective tissue lead to a largely augmented vessel fragility and pathological changes of the skin and skeletal system.

1.2. Acquired Vascular Disorders

The most frequent and important acquired vascular disorders are purpura simplex, senile purpura, Henoch-Schönlein purpura, scurvy, and purpura due to corticosteroids.

1.2.1. Purpura Simplex (Idiopathic Purpura)

Spontaneous easy bruising of the trunk and the lower extremities, especially during the reproductive period without any abnormality of platelet number and function, is a relatively common problem. Sometimes, the patients report a minor trauma with a painful event probably due to a rupture of small vessels. The cause of purpura simplex is unclear, but is probably due to an increased fragility of skin vessels. It is one of the most frequent reasons why patients come for evaluation of their coagulation parameters. From a practical point of view, easy bruising is a cosmetic problem. If the investigation does not reveal an underlying disease, the patient has to be reassured and advised to avoid taking aspirin.

1.2.2. Senile Purpura

Progressive loss of collagen in the dermis and vascular wall may lead to characteristic lesions of old age, senile purpura. The purpura usually occurs on the dorsal side of the hands and wrists and on forearms. The lesions may be quite large and are well demarcated. The skin is very thin, the dorsal veins have fragile walls, and venipuncture may result in rapidly spreading purpura. The lesions resolve slowly. No specific treatment exists. Prolonged pressure should be applied after venipuncture in elderly patients.

1.2.3. Purpura Due to Infections

Infections may cause purpura of the skin and mucous membranes (internal bleeding) by a number of mechanisms, such as direct vessel damage by microorganisms or toxins, vasculitis, thrombocytopenia, or disseminated intravascular coagulation (DIC). There is usually an acute onset of fever, which may be followed by renal failure, rapidly spreading purpura with skin necrosis, and circulatory failure. The treatment of choice is to treat the underlying disorder.

1.2.4. Henoch-Schönlein Purpura (Allergic or Anaphylactoid Purpura)

Henoch-Schönlein Purpura (allergic or anaphylactoid purpura) is a hypersensitivity or acute necrotizing vasculitis involving the skin, kidneys, gut, and joints. Increased permeability of the vessel wall leads to exudation and hemorrhage into the tissue. Streptococcal bacteria have been suspected as offending agents, because the clinical manifestations of the disease often occur 1–3 wk after an upper respiratory tract infection. Drugs such as penicillin and sulfonamides have also been implicated. There is an acute onset of fever with a macular–papular exanthema on the buttocks, legs, and arms. The rash rapidly becomes purpuric and crops of lesions are common. Internal organs (kidneys, gut, joints) are involved in about half of the patients affected. In one half of the patients a cause of the disease cannot be found. Clinical manifestations persist for up to 3 mo. Treatment is symptomatic. Precipitating factors have to be excluded. Corticosteroids may be necessary and are often effective when systemic symptoms are marked. Relapses occur frequently.

1.2.5. MISCELLANEOUS DISORDERS

Purpura due to damage of the vessel wall of the terminal vessels are seen in a number of metabolic disorders such as diabetes mellitus, vitamin C deficiency (scurvy), Cushing syndrome, and uremia, as well as following corticosteroid therapy. Paraproteinemias and amyloidosis may also lead to purpura.

2. PLATELET DISORDERS

Although platelets are classified as cells, they are actually cytoplasmatic fragments derived from megakaryocytes in the bone marrow. Platelet formation and release probably occur through the sinus endothelial cells; however, others postulate that megakaryocytes undergo cytoplasmatic fragmentation in the pulmonary capillary bed. Production and release of platelets from the bone marrow is controlled by thrombopoietin. Platelets remain in the circulation for approx 8–10 d. The normal platelet count ranges from 150,000/μL to 400,000/μL. The diameter of normal platelets is 1–4 μm. At a given point, 70% of the platelets are in the circulation and 30% are in the spleen (splenic pool). The daily platelet production of 40,000/μL can be increased eightfold.

2.1. Quantitative Disorders of Platelets

Thrombocytopenia, by definition, exists when the platelet count drops below 150,000/μL, although bleeding attributable to thrombocytopenia usually never occurs when the platelet count is above 100,000/μL. Spontaneous bleeding usually occurs with platelet counts less than 20,000/μL. Thrombocytopenia is due either to decreased bone marrow production of platelets or increased destruction and sequestration of the platelets from the circulation, or both. A diagnostic approach toward the etiology of thrombocytopenia is shown in Table 2.

2.2. Investigation of Thrombocytopenia

If either bleeding symptoms or an incidentally documented low platelet count lead to the diagnosis of thrombocytopenia, a blood smear must be obtained to rule out the possibility of a pseudothrombocytopenia caused by EDTA (platelet clumps) or a hematological disorder such as acute leukemia. The size of platelets may also give a diagnostic clue, because platelets may be enlarged in hereditary conditions. A drug history must be taken and the patient questioned about symptoms of viral illness. If a hematological systemic disease is suspected, a bone marrow examination will be necessary. Assays for detecting platelet antibodies are quite unspecific and insensitive.

Table 2
Classification of Thrombocytopenias

Decreased platelet production
- Marrow failure (e.g., aplastic anemia)
- Marrow infiltration (e.g., leukemia, MDS)
- Marrow depression—cytotoxic drugs, radiation
- Selective megakaryocyte depression—drugs, ethanol, viruses, chemicals
- Nutritional deficiency—megaloblastic anemia
- Hereditary causes (rare)—Fanconi syndrome, amegakaryocytic hypoplasia, absent radii syndrome, Wiskott-Aldrich syndrome

Increased platelet destruction
- Immune
  - Idiopathic thrombocytopenic purpura
  - Other autoimmune states—SLE, CLL, lymphoma
  - Drug-induced: heparin, quinidine, quinine, gold, penicilline, cimetidine
  - Infectious—HIV, other viruses, malaria
  - Posttransfusion purpura
  - Neonatal purpura
- Nonimmune
  - DIC
  - Thrombotic thrombocytopenic purpura/hemolytic uremic syndrome
  - Cavernous hemangioma
  - Cardiopulmonary bypass
  - Hypersplenism

MDS, myelodysplastic syndrome; SLE, systemic lupus erythematosus; CLL, chronic lymphocytic leukemia; DIC, disseminated intravascular coagulation.

2.3. Thrombocytopenia Due to Decreased Platelet Production

Thrombocytopenia due to decreased platelet production means that the bone marrow is unable to keep up with normal platelet requirements. Table 2 depicts the causes of thrombocytopenia due to underproduction of platelets (e.g., aplastic anemia, leukemia, myelodysplastic syndromes). Thrombocytopenia frequently occurs in patients with underlying malignancies who have received chemotherapy or radiotherapy that destroy the hematological stem cells. These patients require supportive therapy including platelet transfusions if they are bleeding. A permanent normalization of the platelet count is only possible with a successful therapy of the underlying disease. Megaloblastic anemias, including vitamin B_{12} and folic acid deficiencies, can present as isolated thrombocytopenia, although usually, all cell lines are affected. Many patients with acute and chronic disorders of alcohol abuse have thrombocytopenia. Hypersplenism can contribute to the thrombocytopenia if cirrhosis of the liver is present as well. However, for most patients the thrombocytopenia is due to acute alcohol-induced marrow supression. The hereditary causes of thrombocytopenia are quite rare. In amegakaryocytic thrombocytopenia, the platelets are normal to small in size, the platelet life span is normal or only slightly reduced, and the bone marrow biopsy shows a marked reduction in the number of megakaryocytes.

2.4. Thrombocytopenia Due to Increased Platelet Destruction

Isolated thrombocytopenia is, in most instances, caused by increased platelet destruction. In these patients, the rate of platelet destruction cannot be compensated by the bone marrow with increased platelet production. The causes of increased platelet destruction are shown in Table 2. These patients have isolated thrombocytopenia, and the number of megakaryocytes in the bone marrow is normal or increased. The platelet life span is shortened.

2.5. Immune Thrombocytopenia

Immune thrombocytopenia is an increase of platelet destruction caused by immunological mechanisms. The sensitization of platelets by immunoglobulin G (IgG) and IgM antibodies reacting with antigenic sites (usually glycoprotein [GP]IIb/IIIa in idiopathic thrombocytopenic purpura [ITP], platelet alloantigens in post-transfusion purpura, and neonatal isoimmune purpura) on the platelet membrane is the main cause of platelet destruction.

2.6. Idiopathic Thrombocytopenic Purpura

ITP occurs in both children and adults. *Acute ITP in children* is equally common in boys and girls, has its peak incidence at age 2 to 4 yr, and frequently follows a viral infection. More than 80% of these children have a spontaneous remission of their illness in 2 to 4 wk. Serious morbidity or mortality is rare (approx 1%), but the recovery of the platelets can be hastened by the administration of high doses of intravenous IgG (discussed later). The use of corticosteroids without a bone marrow examination is controversial.

The peak incidence of *ITP in adults* is at 20 to 40 yr of age, and the disease is much more common in women than in men (5:1). A number of patients will seek medical attention because of petechiae, purpura, epistaxis, or menorrhagia. In some patients, the hemostatic disorder is unmasked after taking a medication that interferes with platelet function, such as aspirin. However, asymptomatic thrombocytopenia is discovered in a substantial number of patients during routine blood testing. Except for clinical signs of bleeding (petechiae), the physical examination is usually unremarkable. An enlarged spleen usually suggests a disorder other than ITP. In addition to the platelet count, a white blood cell count and hemoglobin level should be measured in adult patients. ITP has normal white blood cells and hemoglobin, unless chronic bleeding would have caused an iron deficiency anemia. A bone marrow study may be useful to exclude other hematological disorders, especially if a splenectomy is planned; however, in a consensus recommendation, it was not generally recommended *(1)*. If it is done, one usually will find megakaryocytes in normal or increased number. As stated earlier, assays for antiplatelet antibodies can no longer be recommended because of the lack of sensitivity and specificity. Other tests may be performed because certain autoimmune diseases are associated with ITP. These tests include those to detect the presence of antinuclear antibodies and rheumatoid factor, thyroid function tests, and serological tests for HIV.

ITP is caused by an autoantibody—almost always IgG—that binds to specific platelet glycoproteins, especially GP IIb, IIIa. These antibodies attached to the platelet membranes may bind complement and cause accelerated platelet destruction through phagocytosis by the reticuloendothelial cells in the spleen and the liver. A compensatory increase in bone-marrow megakaryopoiesis usually occurs, which may initially prevent or delay the development of more severe thrombocytopenia. In a few cases, the measurement of the platelet life-span may be helpful. On rare occasions, platelets of patients with apparent ITP have a nearly normal life-span. The cause of the thrombocytopenia in these patients is unclear, an early myelodysplastic syndrome should be ruled out.

2.7. Treatment in Adults

The first issue is to decide whether a patient requires any specific treatment or not. Patients with moderate thrombocytopenia (platelets >40,000/µL) with no history or signs of bleeding do not require therapy and should just be observed. In contrast, patients with clinical signs of bleeding or very low platelet counts, usually less than 20,000/µL, require therapy. Initial therapy consists of corticosteroids (prednisone or prednisolone 1–2 mg/[kg · d]), which usually will raise the platelet count to safe levels in 70–80 % of the patients within 1 to 2 wk. When the platelet count has risen above 100,000/µL, one can begin to taper the dose of corticosteroids down to 10–15 mg/d. Only a few patients (10–20 %) will have long-lasting remissions following treatment with corticosteroids. Unfortunately, the platelet count of most adults with ITP will fall as the dose of corticosteroids is reduced. Splenectomy is indicated in patients who become unresponsive to corticosteroids or require prohibitively high doses to maintain the platelet count at an acceptable level. Splenectomy will not only remove the major site of platelet destruction but also a source of platelet autoantibody production. Approximately 70–80% of patients will sustain a long-term remission after splenectomy,

and in 60% of patients the platelet count will return to normal. Prior to splenectomy, a vaccination with pneumococcal vaccines is strongly recommended to prevent a life-threatening pneumococcal infection (overwhelming postsplenectomy
infection syndrome [OPSI]) that may occur many years after a splenectomy.
Splenectomy fails to correct the platelet count in about 25% of adults with ITP.
In patients with an initial response to splenectomy followed by a relapse, the
possibility of an accessory spleen should be ruled out. Because subsequent treatments pose increased risks to the patients, it should be decided whether treatment
in failing patients is absolutely necessary. Treatment options for failing patients
include "pulse-dose" dexamethasone (40 mg/d for days 1–4, every 4 wk),
azothioprine, cyclophosphamide, vinca alkaloids, cyclosporine A, and danazole.
The drugs may be effective in a few patients, but they have both considerable
acute and long-term side effects. High doses of intravenous IgG (0.4 g/kg for 2–
5 d or 1 g/kg day 1 [for 1–2 d]) raise the platelet count in about 60–70 % of patients
with ITP. For patients with life-threatening bleeding or preoperatively, if corticosteroids have failed, IgG is the treatment of choice. However, the platelet rise
is of short duration usually lasting only 1–3 wk. The costs of treatment are very
high. For this reason, treatment with intravenous IgG can only be justified in
emergency situations. The anti-D immunoglobulin is effective only in Rh D-
positive nonsplenectomized patients, in whom the antibody binds to the erythrocyte D antigen. The mechanism of action involves immune-mediated clearance
of the opsonized erythrocytes via the Fc receptors of the reticuloendothelial
system, thereby minimizing removal of antibody-coated platelets. Anti-D
(WinRho SDF™) can be administered by intravenous injection over a few minutes. The response rate was 70% in one series, and the increase of platelets lasted
more than 3 wk in 50% of the responders. The standard dosage of 50–75 µg/kg
per day of intravenous anti-D requires 72 h to produce a clinically significant
platelet increase. The great majority of patients who respond to anti-D require
periodic retreatments. Several small studies have investigated the use of
rituximab, a monoclonal antibody directed against the B-cell antigen CD20. The
results were variable, but overall the response rate was about 50%, with 25–30%
sustained responses over 6 mo.

   Because antiplatelet IgG traverses the placenta, about 25% of infants born to
mothers with active ITP will develop this disorder. In some cases, neonatal ITP
also occurs in infants born to women with only a history of a previous ITP.
Prenatal treatment with corticosteroids (prednisone 20–40 mg/d for 10–14 d) is
associated with reduced frequency and severity of thrombocytopenia in the infants. For active ITP associated with bleeding, a cesarean section is recommended. If a fetal scalp sampling reveals a normal or moderately reduced platelet
count of the infant, a spontaneous delivery should be allowed.

2.8. Other Autoimmune Conditions

Immune-mediated thrombocytopenia with elevated levels of platelet-associated IgG occurs as a complication in a number of systemic disorders. It is usually indistinguishable from classic ITP. The association of an immune thrombocytopenia with malignant lymphomas, systemic lupus erythematosus, thyrotoxicosis, infectious mononucleosis, and other severe infections is well known. Also, the thrombocytopenia seen after bone marrow or renal transplantation may be immune mediated. In autoimmune hemolytic anemia, a thrombocytopenia may develop as a parallel event (Evan's syndrome). The secondary thrombocytopenia in these disorders may improve with the treatment of the underlying disease.

2.9. Drug-Induced Thrombocytopenia

A large number of drugs can induce thrombocytopenic purpura. In most cases, isolated thrombocytopenia is caused by immune mechanisms, although few drugs cause direct marrow toxicity in the absence of immune mechanisms. The drugs that commonly cause thrombocytopenia include quinine and quinidine, heparin, H₂-antagonists (cimetidine, ranitidine), gold salts, valproic acid, and certain antibiotics, especially the penicillins and sulfonamides. Clinically, drug-induced thrombocytopenic purpuras are acute in onset, occurring within hours to days after ingesting the offending drug. Chills and fever may precede purpuric and petechial hemorrhage. Historically, the drug-induced thrombocytopenia due to quinine or quinidine has been studied most extensively. The external platelet surface is capable of nonspecifically absorbing certain antibody–drug complexes, which then lead to platelet damage by an "innocent bystander" effect. The administered drug binds as a hapten to a plasma protein or "carrier" to form an antigen. Antibodies stimulated by the immunogen bind to the drug, and these immune complexes secondarily interact with the platelet membrane, leading to cellular damage. Specific metabolic products of certain drugs rather than the primary agent may interact as the offending immunogen. In recent years, heparin has become the most thoroughly studied drug, because it may lead, in up to 5% of patients, to an immune-mediated thrombocytopenia (*see* heparin). In drug-induced thrombocytopenia, all drugs should be discontinued. If absolutely necessary, these compounds should be replaced by pharmacologically equivalent but chemically different preparations. Corticosteroids may be given; their value, however, is disputable. In life-threatening bleeding complications, platelet transfusions should be used.

2.10. Posttransfusion Purpura

The posttransfusion purpura syndrome occurs 1 wk after transfusion of blood or blood products that contain or are contaminated with platelets. In this disorder, platelet-specific alloantigens have been implicated. The PI^{A1} antigen is present in 98% of the population. The other 2% are at risk for the development of posttransfusion purpura if they receive blood products that express PI^{A1}. Thus, the disorder will develop in those patients who have been previously sensitized through blood transfusion or pregnancy. Most cases have developed in multiparous women without prior blood transfusions. The clinical picture resembles that of acute ITP with platelet counts as low as 1000/μL. The diagnosis can be confirmed by demonstrating a platelet-specific antibody from the patient that reacts with PI^{A1}. The antibody will disappear within 1 to 5 wk and the patient usually recovers spontaneously.

2.11. Neonatal Purpura

Neonatal thrombocytopenia may develop due to isoimmunization of the mother against fetal platelets with subsequent transplacental transfer. The incidence of alloimmune neonatal purpura is 1 in 5000 deliveries. The most commonly involved antigen is PI^{A1}, an antigen that is present on platelets of 98% of the population. The infant shows generalized purpura at delivery, and platelet counts are usually below 30,000/μL. Intracranial hemorrhage is a severe complication that occurs in about 10% of affected infants.

2.12. Nonimmune Thrombocytopenia

2.12.1. DISSEMINATED INTRAVASCULAR COAGULATION

This group of disorders is discussed in Chapter 21. It is generally associated with significant thrombocytopenia. The platelets are "consumed" secondary to the generation of excessive amounts of thrombin into the circulation.

2.13. Thrombotic Thrombocytopenic Purpura (Moschcowitz's Disease) and Hemolytic-Uremic Syndrome (Gasser's Syndrome)

In both thrombotic thrombocytopenic purpura (TTP; Moschcowitz disease) and hemolytic-uremic syndrom (HUS; Gasser syndrome), schistocytes (fragmented red blood cells, helmet cells) and low platelets are found. TTP is an acute disease which presents a clinical spectrum, including thrombocytopenic purpura, microangiopathic hemolytic anemia, renal disease, transient fluctuating neurological symptoms, and fever. Neurological symptoms range from transitory bizarre behavioral disturbances with sensorimotor deficits to seizures and coma. The diagnosis is made on clinical grounds and by excluding other causes of schistocytic hemolytic anemia and thrombocytopenia. HUS is a triad of thrombocytopenia, acute renal failure, and intravascular hemolysis with schistocytosis. It is observed mainly in pediatric patients. There is a close clinical, pathophysiological, and therapeutic relationship between TTP and HUS because of similarities of the thrombotic microangiopathy. Clinically, the neurological symptoms of TTP are not present in HUS, whereas the severe renal dysfunction characteristic of HUS is generally not as extreme in TTP. Because the thrombocytopenia is not caused by thrombin, most clotting tests are normal. However, a number of studies have demonstrated abnormalities of the von Willebrand factor (VWF) in patients with TTP. Pathologically, arterioles and capillaries in multiple organs are occluded by hyaline thrombi. This material represents thrombin-induced dense platelet aggregates surrounded by thin layers of fibrin. The exact pathogenesis of the platelet microthrombi has never been clearly elucidated. TTP has been linked to a history of antecedent respiratory tract infections and to the ingestion of certain drugs (antibiotics, oral contraceptives), as well as to the postoperative state, pregnancy, meningococcal and mycoplasma infections, and vaccines. It is speculated that TTP and HUS are the consequence of the intrusion into the circulation of one or more platelet-aggregating agents. The aggregating agent has variously been reported to be a protein(s) with a molecular weight of 37,000 or 59,000 Daltons. This may include a calcium-activated protease (calpain) that has the capacity to cleave VWF multimers into fragments with increased platelet-binding capacity. Also, unusually large VWF multimers that bind to platelet GP Ib-IX and IIb/IIIa with induction of aggregation may be involved. In addition, there is evidence of a VWF depolymerase that reduces the size of the unusually large VWF multimers that are synthesized. Recently it was reported that the VWF-cleaving protease was purified and identified as a new member of the ADAMTS (a disintegrin and metalloprotease with thrombospondin motifs) family of metalloproteinases (ADAMTS13). The gene encoding this protease is located on chromosome 9q34. Autoantibodies to this enzyme were described. These antibodies apparently prevent the formation of small fragments of VWF. During the acute episode, most patients with a single episode of TTP have ultra-large multimers of VWF in plasma, probably because of systemic endothelial cell injury. Serial studies of plasma samples from patients during these episodes have shown that the ultra-large VWF multimers and also the large forms of the multimers disappear as the TTP episode continues and worsens. This is probably due to attachment of the ultra-large VWF multimers to the platelets during intravascular aggregation. There is an increase in large multimers following recovery or between relapses. For confirmation of the diagnosis, biopsies of the gingiva, the bone marrow, skin, or muscle are recommended. These may show hyaline thrombi in 50–60% of patients. In rare cases, familial and chronic relapsing TTP is observed. Such patients have very low levels of ADAMTS13 plasma activity as a result of mutations of the *ADAMTS13* gene. In the more frequent cases of acquired idiopathic TTP, autoantibodies against ADAMTS13 are found. Clinically useful assays to measure ADAMTS13 activity are currently under development.

The treatment of TTP is a hematological emergency. Untreated TTP was fatal in up to 90% of patients. Currently, plasma therapy brings the disease into remission in 80–90% of patients, although relapses occur frequently. The treatment of choice is plasmapheresis and plasma exchange of 3–4 L/d. The rationale behind this treatment is the replacement of platelet-aggregating factors, such as ultra-large VWF multimers and other factors by normal blood components such as the deficient depolymerase. Plasmapheresis and plasma exchange must be continued in some refractory or relapsing patients for up to 4 wk. If plasmapheresis or plasma exchange is not available, the transfusion of larger amounts of fresh frozen plasma may also be effective. This has often been successfully employed with the chronic relapsing form of TTP. Although no sound scientific evidence exists, many clinicians feel that patients with TTP may profit from additional corticosteroid therapy. Plasma exchange with cryoprecipitate supernatant (from which VWF-rich cryoprecipitate has been removed) has been successful in a number of unresponsive patients. Some patients have also improved following intravenous injections of vincristine. There is no evidence that aspirin or dipyridamol are effective, and heparin is probably not only ineffective but also dangerous.

In HUS, a disorder observed mainly in infants and young children, aggressive therapy has reduced mortality to about 5%, although 20–25 % of the patients may suffer permanent renal damage. When anuria is present for less than 24 h, fluid and electrolyte therapy will usually be sufficient. If the HUS is more severe, dialysis is required. This should be started early to prevent permanent renal damage. As yet, it is unclear whether plasma therapy as employed in TTP plays a role in disease management.

2.14. Cavernous Hemangioma (Kasabach-Meritt Syndrome)

Giant cavernous hemangioma is generally detected at birth and is due to abnormal proliferation of capillaries (angiomatoid malformation) that may grow during the first year of life but regress slowly in ensuing years. Thrombocytopenia, which may be severe, results from excessive sequestration and consumption of platelets within the relatively static blood in the vascular network of the tumor. Intravascular coagulation takes place within the tumor. Thrombocytopenia is the most prominent feature of the generalized coagulation disorder. Surgical excision of the tumor, if possible, and radiation therapy have been used successfully in therapy.

2.15. Cardiopulmonary Bypass

During extracorporal perfusion for cardiac surgery, a variable degree of thrombocytopenia almost always occurs. The mechanism of the thrombocytopenia is multifactorial. The drop in platelet number is primarily due to hemodilution. In addition, there is evidence of platelet activation and loss in the plastic tubing. The drop in platelet count generally persists for several days following bypass probably due to increased clearance of damaged platelets. The bypass procedure can also lead to abnormalities in platelet function.

2.16. Hypersplenism

Thrombocytopenia may occur in any disorder associated with an enlarged spleen. Under normal circumstances, approximately one-third of the total body platelet mass is found in the splenic pool, which exchanges with the freely circulating platelets. In patients with splenomegaly, regardless of the cause, the splenic platelet pool may be greatly expanded and up to 90% of the platelets can be trapped at any one time. Thus, a redistribution of platelets will occur, resulting in thrombocytopenia despite normal platelet production and normal platelet survival. The thrombocytopenia secondary to splenomegaly is rarely severe enough to produce hemorrhagic disease.

2.17. Thrombocytosis

Thrombocytosis refers to clinical situations in which the platelet count is significantly elevated. Secondary thrombocytosis usually occurs as a temporary event following splenectomy, or as a response to an acute or chronic inflammatory disease, acute hemorrhage, iron deficiency, or exercise. Asymptomatic secondary thrombocytosis with platelet counts in the range of 600,000 to 1 million µL may be present in a number of patients with untreated carcinoma, Hodgkin's and other lymphomas. The thrombocytosis may be caused by a nonspecific megakaryocytic proliferative response to tissue necrosis. Thrombocytosis has also been noted after the use of drugs such as vincristine, which interferes with microtubules.

Essential thrombocythemia is a chronic myeloproliferative disorder with a sustained increase of platelet production uncontrolled by normal regulatory processes. Essential thrombocythemia is a clonal proliferative disorder primarily affecting megakaryocytes (*see* "Myeloproliferative Disorders"). Hemorrhage and/or thrombosis occur in about one-third of patients. Bleeding is usually from mucosal surfaces and frequently is associated with one or more functional platelet abnormalities.

3. QUALITATIVE PLATELET DISORDERS

Several hemorrhagic disorders can be attributed to abnormalities in platelet function occurring in the presence of adequate numbers of circulating platelets. The abnormalities may result from processes involving adhesion, activation aggregation, or a deficient release reaction. The bleeding time is probably the most useful in vivo test for rapid evaluation of platelet function. In vitro tests to evaluate platelet function include the measurement of adhesiveness to glass bead columns, platelet aggregation tests, and the most reliable system, platelet flow cytometry.

3.1. Bernard-Soulier Syndrome (BSS)

BSS is a rare congenital bleeding disorder transmitted as an autosomal recessive trait. The platelets are usually moderately decreased in number and on review of the blood smear they are large and variable in their morphology. Bleeding from cutaneous and mucous membranes is quite common. The major functional abnormality in this disease is an impaired adhesion of the platelets to the subendothelial matrix causing a markedly prolonged bleeding time. The adhesion defect is due to a deficiency or absence of the GP Ib/IX complex, which results in impaired interaction of platelets with VWF at the vessel wall. Thus, BSS should be suspected when giant platelets are found on the blood smear and when ristocetin is unable to aggregate platelets in the presence of normal VWF. GP Ib/IX is the binding site for VWF when platelets are exposed to ristocetin. The diagnosis is confirmed by quantitation of the GP Ib/IX complex by platelet flow cytometry. Patients with BSS may need platelet transfusions to prevent or treat hemorrhage. However, multiple transfusions will lead to the development of alloantibodies that destroy donor platelets and limit the efficacy of subsequent transfusions. Therapeutic modalities that have been employed with questionable results include desmopressin (DDAVP), corticosteroids, and oral contraceptive therapy to decrease menstrual bleeding. In a life-threatening bleeding complication also the recombinant factor VIIa (NovoSeven™) may be effective (*see* "Hemophilias A and B").

3.2. Thrombasthenia (Glanzmann Disease)

Glanzmann thrombasthenia is an autosomal recessive disorder characterized by moderate to severe mucocutaneous bleeding, including menorrhagia, and postoperative bleeding. In most patients, the bleeding diathesis is severe, although there are exceptions. The hallmarks of the disease are a prolonged bleeding time and an absent aggregation response to all aggregation agonists such as ADP, collagen, epinephrine, thrombin, and arachidonate. The typical form of the disease is marked by a deficiency or absence of the platelet membrane GP IIb/IIIa complex. As a result, the platelets cannot bind fibrinogen following platelet activation and cannot aggregate to form the platelet plug. Thrombasthenic platelets show normal secretory responses and can adhere to the vessel wall. The diagnosis is confirmed by demonstrating the absence of agonist-induced platelet aggregation and the absence or partial deficiency of the GP IIb/IIIa complex by platelet flow cytometry. Glanzmann thrombasthenia is classified into type I patients, who completely lack GP IIb/IIIa and fibrinogen on the surface of their platelets, and type II patients, who have a partial deficiency of GP IIb/IIIa (5–20%) and fibrinogen on the surface of their platelets. In case of bleeding the therapy of choice is platelet transfusions, which are successful initially but are followed as a rule by subsequent immunization. According to recent case reports, the recombinant F VIIa concentrate (NovoSeven™) seems to be a potential alternative to platelet transfusion in Glanzmann's thrombasthenia patients, particularly in those with antiplatelet antibodies and/or platelet refractoriness.

3.3. Abnormalities of Platelet Secretion

Platelet cytoplasma contains four types of granules: dense granules (containing ADP, ATP, calcium, and serotonin), α-granules (containing a variety of proteins), lysosomes (containing acid hydrolases), and microperoxymes (containing peroxidase activity). Following platelet activation, the contents of these granules are secreted in a process called platelet secretion. Inherited disorders of platelet secretion result from the deficiency of one or more of these types of platelet granules or from abnormalities in the mechanism of platelet secretion with a quantitatively normal granule population. These disorders usually cause mild to moderate bleeding manifesting itself by easy bruising, menorrhagia, and excessive postoperative or postpartum blood loss. Patients with a disorder of platelet secretion usually have a moderately prolonged bleeding time, absence of the second wave of platelet aggregation after stimulation with the agonists ADP and epinephrine (δ-granule defect), and decreased aggregation after stimulation with collagen. Similar laboratory patterns may be observed in acquired abnormalities of platelet secretion induced by drugs such as aspirin, or in systemic diseases such as uremia and dysproteinemias.

3.4. α-Granule Deficiency
(Gray Platelet Syndrome, α-Storage Pool Disease)

The gray platelet syndrome is a rare bleeding disorder resulting from the absence of morphologically recognizable α-granules in the platelets of affected patients. The name derives from the large gray platelets that appear on the blood smear. The disorder presumably results from a defect in granule formation or packing within the megakaryocytes. α-granules contain a variety of proteins such as platelet factor (PF)-4, β-thromboglobulin (TG), platelet-derived growth factor (PDGF), thrombospondin, fibrinogen, VWF, and others. The lack of these proteins can cause a life-long history of mild mucocutaneous bleeding and a prolonged bleeding time. The number of platelets is usually decreased (60,000–100,000/μL). Aggregation studies give conflicting results, but usually there is a decrease or absence of collagen-induced aggregation.

3.5. Dense Granule Deficiency (δ-Storage Pool Disease)

The diagnosis of δ-granule deficiency is usually suspected upon finding a reduction in the amount of δ-granule substances (e.g., ADP, serotonin) in the platelets. A defect in the platelet release reaction results in a single reversible aggregation wave, because there are no dense body components to recruit platelets for the second wave.

A hereditary deficiency in dense granules is also a feature of *Hermansky-Pudlak syndrome*, which is associated with oculocutaneous albinism and a ceroid-like pigment in marrow macrophages. Another dense granule deficiency disorder is *Chediak-Higashi syndrome* (oculocutaneous albinism, chronic infections, and hemorrhage). Platelet granule abnormalities have also been reported in *Wiskott-Aldrich syndrome* (thrombocytopenia, infections, eczema). Platelets that have normal dense granule components but are unable to release them have also been classified as having an *"aspirin-like" defect* because the clinical symptoms resemble those following the ingestion of aspirin. Patients with δ-storage pool disease present with a mild to moderate bleeding diathesis characteristic of platelet secretion defects. The number of platelets and their morphology are usually normal, whereas the bleeding time is often, but not always, prolonged.

3.5.1. THERAPY

Severe bleeding episodes may require platelet transfusions, but DDAVP should be tried initially because it may be effective in a number of patients.

Acquired storage pool disease has been described in association with antiplatelet antibodies, in systemic lupus erythematosus, in myeloproliferative disorders, and following tumoricidal doses of mithramycin.

3.6. Acquired Disorders of Platelet Function

Several systemic diseases are complicated by qualitative abnormalities in platelet function. In these systemic diseases, usually external or unphysiological components of the plasma result in partial or complete interference with platelet functions.

3.6.1. UREMIA

Many patients with uremia have a bleeding diathesis characterized by a prolonged bleeding time and abnormal platelet adhesion, aggregation, secretion, and platelet procoagulant activity. The pathogenesis of the platelet defect is not clear. Abnormalities in plasma VWF, reduction in GP Ib, and a decreased adhesion via GP IIb/IIIa have been reported. Uremic platelets exhibit, when stimulated, a reduced release of arachidonic acid from membrane phospholipids. Some of the functional abnormalities may be due to a uremic toxin. Both dialyzable and nondialyzable substances found in uremic plasma can inhibit platelets in vitro at high concentrations. The bleeding diathesis and the prolonged bleeding time in uremia often improve with dialysis. Infusion of DDAVP (0.3 µg/kg) will improve hemorrhage and bleeding times in more than 50% of uremic patients.

3.6.2. MYELOPROLIFERATIVE DISORDERS

Platelet dysfunctions are observed in patients with chronic myeloproliferative disorders (essential thrombocythemia, polycythemia vera), but also in some patients with acute leukemias and myelodysplastic syndromes. The patterns of abnormality vary from patient to patient, and none of the functional defects reliably predicts a potential clinical hemorrhage. In most of these disorders, thrombocytopenia is usually a more significant cause of bleeding than platelet dysfunction. However, in essential thrombocythemia, bleeding may occur with elevated platelet counts, even if the bleeding time is normal. These same patients may also experience vascular ischemic syndromes due to microvascular platelet occlusion.

3.6.3. DYSPROTEINEMIAS

The dysproteinemias (multiple myeloma, Waldenström macroglobulinemia) are another group of systemic disorders in which the hemorrhagic diathesis has multiple causes. One major cause of bleeding complications is due to the blockage of surface-connected platelet functions. Paraproteins adsorbed on platelet and vessel surfaces result in the inhibition of GP IIb/IIIa, platelet adhesion, and clot retraction. Platelet survival is shortened. Additional defects include thrombocytopenia, inhibition of coagulation factors (factor VIII), defective fibrin polymerization, and hyperviscosity.

3.6.4. LIVER DISEASE

Disorders of hemostasis in liver disease are multifactorial. Clotting factor deficiencies, thrombocytopenia, enhanced fibrinolysis, a mild persistent DIC, and dysfibrinogenemia all contribute to bleeding and measurable coagulation defects. Excess fibrinogen/fibrin degradation products that are present in liver disease, adsorb to platelets and may interfere with platelet functions. Bleeding time is frequently prolonged. DDAVP is effective in some patients, but in the case of severe bleeding and platelet counts less than 50,000/µL, platelet transfusions will be necessary.

3.6.5. DRUG-INDUCED PLATELET ABNORMALITIES

Many drugs affect platelet function in vitro, although relatively few of them prolong the bleeding time. Aspirin ingestion results in abnormal platelet function with a moderately prolonged bleeding time and a defective platelet aggregation due to the inhibition of the cyclooxygenase and the thromboxane synthetase (*see* Chapter 19). Large doses of carbenicillin and other penicillins, as well as the cephalosporin moxolactam, prolong the bleeding time in a dose-related fashion. This effect begins within hours after drug administration and may last for several days. All phases of platelet function—adhesion, aggregation, and secretion—may be affected. In vitro, the penicillins impair the interaction of the VWF and aggregation agonists with the platelet surface membrane. The plasma expanders dextran and hydroxyethyl starch can prolong the bleeding time and cause abnormalities of platelet function comparable to those observed in dysproteinemias. Numerous other agents used in clinical medicine adversely affect normal hemostasis. Included among these are the anti-inflammatory agents (diclofenac, indomethacine, and others).

4. INHERITED DISODERS OF BLOOD COAGULATION

Inherited disorders of blood coagulation are due to the lack of synthesis or to the synthesis of a dysfunctional molecule of one and, in rare instances, more than one coagulation factors. Although uncommon, theses disorders have provided a great deal of information about the normal physiology of blood coagulation. Factor VIII and factor IX deficiencies are inherited as a sex-linked trait. Von Willebrand disease (VWD) is inherited in an autosomal dominant manner, whereas all the other abnormalities of coagulation factors show an autosomal recessive pattern of inheritance. Many of the coagulation proteins have been cloned and their amino acid sequences are known.

4.1. Hemophilias A and B

Hemophilia A (factor VIII deficiency) is the most common hereditary disorder of blood coagulation. It is due to the absent or decreased function of coagulation factor VIII, resulting from mutations in the factor VIII gene. The gene for factor VIII is located near the tip of the long arm of the X chromosome (Xq2.8). A rather large number of defects, including many deletions and different point mutations, have been found in the factor VIII gene by mutation analysis. The inheritance is sex-linked, but 30–40% of patients are without a positive family history, thus in these cases, the presence of the factor VIII gene is likely the result of spontaneous mutation. Hemophilia A occurs in approx 1 in 10,000 persons. Because the gene for factor VIII is present on the X chromosome, females are usually not affected because they carry only one defective gene. The inheritance pattern of a case of hempohilia A is shown in Fig. 20.1. Children of a female carrier have a 50% chance of inheriting the abnormal X chromosome.

The inheritance as well as the clinical features of hemophilia B (factor IX deficiency, Christmas disease) are identical to those of hemophilia A. The inci-

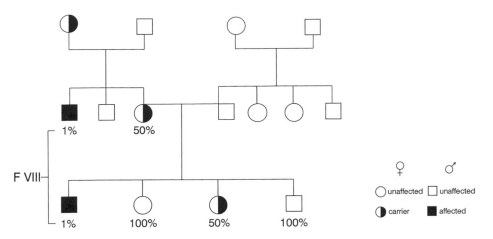

Fig. 20.1. Sex-linked pattern of inheritance in hemophilia A and B.

dence is one-fifth of that of hemophilia A. The two disorders can only be distinguished by coagulation factor assays. The factor IX gene is close to the gene for factor VIII near the tip of the long arm of the X chromosome (Xq2.6). It is about one-fifth the size of the factor VIII gene. Molecular probes have demonstrated point mutations or deletions within the gene in a number of families.

4.1.1. CLINICAL PRESENTATION

Excess bleeding is relatively uncommon at birth. The first bleeding problems usually start when a child starts crawling, and this may be from 9 mo to 1 yr of age. Bleeding, however, can occur after surgery, i.e., circumcision. The first signs that parents may notice are large skin bruises. Abnormal and recurrent bleeding can then occur from any part of the body. A dominant feature of the severe form of the disorder is recurrent painful bleeding into the joints (hemarthrosis) and into the muscles (muscle hematomas). Joint bleeding usually involves the large joints (knees, ankles, ellbows), and the accumulation of blood in the joint space leads to severe pain. If left untreated, the recurrence of the bleeding episodes will lead to progressive deformity and crippling in severely affected patients (Fig. 20.2). Soft tissue and intramuscular bleeding may lead to considerable blood loss, particularly in the retroperitoneum and the thigh. Repeated subperiostal hemorrhage with bone destruction, new bone formation, and expansion of the bone may result in large pseudotumors. Bleeding in the pharyngeal area may be life-threatening because of potential airway obstruction. Minor head traumas may cause serious CNS bleeding leading to death or permanent disability. The severity of the bleeding manifestations depends on the remaining activity of factors VIII or IX measured in clotting assays (*see* Table 3).

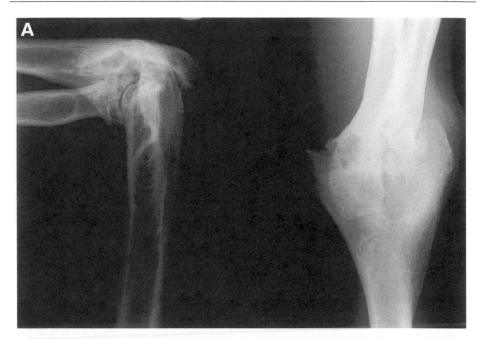

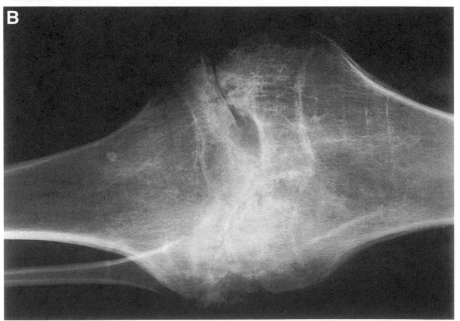

Fig. 20.2. Repeated hemarthroses result in chronic synovitis, destruction of cartilage, and progressive flexion contractures. **A** and **B** are X-rays depicting the elbows and the knee of a 35-yr-old patient with hemophilia.

Table 3
Correlation of Factor VIII or IX Activity and Disease Severity

Coagulation factor activity (%)	Clinical manifestations
>1	Severe disease
	Recurrent spontaneous bleeding episodes
	Joint deformities and crippling, if insufficiently treated
1–5	Moderate disease
	Occasional spontaneous bleeding
	Postsurgical or posttraumatic bleeding
5–20	Mild disease
	Postsurgical or posttraumatic bleeding

4.1.2. LABORATORY DIAGNOSIS

The laboratory diagnosis of the hemophilias is straightforward, as often the family history and the clinical manifestations suggest the diagnosis. Of the screening tests, only the activated partial thromboplastin time (aPTT) is prolonged. With the severe form of hemophilia, a prolongation in the range of 90–100 s can be expected. Subsequent testing with a specific, factor VIII- or IX-deficient plasma can prove the suspected diagnosis of hemophilia A or B. The bleeding time, the prothrombin time, and also the VWF activity should be normal.

Diagnosis of carrier status with DNA analysis is more predictive if a restriction-length polymorphism can be established for the affected family. Until recently, the ratio of factor VIII to VWF was used to predict a carrier status. This ratio is 0.5 in the carrier status as opposed to 1.0 in normal females. However, the normal range of factor VIII is broad, which makes this method unreliable. For antenatal diagnosis, chorionic biopsies at 8–10 wk gestation will provide sufficient DNA from fetal cells for analysis using PCR technology. Caution should be used in making a diagnosis of moderate or mild hemophilia B in the neonatal period because normal levels of factor IX in full-term infants are not reached until 6–9 mo. Factor VIII levels, on the other hand, are in the normal adult range by 28 wk of gestation. Thus all forms of hemophila are distinguishable by assay in both premature and full-term infants.

4.1.3. TREATMENT

Acute bleeding episodes are treated with concentrates of clotting factor VIII in hemophilia A and clotting factor IX in hemophilia B. The plasma concentrates are derived from the plasma donations of 10,000 or more individuals. Since the mid-1980s, all commercial concentrates have been subjected to virucidal techniques to eliminate the transmission of pathogenic blood borne viruses (*see* "Treatment-Related Problems"). Since the mid-1990s, recombinant factor VIII concentrates have also been included in the treatment regimens, mainly for previously untreated persons ("PUPs"). Spontaneous bleeding (joints, muscles) is usually controlled if the patient's factor level is raised to 20% of the normal level. If the hemorrhage is occurring at critical sites (CNS, nasopharyngeal area), before major surgery, or after serious posttraumatic bleeding, the factor VIII or IX level should be elevated to 100% and then maintained above 50% until healing has occurred. The amount of clotting factor needed can be calculated as follows:

1 unit of factor VIII/kg will raise the blood level by 1%

1 unit of factor IX/kg will raise the blood level by 1–2%

However, it must be taken into consideration that, in the event of acute bleeding, the rise of the factor level may be only half of the amount calculated for more stable situations.

DDAVP provides an alternative treatment for increasing the factor VIII levels in patients with a mild form of hemophilia A. A residual factor VIII activity (usually >10%) is required to obtain a moderate rise in the patient's factor VIII level following the intravenous administration of 0.3 µg/kg DDAVP.

Local supportive measures in treating hemarthrosis and hematomas include resting the affected extremity and administration of systemic nonspecific drugs such as antifibrinolytic agents (e.g., tranexamic acid), which may be helpful in prevention or treatment of mucocutanous hemorrhage and after dental procedures.

Most patients attend specialized hemophilia centers where they are educated and trained on the management of bleeding complications including home treatment. The coagulation factor concentrates may be stored in domestic refrigerators and, at the earliest suggestion of bleeding, the affected hemophiliac can be treated at home. This early home treatment reduces the occurrence of crippling hemarthrosis and also saves a great number of hospital days. Treatment of hemophilia involves not only replacement therapy but an overall approach to the patient and his family with regard to education, psychosocial care, and periodical dental and orthopedic evaluation. With modern treatment, the daily life of a child with hemophilia can be almost normal, although certain activities (body contact sports) should be avoided.

4.1.4. TREATMENT-RELATED PROBLEMS

A serious problem in the management of hemophilia is the development of inhibitors (usually IgG antibodies), which occur in 20% of patients with hemophilia A but only in 1% of patients with hemophilia B. As a result, the infusion of the usual dose of factor VIII is no longer effective. The level of the inhibitors is expressed in Bethesda Units (BU). In the event of bleeding, "low responders" (<5 BU) are usually treated with very high doses of factor VIII concentrates, whereas for "high responders" (>5 BU) alternative treatment modalities are required. These include certain factor IX concentrates containing activated factors that "bypass" the need for factor VIII (known as factor VIII inhibitor bypassing activity or FEIBA), or a recombinant activated factor VII concentrate (NovoSeven™).

Many hemophiliacs have features of subclinical liver disease and a few have overt chronic hepatitis, due to the many infusions of clotting factor products that had not been strictly subjected to virucidal techniques before the mid-1980s. A fact is that transmission of hepatitis B or, more frequently, hepatitis C had occurred in a great number of patients prior to 1985. This also accounts for the transmission of AIDS, which was for a number of years the most common cause of death in severe hemophilia. As a result of HIV in clotting concentrates infused before 1985, more than 50% of the hemophiliacs treated in the United States or western Europe were HIV positive. The incidence of clinical AIDS had been steadily increasing. Fortunately, the new virucidal techniques (pasteurization, terminal high temperature heating of lyophilized concentrates, and/or solvent/detergent methods) have effectively eliminated new HIV transmissions and have virtually prevented transmission of the lipid-enveloped hepatitis B, C, and D viruses. In the 1990s, the safety has further increased by the introduction of genetically engineered recombinant factor VIII concentrates.

4.2. Von Willebrand Disease

VWD is characterized by an abnormal platelet adhesion with or without a low factor VIII activity. VWF promotes platelet adhesion and is also the carrier for factor VIII, protecting the latter from premature destruction. This explains the combination of defective platelet adhesion and reduced levels of factor VIII.

4.2.1. GENETICS

VWD is a bleeding disorder inherited in an autosomal dominant disorder. The penetrance is high, but the expression is quite variable from family to family and also within families. Severe type 3 VWD is inherited in an autosomal recessive manner and is associated with very low or undetectable levels of VWF. A large number of molecular defects have been identified in VWD, including point mutations and major deletions.

4.2.2. PREVALENCE AND CLINICAL PRESENTATION

VWD is clearly the most common genetic bleeding disorder to be encountered in clinical practice, although its estimated incidence varies widely from 0.1% to as high as 1% of the general population. The most common variant, type 1 VWD, characterized by a moderate quantitative deficiency of functionally normal VWF, accounts for about 70% of patients. The most common clinical features in VWD are mucocutanous episodes, including epistaxis, easy bruising, hematomas, and menorrhagia. Postoperative bleeding occurs after tooth extraction, tonsillectomy, and, naturally, following major operative procedures. Bleeding is quite variable in each patient and within the same family, and menstrual blood loss in females varies widely in the same family. An unexplained observation is the tendency of clinical symptoms to decrease after the patient enters the second decade of life.

4.2.3. LABORATORY DIAGNOSIS

Initial diagnostic tests should include the bleeding time, a factor VIII assay, and measurement of the levels of VWF. Bleeding time varies from abnormal in moderately and severely affected patients to normal in patients with mild forms of VWD. Bleeding time correlates well with the clinical symptoms. Because bleeding time performed on the skin is quite insensitive, the automatic platelet function analyzer (PFA-100®, Dade International) has become popular. Anticoagulated fresh whole blood passes at a high shear rate through a capillary tube through a membrane coated with collagen, in the presence of ADP or epinephrine, to an aperture. Formation of a platelet plug is signaled by a closure time (CT). CT is more sensitive in VWD than bleeding time. Decreased factor VIII activity will be detected only in patients with a moderate or severe form of VWD. aPTT may be prolonged in those patients whose factor VIII activity is decreased to less than 40% of normal. There is a defective platelet aggregation with ristocetin in most patients with a moderate or severe form of VWD. Aggregation to the other agonists (ADP, collagen, epinephrine) is normal. The VWF or ristocetin co-factor assay uses washed or formalin-fixed normal platelets and compares the rate of platelet aggregation using patient vs normal plasma in the presence of ristocetin. This test measures the patient's plasma VWF activity in a quantitative manner.

Agarose gel electrophoresis allows visualization of different sizes of the VWF multimers. This assay identifies the variant forms of VWD and helps to subdivide the disorder into three major subtypes. Type 1 VWD refers to a partial quantitative deficiency of VWF. Type 2 VWD refers to qualitative deficiency of VWF. Type 3 VWD refers to a virtually complete deficiency of VWF. The qualitative type 2 VWD is divided further into four variants—2A, 2B, 2M, and 2N—based on the phenotype.

4.2.4. TREATMENT

Most patients with moderate disease (usually type 1) and mild bleeding symptoms or bleeding after minor surgery will respond to DDAVP (deamino-8-D-arginine-vasopresssin, desmopressin, Stimate®), a synthetic analog of the natural hormone vasopressin, which releases factor VIII, VWF, and plasminogen activator from storage sites. It is given in a dosage of 0.3 µg/kg i.v. over 30 min. DDAVP probably releases the very large VWF multimers from the endothelial cells or platelets and thus corrects the prolonged bleeding time. The effect extends over several hours, the response decreases if treatment is repeated over a period of several days. It is helpful to determine the response to DDAVP at diagnosis or before an elective procedure. The levels of factor VIII and ristocetin co-factor activity should be determined 1 and 4 h after a test is done. DDAVP should not be given in type 2B (may cause platelet agglutination and thrombocytopenia) and type 3 VWD (it is ineffective). In these subtypes bleeding episodes must be treated with plasma, cryoprecipitates, or intermediate-purity factor VIII concentrates, which contain VWF and factor VIII (e.g., Humate P®, licensed in the United States for treatment of VWD). Factor VIII infusions may be associated with sustained increases of factor VIII activity due to the fact that the infused VWF in the factor VIII concentrate prolongs the survival of the patient's own factor VIII. Fibrinolytic inhibitors (tranexamic acid) have proved useful in reducing bleeding from the mouth, nose, or uterus. In type 1 VWD, estrogens or oral contraceptives, as well as pregnancy, increase the level of both factor VIII and VWF. During and after delivery, care should be taken to minimize bleeding. In types 1 and 2, factor VIII levels should be monitored for up to 2 wk. Alloantibodies to VWF develop in 10–15% of patients with type 3 disease. In this situation, very high doses of recombinant factor VIII can be infused until hemostasis is obtained. Acquired von Willebrand syndrome is due to an accelerated clearance of VWF secondary to its binding to abnormal cells or surfaces. This is observed in lymphomas, essential thrombocythemia, and valvular heart disease.

4.3. Other Inherited Disorders of Coagulation Factors

All other inherited disorders (deficiency of fibrinogen, and factors II, V, VII, X, XI, XII, and XIII) are very rare. In most instances the inheritance is autosomal recessive and there is a clear correlation between the patient's symptoms and the severity of the coagulation factor deficiency. The conditions rarely produce hemarthrosis and many patients with these inherited coagulation deficiencies will not bleed unless they are exposed to surgery or trauma.

Inherited defects of fibrinogen are quantitative or qualitative. Quantitative defects include heterozygous hypofibrinogenemia or homozygous afibrinogenemia. Qualitative defects—the dysfibrinogenemias—are inherited as incompletely autosomal dominant traits with more than 200 reported fibrinogen variants. Defective fibrin polymerization or fibrinopeptide release may occur. The diagnosis should be suspected when the aPTT, the prothrombin time, and thrombin time are prolonged.

Deficiencies of the vitamin K-dependent factors II, VII, and X are associated with spontaneous hemorrhages only in homozygotes, which is also true for patients with factor V deficiency. Screening studies show a prolonged prothrombin time in all four deficiency states, but also the aPTT may be prolonged if the factor activity is below 30% of normal.

Factor XI deficiency is remarkable for the variability in bleeding symptoms associated with it. Although rare in the general population, the incidence is much higher in Ashkenazi Jews, in which as many as 5–10% have been estimated to be heterozygotes. The diagnosis is made when a prolonged aPTT and a decreased factor XI level are present.

Factor XIII deficiency is rare and is usually manifest clinically only in homozygotes. Symptoms include delayed postoperative bleeding with abnormal scar formation. The coagulation screening tests are normal, but clot solubility (e.g., in 5 mol/L urea) is not.

Deficiencies of the contact phase coagulation factors (factor XII, prekallikrein, high-molecular-weight kininogen) are not associated with a clinical bleeding diathesis. All three factor deficiencies may be suspected in the presence of a long aPTT in the absence of bleeding symptoms. In factor XII (Hageman factor) deficiency a latent hypercoagulability is probably present.

Therapeutic recommendations for the treatment of the rare autosomal-recessive coagulopathies described previously are outlined in Table 4.

5. ACQUIRED COAGULATION DISORDERS

Acquired disorders of blood coagulation are much more common than the inherited disorders and occur in a variety of clinical situations. Multiple coagulation factor deficiencies are usual, which is not the case for the inherited disorders. Many of these abnormalities are associated with the potential for significant bleeding, others are associated with bleeding and/or thrombosis, and still others are primarily laboratory phenomena. Routine screening tests of blood coagulation can establish a presumptive diagnosis in most cases.

5.1. Vitamin K Deficiency

Vitamin K is a fat-soluble vitamin obtained by dietary intake of vegetables and liver and absorbed in the small intestine, or produced by bacterial synthesis in the small intestine. Vitamin K plays an important role in the posttranslational synthesis of the vitamin K-dependent coagulation factors. Inadequate diet, malabsorption, or intake of drugs such as warfarin, which act as vitamin K antagonists, can cause a deficiency of vitamin K. This in turn leads to a decrease in the functional activity of the clotting factors II, VII, IX, and X, and the coagulation antagonists protein C and S. Immunological methods show normal levels of

Table 4
Therapeutic Recommendations for Other Inherited Coagulopathies

Factor	Half-life (h)	Required blood level	Source
II	41–72	20%	Plasma, complex concentrate
V	24–36	10–15%	Plasma
VII	2–5	10%	Plasma, complex concentrate, factor VII concentrate
X	20–42	20%	Plasma, complex concentrate
XI	60–70	15–20%	Plasma
XIII	100–120	2–3%	Plasma, factor XIII concentrate

these factors. These nonfunctional proteins are called PIVKA (proteins formed in vitamin K absence). Conversion of the PIVKA factors to their biologically active forms is a posttranslational event involving the insertion of carboxyl groups at the γ carbon glutamic acid residues in the N-terminal region. γ-Carboxylated glutamic acid plays an essential role in the binding of the zymogen to calcium—a step that is required for the activation of these zymogens to serine proteases. In the process of carboxylation, vitamin K is converted to vitamin K epoxide, which is converted back to the reduced form by reductases. Oral anticoagulants are thought to interfere with the reduction of vitamin K epoxide leading to a functional vitamin K deficiency.

5.1.1. Clinical Manifestations

5.1.1.1. Deficiency in the Newborn. The vitamin K-dependent factors are low at birth and there is a further drop in breast-fed children during the first days of life due to the immaturity of liver cells and the low quantities of these factors in breast milk. Less than 1% of newborns may develop hemorrhages, usually between the second and fourth day of life. The diagnosis is based on a low prothrombin time. The therapy of choice is vitamin K (phytomenadione) at a dosage of 1 mg given orally or intramuscularly. Children who are bleeding should receive vitamin K every 6 h, and if the hemorrhage is more severe, fresh frozen plasma should be given as well.

5.1.1.2. Deficiency in Adults. Because body stores are limited, dietary deficiency may arise within a few weeks in patients who are not eating properly. Systemic illnesses, parenteral nutrition, hepatic failure, malabsorption due to small bowel disease, obstruction of bile flow, and antibiotic treatment may be compounding factors causing vitamin K deficiency and associated with overt bleeding. Both the prothrombin time and aPTT are prolonged and clotting factor analysis reveals low levels of factors II, VII, IX, and X in plasma. In liver disease, additional coagulation defects are present. Most patients with mild to moderate deficiencies do not have bleeding problems. Vitamin K, 10 mg administered intravenously over 3–5 min, should shorten or correct the abnormal prothrombin time within 6–8 h. Oral or parenteral treatment should be continued until the basic disorder is corrected.

5.2. Liver Disease

Patients with liver disease may have multiple coagulation abnormalities that predispose them to bleeding. The liver plays an important role in hemostasis because hepatocytes synthesize coagulation factors I (fibrinogen), II, V, VII, IX, X, XI, XII, and XIII, as well as the coagulation inhibitors antithrombin, protein C and S, and components of the fibrinolytic system. As hepatic disease progresses, deficiencies of some or, in severe disease, of all factors may occur. Liver disease also leads to a reduced clearing of activated clotting factors and plasminogen activators. Finally, as a result of very low thrombopoietin levels and splenomegaly, thrombocytopenia is a common feature in advanced liver disease. Biliary obstruction can result in impaired absorption of vitamin K, causing a further drop in factors II, VII, IX, and X due to decreased synthesis. All of these defects can cause a multiplicity of coagulation abnormalities, making the precise mechanism leading to the abnormal tests difficult to interpret. Prolongation of the prothrombin time is usually the earliest abnormality. A prolonged aPTT, hypofibrinongenemia, a prolonged thrombin time, and thrombocytopenia occur as the disease progresses. The great majority of bleeding complications are secondary to preexisting anatomic lesions such as esophageal varices or gastritis and peptic ulcers related in part to portal hypertension. Patients with overt bleeding may be at additional risk to develop intravascular coagulation and fibrinolysis.

In general, fresh-frozen plasma containing all coagulation factors may be useful in treating bleeding complications. Large volumes would be necessary to correct the multiple coagulation defects. However, most patients would not be able to tolerate large volume loads. Thus, the efficiency of fresh-frozen plasma is of questionable benefit. Vitamin K may be of value in some patients. Prothrombin concentrates, theoretically of value, carry the risk of enhancing pre-existing intravascular coagulation and inducing thrombotic complications. Heparin may prolong the half-life of some coagulation factors, but often increases the hemorrhages and should not be given.

5.3. Disseminated Intravascular Coagulation

The common denominator in DIC is the pathological generation of thrombin, which leads to widespread intravascular deposition of fibrin and to the consumption of coagulation factors and platelets ("consumption coagulopathy"). DIC is

Table 5
Causes of Disseminated Intravascular Coagulation

Obstetric complications
    Amniotic fluid embolism
    Retained dead fetus
    Premature separation of placenta
    Eclampsia
Malignancy
    Acute promyelocytic leukemia
    Pancreatic carcinoma and other neoplasms
Infections
    Gram-negative septicemia
    Meningicoccal septicemia
    Septic abortion
    Falciparum malaria
Hypersensitivity reactions
    Incompatible blood transfusion
    Anaphylaxis
Miscellaneous
    Heat stroke
    Hypothermia
    Snake bites
    Severe burns
    Vascular malformations (Kasabach-Merritt syndrome)
    Acute liver failure

as such not a disease entity, but the consequence of a variety of disorders that diffusely lead to the activation of coagulation mechanisms within the bloodstream. The formation of thrombi in the microcirculation activates the fibrinolytic process as a compensatory mechanism to lyse the clots. This mechanism generates circulating fibrin degradation products, which in concert with the coagulation deficiencies and thrombocytopenia results in bleeding.

DIC occurs in a wide spectrum of diseases. DIC may be triggered by the liberation and entry of procoagulant material into the circulation, which may occur after premature separation of the placenta, in widespread metastatic carcinoma, or in acute promyelocytic leukemia (M3-leukemia). Another mechanism potentially triggering DIC is the widespread endothelial damage occurring in endotoxinemia, meningococcal septicemia, or following severe burns or hypothermia. Vascular stasis as in circulatory shock and severe pulmonary embolism can also precipitate DIC.

Table 5 lists the most common disorders associated with DIC.

Table 6
Tests of Hemostasis in Suspected Disseminated Intravascular Coagulation

Platelets[a]
Fibrinogen[a]
Activated partial thromboplastin time
Prothrombin time
Thrombin time
Fibrinogen/fibrin split products (D-dimer)
Fibrin–monomer complex
Antithrombin, protein C

[a]**Important:** Take serial measurements of platelets and fibrinogen.

5.3.1. CLINICAL FEATURES

The most common signs of hemorrhages are petechiae, ecchymosis, oozing from venipuncture sites and catheter sites, as well as bleeding from surgical incisions. Thrombosis, which occurs in acute, very severe DIC, may lead to cutaneous acrocyanosis or gangrene, oliguria, acute respiratory distress, and neurological changes. The thrombotic changes are prominent in patients with septicemia and hypoperfusion.

Not all patients experience severe bleeding and thrombotic complications. Patients with a more chronic form of DIC, as commonly observed in malignancy, have mild or no clinical symptoms at all and DIC becomes evident only by laboratory analysis. However, these patients may become symptomatic after stress situations such as surgery or severe infection.

5.3.2. LABORATORY FINDINGS

Because DIC is an acute emergency that may occur during the nighttime or on weekends, the physician should have access to a simple panel of laboratory tests that are available 24 h a day in the hospital laboratory. More sophisticated tests are important for scientific questions. Table 6 lists a panel of tests that should be requested if DIC is suspected.

The most common laboratory findings are thrombocytopenia, decreased fibrinogen level, prolonged aPTT, prothrombin time and thrombin time, elevated fibrinogen/fibrin split products or elevated D-dimers, and positive testing for fibrin-monomer complexes. The inhibitors of coagulation, antithrombin, and protein C are also likely to be depressed.

5.3.3. TREATMENT

Most important in the management of DIC is the treatment of the underlying cause. All additional therapeutic recommendations are primarily empirical and often not based on scientific evidence. Supportive therapy with fluid, blood, fresh frozen plasma, platelet concentrates, and fibrinogen are indicated in patients with dangerous or extensive bleeding. The use of heparin to reduce thrombin generation and interrupt the consumption of coagulation factors leading to fibrin formation and microthrombi may be theoretically convincing, but is highly controversial among experts. Many clinicians have observed that the use of heparin has even aggravated bleeding in a number of cases. It may have its place, however, at the very beginning of DIC in the absence of bleeding and in the more chronic forms of DIC. Because the inhibitor antithrombin, which is consumed during the process of DIC, acts as a direct inhibitor of thrombin, some smaller study groups tried to evaluate antithrombin concentrates as a therapeutic agent in the management of in acute DIC. In these small studies conducted in Europe, it could be shown that antithrombin was able to shorten the duration of DIC, but did not contribute to a prolonged survival of the patients studied. This may be due to the small number of patients studied. In a large multicenter study in the United States (KyberSept Trial), high-dose antithrombin therapy had no effect on 28-d all-cause mortality in adult patients with severe sepsis and septic shock (usually associated with DIC) when administered within 6 h after onset. High-dose antithrombin was associated with increased risk of bleeding when administered with heparin. There was some evidence to suggest a treatment benefit of antithrombin in the subgroup of patients not receiving concomitant heparin (2).

Drotrecogin alfa (activated) is a recombinant human activated protein C preparation caused a reduction of the relative risk of death of 19.4% in a large double-blind phase III sepsis study, at the cost of a slight increase in bleeding complications. Other effects apart from coagulation inhibition seem to be involved in the clinical benefit of this treatment. The approved indication for treatment with drotrecogin alfa (activated) is severe sepsis associated with organ dysfunction, independent of the presence of DIC. Patients are treated with 24 µg/kg body weight per hour for 96 h (Tayler et al.).

5.4. Acquired Inhibitors

Acquired inhibitors of coagulation factors can result in bleeding or thrombosis. Most of these inhibitors are IgG or IgM antibodies. They may develop in response to a specific antigen exposure, as in patients with hemophilia A who are treated with factor VIII concentrate (see"Hemophilias A and B," and "Treatment-Related Problems"). Factor VIII antibodies may also arise in a number of other clinical settings, such as in the postpartum period, in certain immunological disorders (lupus erythematodes, rheumatoid arthritis), following menopause, and after exposure to certain drugs. They also may occur in healthy persons.

These inhibitors usually prolong the aPTT or the prothrombin time if they are directed against factor II, V, VII, or X. They may be identified in vitro by the inability of normal plasma at a ratio of 1:1 with patient plasma to correct the coagulation deficiency. Antibodies against VWF have also been described, usually associated with chronic myelogenous leukemia ("acquired VWD").

If the patient is not bleeding, then no therapy is required. Clinical bleeding requires replacement therapy. The infused coagulation factor may be ineffective because of the rapid in vivo inactivation by the antibody. With effective treatment of the underlying disease, the antibody may disappear. In postpartum or menopausal women with acquired inhibitors and bleeding manifestations, an immunosuppressive treatment (azothioprin, cyclophosphamide, anti-IgG-columns) may be necessary.

Another inhibitor known as lupus anticoagulant interferes with phospholipid-dependent stages in coagulation and is usually detected by a prolongation of the aPTT. This inhibitor is detected in more than 10% of patients with systemic lupus erythematosus and in patients with other autoimmune diseases. Frequently, the patients also have antibodies to other lipid-containing antigens, such as cardiolipin. Because the lupus anticoagulant interferes with phospholipids, all tests that depend on coagulation factor–phospholipid interactions are prolonged. The lupus anticoagulant is not associated with a bleeding tendency, but the risk of thrombosis and recurrent abortion is increased. Because the lupus anticoagulants and/or antiphospholipid antibodies may be associated with a variety of clinical presentations, therapeutic recommendations for individual patients will depend on the predominant clinical manifestations (*see* Chapter 21).

5.5. Massive Transfusions

The transfusion of large amounts of blood within a few hours may lead to severe coagulation disturbances and consequently to severe bleeding, requiring even more transfusions. The extent of these disturbances is dependent on the amount of transfused units of blood, the duration of storage of the blood, the proteases derived from the leukocytes within the stored blood, the amount of additional plasma expanders transfused, and, of course, the underlying disease and its complications. Blood loss results in reduced levels of platelets, coagulation factors, and inhibitors. Further dilution of these factors occurs during replacement therapy with stored blood and plasma expanders. After 24–48 h storage at 4°C, the platelet count falls progressively and the function of platelets also deteriorates. In addition, the labile factors V and VIII lose activity because of their short half-lives. A latent DIC may be aggravated by microaggregates of platelets and degenerate leukocytes. Established bleeding with abnormal coagulation tests (aPTT, prothrombin time) and low platelets should be treated by administration of fresh-frozen plasma, platelet transfusions, and erythrocyte concentrates as needed. The value of transfusion of fresh whole blood or "warm blood" has never been proven.

REFERENCES

1. George JN, Woolf SH, Raskob GE, et al. Idiopathic thrombocytopenic purpura: a practical guideline developed by explicit methods of the American Society of Hematology. *Blood* 1996;88:3–40.
2. Warren BL, Eid A, Singer P, et al. High-dose antithrombin III in severe sepsis. *JAMA* 2001;286:1869–1878.

SUGGESTED READING

Andersen J. Response of resistent idiopathic thrombocytopenic purpura to pulsed high-dose dexamethasone therapy. *N Engl J Med* 1994;33:1560–1564.

Bick RL. Disseminated intravascular coagulation: pathophysiological mechanisms and manifestations. *Semin Thromb Hemost* 1998;24:3–18.

Dempfle CE. Coagulopathy of sepsis. *Thromb Haemost* 2004;91:213–224.

Goodnight SH. Primary vascular disorders. In: Colman RW, Hirsh, J, Marder, Clowes AW, George JN, eds. *Hemostasis and Thrombosis. Basic principles and clinical practice*, 4th ed. Philadelphia: Lippincott Williams & Wilkins, 2001:pp. 945–953.

Cattaneo M. Inherited platelet-based bleeding disorders. *J Thromb Haemost* 2003;1:1628–1636.

Furie B, Limentani SA, Rosenfield CG. A practical guide to the evaluation and treatment of hemophilia. *Blood* 1994;84:3–9.

Sadler JE, Mannucci PM, Berntorp E, et al. Impact, diagnosis and treatment of von Willebrand disease. *Thromb Haemost* 2000;84:160–174.

Sadler JE, Moake JL, Miyata T, George JN. Recent advances in thrombotic thrombocytopenic purpura. *Hematology (Am Soc Hematol Educ Program) 2004;*407–423.

Kaufman DW, Kelly JP, Johannes CB, et al. Acute thrombocytopenic purpura in relation to the use of drugs. *Blood* 1993;82:2714–2718.

Mannucci PM. Hemophilia: treatment options in the twenty-first century. *J Thromb Haemost* 2003;1(7):1349–1355.

Mannucci PM. Treatment of von Willebrand's disease. *N Engl J Med* 2004;51:683–694.

Nurden AT, George JN. Inherited disorders of platelet membrane: Glanzmann thrombasthenia, Bernard-Soulier-Syndrome, and other disorders. In: Colman RW, Hirsh J, Marder VJ, Clowes AW, George JN, eds. *Hemostasis and Thrombosis. Basic principles and clinical practice*, 4th ed. Philadelphia: Lippincott Williams & Wilkins, 2001:pp. 921–944.

Ratnoff OD. Hemostatic defects in in liver and biliary tract disease and disorders of vitamin K metabolism. In: Ratnoff OD, Forbes CD, eds. *Disorders of Haemostasis,* 3rd ed. Philadelphia: WB Saunders, 1996:pp. 422–442.

Rao AK. Congenital disorders of platelet secretion and signal transduction. In: Colman RW, Hirsh J, Marder VJ, Clowes AW, George JN, eds. *Hemostasis and Thrombosis. Basic principles and clinical practice*, 4th ed. Philadelphia: Lippincott Williams & Wilkins, 2001:pp. 893–904.

Riewald M, Riess H. Treatment options for clinically recognized disseminated intravascular coagulation. *Semin Thromb Hemost* 1998;24:53–59.

Rock GA, Shumak, KH, Buskard NA, et al. Comparison of plasma exchange with plasma infusion in the treatment of thrombotic thrombocytopenic purpura. *N Engl J Med* 1991;325:393–397.

Shapiro SS, Siegel JE. Hemorrhagic disorders associated with circulating inhibitors. In: Ratnoff
    OD, Forbes CD, eds. *Disorders of Haemostasis*, 3rd ed. Philadelphia: WB Saunders, 1996, pp.
    208–227.
Stasi R, Provan D. Management of immune thrombocytopenic purpura in adults. *Mayo Clin Proc*
    2004;79:504–522.
Tayler FB, Kinasewitz G. Activated protein C in sepsis. *J Thromb Haemost* 2004;2:708–717.

21

Thrombophilia, Thromboembolic Disease, and Antithrombotic Therapy

Erhard Hiller, MD

CONTENTS

1. THROMBOPHILIA (HYPERCOAGULABILITY)

Patients with a tendency to thrombosis are defined as having thrombophilia. The term "inherited thrombophilia" should be used for individuals with predisposing genetic defects. Hypercoagulability and thrombophilia are synonymous. Thrombophilia is usually suspected in patients with one or more of the following clinical features: idiopathic thrombosis, thrombosis at a young age, recurrent thrombosis, and thrombosis at an unusual site. Individuals who have laboratory abnormalities or clinical disorders that are known to predispose to thrombosis, but have not had an episode of thrombosis, are potentially thrombophilic. Prior to 1993, the diagnosis of a hereditary disorder could be established in only 10–15% of younger patients presenting with venous thromboembolism (VTE). The only disorders known at this time were deficiencies of antithrombin (AT), protein C, and protein S. With the discovery of the factor V Leiden mutation (activated protein C [APC] resistance; *see* "Inherited Hypercoagulable States") and, more recently, the prothrombin gene mutation, it is currently possible to define genetic risk factors in many younger patients with idiopathic venous thrombosis.

From: *Contemporary Hematology: Modern Hematology, Second Edition*
Edited by: R. Munker, E. Hiller, J. Glass, and R. Paquette © Humana Press Inc., Totowa, NJ

Table 1
Inherited and Acquired Hypercoagulable States

Inherited hypercoagulable states
    Activated protein C resistance due to factor V Leiden mutation
    Prothrombin gene mutation
    Antithrombin deficiency
    Protein C deficiency
    Protein S deficiency
    Elevated factor VIII level
    Dysfibrinogenemia (rare)
    Hyperhomocysteinemia
Acquired hypercoagulable states
    Antiphospholipid syndrome (Lupus anticoagulant)
    Malignancy
    Nephrotic syndrome
    Paroxysmal nocturnal hemoglobinuria
    Postoperative state
    Immobilization
    Old age
    Pregnancy
    Oral contraceptives or other estrogen use

The main acquired thrombophilic disorders are antiphospholipid antibodies and/ or lupus anticoagulant (LA), malignancy, nephrotic syndrome, myeloproliferative disorders, paroxysmal nocturnal hemoglobinuria (PNH) and induction of cancer chemotherapy. In Table 1, patients with thromboses are placed into two major categories. The first group has the characteristics suggesting an inherited thrombotic disorder, whereas the second group describes acquired or secondary hypercoagulable states arising in a heterogenous group of disorders.

1.1. Inherited Hypercoagulable States

1.1.1. Factor V Leiden Mutation (APC Resistance)

Resistance to the anticoagulant APC was first reported by Dahlbäck (1) to be a major cause of hereditary thrombophilia. It is inherited as an autosomal trait and associated with the disease in some 40% of thrombophilic families. The frequency of APC resistance in unselected white patients with thromboembolism has been found to be between 20 and 30%. The probability of developing a thrombosis during lifetime is sevenfold as compared to controls. Dutch investigators from Leiden subsequently showed that a defect in factor V (i.e., the mutation of argine 506 to glutamine 506 [Arg506Glu, Factor V Leiden]), is the cause of APC resistance in 90% of the cases. This is the site at which factor Va is inactivated by APC through the degradation of the factor Va heavy chain. The alteration Arg506Glu makes the mutant factor Va molecule resistent to inactivation by APC. Most patients with APC resistance are heterozygous for the factor V Leiden mutation and are at a relatively low thrombotic risk, whereas homozygotes are at a much higher thrombotic risk. The factor V Leiden-associated thrombotic risk depends very much on the additional underlying clinical setting. Thus, oral contraceptives and pregnancy may significantly increase the risk for venous thrombosis in women with the mutation, whereas a statistical significant increased risk with preexistent cancer or recent surgery could not be demonstrated (only 1.7-fold increase). The latter may be due to the prophylactic heparin treatment given during surgery *(2)*. The prevalence of heterozygosity for factor V Leiden ranges between 5 and 7% in Caucasians. The mutation is apparently not present in African blacks, Chinese, Japanese, or native American populations.

1.1.2. Prothrombin Gene Mutation

In 1996, investigators in Leiden also reported that a G to A substitution at nucleotide, 20210 in the 3'-untranslated region of the prothrombin gene leads to elevated plasma prothrombin levels and an increased risk of venous thrombosis. In the Leiden Thrombophilia study, 6.2% of patients with venous thrombosis and 2.3% of matched controls had this prothrombin gene mutation. The mutation is associated with a 2.8-fold increased risk of venous thrombosis. Among the patients with thrombosis, 40% also carried the factor V Leiden mutation, which supports the view of venous thrombosis as a multigene disorder. The prothrombin gene mutation is the second most common genetic risk factor for venous thrombosis.

1.1.3. AT Deficiency

AT inhibits blood coagulation by inactivating thrombin and the other serine proteases, i.e., factors XIIa, XIa, Xa, and IXa. AT deficiency is an autosomal-dominant disorder with reduced and highly variable penetrance. Thus, between 15 and 100% of the AT-deficient members of affected families suffer from thromboembolic disease. It is estimated that the lifetime thrombotic risk for heterozygotes is 80–90%. Symptomatic AT deficiency has a prevalence of 0.02–0.05% in the general population, but asymptomatic deficiency is propably up to ten times more frequent (0.17%). The risk of developing thrombosis is low until the age of 15, and then occurs at a rate of approx 2–4% per year. Patients with AT deficiency are at a higher thrombotic risk to develop thrombosis than those with other defects. A number of molecular variants has been described in different affected families. AT concentrates are available for acute thrombotic episodes and for prophylaxis during surgery or delivery.

1.1.4. PROTEIN C AND S DEFICIENCIES

Protein C is a vitamin K-dependent protein, which acts as inhibitor of the activated factors V and VIII. Deficiency of protein C accounts for 3% of cases of hereditary thombophilia. Inheritance is autosomal dominant with variable penetrance. The rare homozygous patient presents with severe purpura fulminans in infancy. A number of patients develop "coumarin necrosis" of the skin when treated with oral anticoagulants, thought to be due to reduction of protein C levels in the first two days of oral anticoagulant treatment before the reduction in the levels of factors II, VII IX, and X. According to a large collaborative Austrian/German study a lifetime thrombosis risk of 80% or higher was calculated for heterozygous relatives with an annual incidence rate of 2.5%.

Protein S is a co-factor of APC in the inactivation of factors Va and VIIIa. Protein S exists in a free form (30–40%) and in a complex with the C4b-binding protein. Only the free form has APC co-factor activity. The inheritance of protein S deficiency is autosomal dominant. The thrombotic risk profile of deficient individuals is similar to those with protein C and AT deficiency. Data on the prevalence of protein S deficiency in the general population are lacking. An acquired decrease in protein S levels occurs in pregnancy and under oral contraceptives.

1.1.5. HYPERHOMOCYSTEINEMIA

Hyperhomocysteinemia was found in one study in 10% of patients with a first episode of venous thrombosis. In comparison with sex-matched controls, a relative risk of 2.3 was calculated, a figure which was confirmed in other studies. Similar to venous thrombosis, hyperhomocysteinemia is also a common finding among patients with arteriosclerosis, particularly among those who suffer from clincal events at young age. A common genetic mutation may contribute to an elevation of plasma homocysteine. A missense mutation in methylentetrahydrofolate reductase (*MTHFR*) at bp 677 that converts alanine to a valine codon was confirmed as a genetic risk factor for mild homocysteinemia, primarily when folate levels are low. Additional genetic variants in *MTHFR* and in other enzymes of homocysteine metabolism are being identified.

1.1.6. HIGH PLASMA CONCENTRATIONS OF FACTOR VIIIC

Studies have shown that an elevated level of factor VIII procoagulant activity (factor VIIIc) is likely an independent, relatively prevalent risk factor for venous thrombosis. The cause and the precise pathogenetic mechanism of the elevated factor VIIIc, a known acute phase protein, is not understood. It is unclear whether an increased factor VIIIc concentration is familial. It also remains unclear whether there is a critical cut-off value of factor VIIIc plasma concentration or that there exists a dose-dependent relationship with the risk of thrombosis. According to one study increased factor VIIIc levels (>175 IU/dL) may be found in approximately one-fourth of unselected patients with symptomatic VTE *(3)*.

1.1.7. LABORATORY DIAGNOSIS OF INHERITED THROMBOPHILIA

Patients suspected of having an inherited thrombophilia should be referred to a specialized coagulation laboratory. An important consideration in the laboratory evaluation of these patients is the timing of testing. Incorrect diagnoses can be made as a result of the influence of acute thrombosis, anticoagulant treatment, or co-morbid illnesses. Coagulation assays with high sensitivity and specificity for the factor V Leiden mutation are now widely available. These tests are based on the resistance of the mutant factor Va molecule to inactivation by APC. They can not be done while a patient is under oral anticoagulant treatment. However, testing for the factor V Leiden mutation can be performed by analyzing DNA obtained from blood mononuclear cells regardless of whether or not the patient is under oral anticoagulant treatment. The best screening tests for deficiencies of AT, protein C, and protein S are functional assays that detect both quantitative and qualitative defects. The prothrombin gene mutation can only be tested genetically.

1.2. Acquired Hypercoagulable States

The risk of postoperative venous thrombosis has been a well-known fact for many decades. Thrombosis is more likely to occur in the aged, obese, those with a previous history of thrombosis, and in those in whom surgery for malignancy, hip, or knee surgery is performed.

Venous stasis and immobility are factors responsible for the high incidence of postoperative venous thrombosis and for venous thrombosis associated with congestive heart failure and varicose veins.

Patients with *malignancy*, especially gastrointestinal carcinomas and carcinoma of the breast, lung, and prostate have a continuous increased risk of thromboembolism. This is due to liberation of tissue factor from the tumor activating the extrinsic pathway of coagulation, as well as to direct activation of factor X by a cancer procoagulant (CP) from mucous adenocarcinomas independent of the presence of factor VII.

Myeloproliferative disorders, such as polycythemia vera and essential thrombocythemia, are associated with a relatively high risk of thromboembolism and arterial thrombosis due to increased viscosity, elevated number of platelets, and increased activity of platelets. Thromboses at atypical sites like hepatic and cerebral veins are not uncommon. PNH and sickle cell anemia are complicated by an increased number of venous thromboses, which also may occur at unusual sites.

A high incidence of postoperative venous thrombosis exists for women on *high-dose estrogen* therapy and full-dose estrogen-containing oral contraceptives. Estrogen therapy is associated with increased plasma levels of a number of coagulation factors and decreased levels of AT and tissue-plasminogen activator (t-PA) in the vessel wall. Presently, there is controversial discussion as to whether the new low-dose estrogen contraceptives are associated with a lower number of thrombotic complications.

The *LA,* often associated with antiphospholipid antibodies (*see* Chapter 20), is found in systemic lupus erythematosus, but also in other autoimmune disorders, in lymphoproliferative disease, postviral infections, after certain drugs, and for unknown reasons (postpartum, with menopause). It is often, but not necessarily, identified by a prolonged activated partial thromboplastin time (aPTT). This phenomenon is caused by an antibody that is directed against membrane phospholipids causing a prolongation in all coagulation reactions in which phospholipids are involved. Patient with LA have an increased risk to develop venous and arterial thrombosis and pregnant women are at high risk for recurrent abortion due to placental infarction.

1.3. Management of Thrombophilia

The acute management of an initial thrombosis or pulmonary embolism (PE) in patients with hereditary or acquired thrombophilia is generally not different from that of patients without thrombophilia (*see* "Thromboembolic Disease"). Because recent data indicate that the risk of recurrence is greater in patients with ongoing as opposed to temporary risk factors, it is reasonable to continue anticoagulant treatment in patients with inherited thrombophilia but no additional exogenous risk factor (e.g., pregnancy, surgery) for at least 6 mo and no shorter period. After 6 mo, an assessment must be made as to the relative benefit of long-term anticoagulant therapy vs the potential side effects, inconvenience for the patient, and costs. According to one study, testing for thrombophilia in unselected patients who have had a first episode of VTE does not allow prediction of recurrent VTE in the first 2 yr after anticoagulant therapy is stopped *(4)*.

2. THROMBOEMBOLIC DISEASE

Thrombosis can occur in either the arterial or venous system, but the thrombi differ in their structure and clinical significance. Arterial thrombi usually form at the site of pre-existing vascular lesions causing platelet reaction and accumulation, and leading to the development of a "white" platelet thrombus. In veins, thrombus formation is the consequence of increased thrombin formation in areas of retarded blood flow and coagulated blood leads to the development of a "red" thrombus.

2.1. Venous Thrombosis

2.1.1. PATHOGENESIS

The complexity of venous thrombosis was already apparent to Virchow, who stated in 1856 that the pathophysiology of thrombosis involved three factors: (1) damage to the vessel wall, (2) stasis, and (3) increase in blood coagulability (*"Virchow's triad"*). None of these factors alone is usually capable of causing thrombosis. It is the coincidence of activation of blood coagulation at the time of surgery, the immobile leg veins, and possibly the damaged vessel wall, which cause thrombosis. Whereas the first two components of Virchow's triad represent acquired conditions, blood hypercoagulability is a result of both endogenous (inherited) and exogenous (acquired) factors as outlined in the previous chapter on thrombophilia.

2.1.2. CLINICAL MANIFESTATIONS AND DIAGNOSIS

Thrombosis in veins occurs most commonly in deep and superficial veins of the lower extremities. Deep vein thrombosis (DVT) usually begins in the soleal arcade of the calf muscles where they may resolve, organize, or extend. When extension occurs, the thrombus involves the popliteal, superficial femoral, common femoral, and iliac veins; more rarely the inferior vena cava is affected. Once extension into the major deep vessels of the leg has occurred, the patient is at significant risk for circulatory obstruction, valve damage, and PE (*see* "Prophylaxis"). Damage to the venous valves may cause venous stasis and insufficiency; possibly leading to chronic edema, fibrosis, pigmentation, and trophic ulceration of the extremity. In a particularly serious form of DVT called *phlegmasia cerulea dolens*, cyanosis and swelling of the extremity are associated with the disappearance of the arterial pulses. The massive venous occlusion involving the deep, superficial, and intercommunicating veins will lead to a total outflow obstruction. The leg becomes cold and without immediate surgical intervention gangrene and circulatory shock may follow.

Superficial thrombophlebitis usually is diagnosed clinically, because the thrombosed vessel can be palpated beneath the skin as a tender cord. DVT is much more difficult to diagnose, because it may or may not be accompanied by local symptoms and signs. The most useful noninvasive technique is compression ultrasonography. The sensitivity and specificity for proximal DVT are more than 95%. However, for isolated DVT in the calf, the sensitivity of ultrasonography is lower. Venography, though most specific, is no longer used often clinically because of its invasive nature, its technical demands, and potential risks, such as allergic reactions and renal dysfunction.

2.1.3. PROPHYLAXIS

Stasis should be eliminated whenever possible. This includes the wearing of elastic stockings or a supportive hose and also intermittent pneumatic compression. Early ambulation is encouraged after surgery or illness. Prophylactic heparin therapy must be considered in high-risk groups and is mandatory for surgical patients during the peri- and postoperative period. Heparin and its derivative, low-molecular-weight heparin (LMWH), are the anticoagulants of choice for prophylaxis and treatment of DVT. Both types of heparin are given in lower doses when employed for primary prophylaxis than when used for the treatment of DVT. Their major anticoagulatory effect is produced by activating AT. For general surgical patients, 5000 U of standard heparin is administered subcutaneously two or three times daily and LMWH is administered once daily by subcutaneous injection in a fixed standard dose. Laboratory monitoring is not necessary, because the low-dose heparin or LMWH used for prophylaxis usually do not lead to a prolongation of the clotting times, such as the aPTT. In high-risk situations, the dosage may have to be increased.

2.1.4. TREATMENT

The continous intravenous infusion of heparin has been, until recently, the preferred mode of therapy in the treatment of DVT or PE. In adult patients with an average weight of 70 kg, doses of 30,000–40,000 U over 24 h (1200–2000 U/ h with a loading dose of 5000 U) are usually required. Subcutaneous heparin (e.g., 15,000 U every 12 h) can be used as an alternative to the intravenous route. The therapy must be monitored by maintaining the aPTT between 1.8 and 2.5 times the normal time. Multicenter studies and meta-analyses have shown that LMWH is as safe and effective as normal heparin in preventing recurrent VTE, and causes less bleeding. LMWH must be administered in a weight-adjusted fashion and does not require laboratory monitoring. Estimates of the number of hospital days that would be saved by outpatient administration of initial therapy average 5 to 6 d for each patient. Warfarin therapy can be started on day 2 after the initiation of heparin therapy. Thus on days 5–7, one can expect that warfarin is in the therapeutic range (international normalized ratio [INR] > 2) (*see* p. 341) and heparin can be discontinued. Oral anticoagulant therapy should be continued for at least 3 mo and longer than 3 mo when the thrombophilic state persists. In recent studies, it was shown that long-term, low-intensity warfarin therapy was highly effective in preventing recurrent thromboembolism *(5)*.

The anticoagulants heparin and warfarin prevent additional thrombus formation and PE. However, after anticoagulant treatment, venous valve function and venous pressure seldom normalize, thus predisposing to the postthrombotic syndrome. Thrombolytic agents potentially dissolve the preformed thrombus and restore the venous flow more promptly. In the treatment of DVT, it appears that the early use of thrombolytic agents, such as streptokinase or urokinase, decrease pain, swelling, and loss of venous valves; in some studies, it reduced the incidence of the postphlebitic syndrome. However, this syndrome develops late and is variable in its manifestation, and there are conflicting findings as to the long-term benefit. Because of the potentially severe bleeding complications and the uncertain long-term benefit, thrombolytic therapy should be reserved for selected younger patients with massive DVT involving the femoral and iliac veins (for dosage, *see* "Thrombolytic Therapy").

Inferior vena caval filter placement is recommended when there is a contraindication or complication of anticoagulant therapy in a patient with or at high risk for proximal vein thrombosis or PE. It is also recommended for recurrent embolisms that occur despite adequate anticoagulation and for chronic recurrent embolism with pulmonary hypertension.

2.2. Pulmonary Embolism

PE is a common complication of DVT that originates in the deep veins of the leg in more than 90% of the cases. Most PEs are clinically silent. Dyspnea is the most frequently reported symptom. Massive PE causes tachypnoe, tachycardia, cyanosis, and hypotension. The diagnostic tests for PE include pulmonary angiography, ventilation/perfusion lung scanning, and, more recently, spiral computed tomographic scanning. An elevated level of the D-dimer is well compatible with a clinically suspected PE, whereas negative or normal D-dimers make a diagnosis of PE very unlikely.

Anticoagulants as previously outlined for treatment of DVT are definitely effective in reducing morbidity and mortality from PE. Thrombolytic therapy with streptokinase or recombinant tissue plasminogen activator (rt-PA) is more effective than heparin alone in improving the angiographic defects produced by PEs and may be better than heparin at preventing death in patients with massive PE associated with shock. Based on these findings, thrombolytic therapy is the treatment of choice for patients with massive PE. Massive emboli may be defined as two lobar arteries completely obstructed with thrombus or several smaller thrombosed vessels. The optimal treatment requires immediate start of infusion upon diagnosis. Recent new therapeutic schedules have employed large doses of thrombolytic agents as employed in cases of acute myocardial infarction. Thus 1.5 to 3×10^6 U of streptokinase or 100 mg of rt-PA are infused over 60 to 120 min leading frequently to prompt reperfusion of blood flow in the obstructed vessels.

2.3. Arterial Thrombosis

Atherosclerosis is the most common underlying cause of coronary heart disease, cerebrovascular disease, and peripheral arterial disease. Arterial thrombosis usually is a complication of atherosclerosis. Endothelial lesions due to atherosclerosis of the arterial walls and plug rupture expose the blood to tissue factor and subintimal tissue, such as collagen. This may initiate the adhesion of platelets to the site of endothelial damage and the subsequent formation of a platelet plug, which incorporates fibrin strands. Further aggregation is enhanced by the liberation of adenosine diphosphate (ADP) and thromboxane A_2 (TxA_2) from the activated and damaged platelets. The platelet plug may organize and becomes incorporated into the atherosclerotic plaque. With more marked arterial narrowing, shear rates increase and promote more extensive platelet and fibrin deposition, which can result in the formation of an occlusive thrombosis.

The most effective means of preventing arterial thrombosis is to prevent atherosclerosis. A discussion of the risk factors and conditions and the reversal of these conditions is beyond the scope of this chapter. At this point only the three forms of medical therapy used in the treatment of arterial thrombosis—antiplatelet drugs, anticoagulants, and thrombolytic agents—will be discussed shortly.

2.3.1. ANTIPLATELET DRUGS

Two antiplatelet drugs, aspirin and ticlopidine, have been shown to be effective in preventing and treating arterial thromboses. During recent years, glycoprotein (GP) IIb/IIIa-receptor antagonists have also been introduced and show great promise.

2.3.1.1. Aspirin. The antithrombotic effects of aspirin are attributed to its ability to irreversibly inhibit platelet cyclooxygenase, thus reducing the synthesis of TxA_2, a potent inducer of platelet aggregation and vasoconstriction. The inhibitory effects of aspirin persist for the life span of platelets, because the drug irreversibly acetylates cyclooxygenase. The recommended oral dose is beween 100 and 300 mg daily. In a number of studies, it has been demonstrated that aspirin has a mild to moderate benefit in reducing the incidence of further myocardial infarction and sudden death in patients with coronary artery disease. Aspirin also reduces the risk of stroke in patients with cerebral ischemia, particularly in men, and decreases the risk of acute thrombosis after aortocoronary bypass or coronary angioplasty. It may be useful in patients with thrombocytosis.

2.3.1.2. Ticlopidine and Clopidogrel. Ticlopidine and clopidrogrel inhibit platelet aggregation induced by ADP and a variety of other agonists. Unlike aspirin, the inhibitory effects on platelet function are delayed for 24–48 h after administration, limiting the potential value when rapid antithrombotic action is required. Ticlopidine has been shown to be more effective than aspirin in reducing strokes in patients who have suffered from transient cerebral ischemia (TIA) or a minor stroke. Ticlopidine is also effective in reducing acute occlusion of coronary bypass grafts and stents following angioplasty. In the latter setting, it is often given in combination with aspirin. The recommended dose of ticlopidine is 200 mg as tablets twice daily. The most serious side effect is neutropenia occurring in 1–2%, less serious side effects are diarrhea and skin rashes. For this reason, clopidogrel has been introduced, which has the same antithrombotic properties as ticlopidine without the side effects. The recommended dose is a 75-mg tablet, once daily.

2.3.1.3. GP IIb/IIIa-Receptor Antagonists. GP IIb/IIIa antagonists inhibit platelet aggregation in response to all agonists, including collagen and thrombin, because they block fibrinogen bridging between platelets, the final common pathways of platelet aggregation. Three GP IIb/IIIa receptor antagonists have been approved as adjunctive therapy to decrease the ischemic complications of percutaneous coronary interventions (PCI) and/or unstable angina. They include the chimeric murine/human monoclonal antibody 7E3 Fab fragment abciximab Reopro™, eptifibatide (Integrilin™), a cyclic hexapeptide, and tirofiban (Aggrastat™), a nonpeptidyl GPIIb/IIIa antagonist. Abciximab is administered as an intravenous bolus of 0.25 mg/kg followed by an infusion rate of 10 µg/min for 12 h. Abciximab is currently approved for high-risk coronary ballon angioplasty. It has also been used with a favorable clinical experience in stent implantation. The agents are very effective in providing both short-term and long-term benefit after PCI. Severe thrombocytopenia is an infrequent but potentially serious complication of therapy with all the agents.

2.3.2. ANTICOAGULANTS

The role of anticoagulants in the treatment of arterial thrombosis is controversial. In patients with acute myocardial infarction, heparin in moderate doses (12,500 U subcutaneously twice daily) may reduce reinfarction and death, and will reduce the incidence of mural thrombosis. Heparin also prevents early reocclusion of the infarct-related artery after successful thrombolysis. Oral anticoagulants are probably effective in the long-term treatment of patients with myocardial infarction as several studies have shown.

2.3.3. THROMBOLYTIC THERAPY

More than 80% of patients with acute myocardial infarction have thrombotic occlusion of the infarct-related coronary artery. Thrombolytic therapy will produce rapid lysis of these thrombi in 50–75% of the cases. t-PA has been found to be more effective than streptokinase in achieving early coronary lysis, but both drugs improve left ventricular function and reduce mortality. In combination with aspirin both agents reduce mortality by 40–50%. In the Global Utilization Strategy for Thrombolysis of Occluded Arteries (GUSTO) study, an accelerated t-PA regimen resulted in a 14% greater reduction of mortality than was achieved with streptokinase. For dose recommendations, *see* the next section.

3. ANTITHROMBOTIC THERAPY

The conventional anticoagulant therapy with unfractionated heparin and oral anticoagulants is based on indirect inhibition of coagulation factors. It is widely used in the prophylaxis and treatment of thromboembolic disease. Its value in the treatment of arterial thrombosis is less well established.

3.1. Unfractionated Heparin

Unfractionated heparin (UFH) is a mucopolysaccharide from either porcine or bovine sources with an average molecular weight (MW) of 15,000 Daltons. The anticoagulant effect is produced by its interaction with AT. Binding of a pentasaccharide sequence to AT causes a conformational change that accelerates its interaction with thrombin and the other serine proteinases (i.e., factors Xa, IXa, XIa, and XIIa). UFH can be administered by intravenous or subcutaneous route. The biological half-life is 1–1.5 h. The bioavailability is only 30% after subcutaneous administration. This is due to binding to a number of plasma proteins, endothelial cells, von Willebrand factor, and neutralization by platelet factor (PF) 4. For this reason the LMWH were introduced (discussed later).

The main indications for heparin are the treatment of DVT, PE, acute myocardial infarction, and unstable angina pectoris. It is also used in cardiopulmonary bypass surgery and for anticoagulation during pregnancy as it does not cross the placenta.

For treatment of acute thromboembolic events, continuous intravenous infusion with a perfusion pump has been the standard treatment for decades until the LMWHs were introduced. For adult patients with a weight of 70 kg, doses of 30,000–40,000 U over 24 h (1200–1800 U/h) with a loading dose of 5000 U are usually required. Subcutaneous heparin in a dose of 15,000–18,000 U every 12 h is equally effective. Therapy is monitored by maintaining the aPTT between 1.5 and 2.5 times the normal value. It is usual to start warfarin therapy after 1–3 d of heparin treatment and overlap with heparin until an INR in the therapeutic range (2.5–3.5) has been reached.

In peri- and postoperative thrombosis, prophylaxis with UFH is given every 8 (high risk) or every 12 (normal risk) h in a dose of 5000 U subcutaneously. It is not necessary to monitor the prophylactic dose.

3.2. Low-Molecular-Weight Heparins

LMWH is manufactured from UFH, usually of porcine origin, by controlled depolymerization using either chemical or enzymatic techniques. LMWH-fractions have an MW of about one-third of UFH (MW 5000). The smaller size with its reduced negative charge causes less binding to plasma proteins and endothelial cells, resulting in a much better bioavailability and more predictable anticoagulant response than UFH. The longer half-life allows a single daily subcutaneous dosage as thrombosis prophylaxis. The various LMWHs differ in mean molecular weight, aminoglycan content, and anticoagulant activity, which is usually expressed as anti-Xa activity. In contrast to UFH, LMWH have only minor anti-IIa activity. Thus, even when used in higher therapeutic doses, the aPTT will not be prolonged and cannot be used for monitoring. Currently, three LMWH preparations, enoxaparin (Lovenox®), dalteparin (Fragmin®), and ardeparin (Normiflo®)

have been approved in the United States, and probably additional LMWH prepa-rations—as is the case in Europe—will be approved in the near future. Because evidence is accumulating that LMWHs have fewer serious complications than UFH, such as bleeding, heparin-induced immune thrombocytopenia (HIT), and osteoporosis, UFH has been replaced by LMWH in thrombosis prophylaxis in many institutions. Recent randomized trials have shown that LMWHs are also safe and effective in the treatment of uncomplicated DVT and even PE at home as compared to intravenous UFH in the hospital. The rates of recurrent throm-boembolism and major bleeding did not differ in the two treatment approaches. The dose is weight-adjusted and laboratory monitoring is not required. The positive results of a number of studies and one or two daily doses of LMWH required will likely lead to the use of LMWHs in outpatient treatment of uncom-plicated VTE in the majority of patients.

3.3. Complications of Heparin Therapy

The main adverse effects of UFH include bleeding, thrombocytopenia, and osteoporosis after prolonged therapy. Patients predisposed to bleeding (peptic ulcer, malignancy, liver disease, postoperatively) must be carefully monitored and the dose of heparin reduced, unless a life-threatening clinical event (serious PE) justifies a full heparin dose in spite of a high bleeding risk. If life-threatening hemorrhage occurs, the effects of heparin can be reversed quickly by intravenous infusion of protamine sulfate. The usual dose of protamine sulfate is 1 mg/100 U of heparin. The drug can be also used to reverse some of the action of LMWH.

Heparin-induced immune thrombocytopenia (HIT) is a quite frequently rec-ognized complication of heparin therapy that usually occurs within 5–10 d after initiation of heparin treatment. Of patients who receive UFH, 0.1 to 1% develop immune thrombocytopenia mediated by immunoglobulin (Ig)G antibody di-rected against a complex of PF 4 and heparin. This may be accompanied by arterial or venous thrombosis ("white clot syndrome") with potentially serious complications, such as limb amputation, cerebral infarction, or death. For this reason platelet counts determined two to three times weekly are required during the first 3 wk of treatment. When HIT is diagnosed, heparin in all forms must be discontinued immediately. For patients requiring ongoing anticoagulation, two alternatives are possible:

1. Danaparoid (Orgaran, N.V. Organon Oss, The Netherlands)
2. Hirudin or argatroban, both are direct thrombin inhibitors (*see* following)

LMWHs may also cause HIT, but as compared with UFH, the incidence of HIT is definitely lower.

Osteoporosis and fractures of vertebral bodies have been observed in patients who have been treated with daily UFH doses of 20,000 U or more over a period of several months. It is believed that this complication does not occur with LMWH.

3.4. Oral Anticoagulants

Oral anticoagulants produce an anticoagulant effect by inhibiting the vitamin K-dependent γ-carboxylation of coagulation factors II, VII, IX, and X. This leads to biological inactive forms of these coagulation proteins (*see* Chapter 19). By the same mechanism, synthesis of the inhibitors proteins C and S is impaired. Currently, the following compounds, all 4-hydroxy coumarins, are in use: warfarin (Coumadin®) mostly used in the United States, Canada, and Scandinavia; phenprocoumon (Marcumar®), acenocoumarol (Sintrom®), and bishydroxy-coumarol (dicoumarol), used in other European countries. Oral anticoagulants have a very good bioavailability. Once absorbed from the intestinal tract, they are bound to plasma proteins (97–99%), primarily to albumin. Therefore, interactions with other drugs capable of displacing these agents from binding sites must be taken into consideration. Changes in blood coagulability do not occur before 12 h after administration. It takes several days until the 4-hydroxy coumarins are clinically fully effective and heparin can be discontinued. Laboratory monitoring is mandatory throughout the course of treatment. Most commonly the prothrombin time (PT) is used. It is sensitive to reduced activity of factors II, VII, and X, but insensitive to a reduced factor IX. To standardize the monitoring of oral anticoagulant therapy, the World Health Organization has developed an international reference thromboplastin from human brain tissue and has recommended that the PT ratio be expressed as the INR (*see* Chapter 19). The therapeutic range corresponds to an INR of 2–3.5. It is usual to start warfarin treatment with 10 mg on days 1 and 2, 5 mg on day 3, and then alter the dose according the results of the PT. The usual maintenance dose of warfarin is 3–9 mg daily, but individual responses vary greatly.

3.5. Complications and Interactions

Bleeding complications are observed in 10–20% of patients treated with oral anticoagulants. Half of these complications occur because the therapeutic range of the PT or INR has been exceeded. Most bleeding complications are mild (epistaxis, hematuria), but more serious bleeding, such as retroperitoneal hematomas, gastrointestinal bleeding, or even cerebral bleeding, may occur. In keeping within the therapeutic INR range of 2.0 and 3.0 for most indications, the hemorrhagic complications have decreased. Patients with life-threatening hemorrhage or overdosage (error, suicidal) require immediate correction of the PT. The administration of prothrombin complex preparations simultaneously with vitamin K is necessary.

Drug interactions that affect the albumin-binding or excretion of oral anticoagulants, or those that decrease the absorption of vitamin K interfere with the control of therapy and may either increase the risk of bleeding or render the

Table 2
Drugs and Other Factors That Interfere With the Control of Anticoagulant Therapy

Potentiation of oral anticoagulants
Reduced coumarin binding to albumin
    Phenylbutazone
    Sulfonamides
Inhibition of microsomal degradation
    Allopurinol
    Metronidazole
    Cimetidine
    Tricyclic antidepressants
Alteration of hepatic receptor site
    Quinidine
    Thyroxin
Diminished vitamin K uptake
    Malabsorption
    Antibiotic therapy (moxalactam)
Depression of the effects of oral anticoagulants
Acceleration of microsomal degradation
    Barbiturates
    Rifampicin
Increased synthesis of clotting factors
    Estrogen
    Oral contraceptives
    Pregnancy

treatment ineffective because of an insufficient anticoagulation. Table 2 lists a number of drugs that either potentiate or depress the effects of oral anticoagulants.

Warfarin-induced skin necrosis is a rare complication. During initiation of warfarin therapy, usually between days 2 and 7, the patient develops a bluish purple lesion on the buttock, breast, or thigh. Over several days this lesion becomes increasingly necrotic while the surrounding tissue becomes erythematous and inflamed. Thrombi in the microvascualture can be demonstrated histologically. This skin necrosis is often due to a hereditary protein C deficiency. After the onset of warfarin therapy, the activity of protein C, which has a short half-life, drops to low levels before the other vitamin K-dependent coagulation factors reach an anticoagulant level. Thus, protein C, already at a reduced level due to the hereditary deficiency, is inappropriately low for 1–2 d following the onset of warfarin therapy. For this reason, heparin must be simultaneously given during the first 5 d.

Teratogenic effects have been described with coumarin derivatives. Fetal exposure during the first trimester may result in embryopathies (nasal hypoplasia, epiphyseal abnormalities). Oral anticoagulants are therefore contraindicated in the first trimester of pregnancy. LMWH is recommended throughout the pregnancy, if anticoagulation is mandatory.

3.6. Direct Thrombin Inhibitors (Hirudin)

In contrast to UFH and LMWH, direct thrombin inhibitors inactivate not only free thrombin, but also thrombin bound to fibrin. Hirudin (Desirudin, Lepidurin), a polypeptide obtained by recombinant technology, and its synthetic derivative hirulog interact with both the active site of thrombin and the substrate recognition site. From a theoretical point of view, the direct thrombin inhibitors should be superior to heparin, which is an indirect thrombin inhibitor. However, randomized controlled trials conducted in patients with acute coronary syndromes reported no significant evidence for a superiority of the direct thrombin inhibitors (desirudin) over UFH.

Lepirudin was extensively studied in heparin-induced thrombocytopenia, and appears effective and safe, allowing platelet count recovery and providing adequate anticoagulation.

In a study in patients undergoing hip replacement, desirudin significantly reduced the frequency of postoperatice DVT compared with LMWH therapy without an increased incidence of bleeding.

aPTT is largely used to monitor therapy with direct thrombin inhibitors. However, aPTT is insensitive at plasma levels higher than 0.6 mg/L of hirudin, so that overdoses may be missed despite monitoring. Therefore, therapy with direct thrombin inhibitors should be monitored with the ecarin clotting time. Renal insufficiency causes accumulation of the blood levels of hirudin and a high risk of bleeding because the drug is exclusively excreted by the kidney.

3.7. New Antithrombotic Drugs

Two new antithrombotic drugs have been investigated in a number in large-scale clinical studies and have the potential of improving the treatment of thrombotic disorders. One of them, fondaparinux, has already been introduced in Europe.

3.7.1. Fondaparinux (Arixtra®)

Fondaparinux is a pentasaccharide and is a synthetic antithrombotic agent. To inhibit thrombin, UFH must bind not only to AT but also to thrombin itself, whereas fondaparinux binds only to AT and is therefore a specific inhibitor of factor Xa. Its pharmacokinetic properties allow for a simple, fixed-dose, once-daily regimen of subcutaneous injection without the need for monitoring. In a dosage of 2.5 mg s.c. once daily, it was found to be superior to enoxaparin in thrombosis prophylaxis in high-risk patients undergoing orthopedic surgery for hip and knee replacement. Also, in a dose-ranging trial involving patients with symptomatic proximal DVT, 7.5 mg of fondaparinux appeared to have efficacy and safety similar to those of LMWH (dalteparin). In a clinical trial of initial antithrombotic therapy for acute symptomatic PE, therapy with fondaparinux was equal to therapy with UFH. It probably does not cause HIT.

3.7.2. New Direct Thrombin Inhibitors (Argatroban, Ximelagatran)

As a result of better understanding the interaction of hirudin with thrombin, other direct thrombin inhibitors such as argatroban and melagatran, both of which can neutralize clot-bound thrombin, have been developed. Argatroban is is approved in the United States and Canada for both prophylaxis and treatment of thrombosis in patients with HIT and in the United States as an antithrombotic agent during percutaneous coronary interventions in patients with HIT or a history of HIT. The therapeutic half-life is 46 ± 10 min. Treatment is initiated at a dose of 2 μg/kg/min. The aPTT is checked 2 h later, and the dose is adjusted to prolong the aPTT one-and-a-half to three times the baseline (maximum 100 s). There is no antidote for bleeding. Melagatran is poorly absorbed, but has been chemically modified and, in the form of ximelagatran, is the first new oral anticoagulant since warfarin. Ximelagatran is metabolized to melagatran and, like fondaparinux, does not require laboratory monitoring. It has been tested in a number of major clinical trials and was equal and in some trials even superior to the conventional antithrombotic drugs such as heparin and warfarin. In a study for the prevention of VTE after total hip- and knee-replacement surgery, two daily oral doses of 36 mg were superior to enoxaparin. In prevention of arterial thromboembolism in atrial fibrillation, ximelagatran was as effective as oral anticoagulation with warfarin. Ximelagatran is not approved by the US Food and Drug Administration and suspended in Europe in 2006 as a result of liver toxicity.

3.8. Fibrinolytic Therapy

Fibrinolytic agents, in contrast to anticoagulants, digest and dissolve arterial and venous thrombi and emboli and thus reinstitute blood flow distal to the site of obstruction. They have been used systemically for patients with acute major PE, ileofemoral DVT, acute myocardial infarction, and locally in patients with acute peripheral arterial occlusion.

To date, four different fibrinolytic agents have been approved for clinical use: streptokinase , urokinase , rt-PA, and acylated plasminogen-streptokinase activator complex (APSAC). Fibrinolytic agents are administered by intravenous systemic infusion and by local intravenous or intraarterial perfusion. Thrombolytic therapy should be initiated as early after diagnosis as possible. However,

Table 3
Contraindications to Fibrinolytic Therapy

Absolute contraindications
    Established hemorrhage
    Cerebrovascular accident, head injury in the past 2 mo
    Neurosurgery during past 2 mo
    Intracranial aneurysm or neoplasm
    Aortic dissection
    Proliferative diabetic retinopathy
Relative contraindications
    Surgery during past 10 d
    Arterial puncture previous 7 d
    Prior organ biopsy
    Recent obstetric delivery
    Past history of gastrointestinal bleeding
    Severe hypertension (systolic > 200 mmHg, diastolic > 110 mmHg)

certain clinical situations or complications exclude the use of thrombolytic agents (*see* Table 3).

For most indications, administration of standardized dosage regimens of the thrombolytic agents is common practice. Studies comparing mortality reductions between various thrombolytic agents in coronary thrombolysis have generally shown no significant differences.

3.8.1. STREPTOKINASE

Derived from β-hemolytic streptococci; indirect plasminogen activator; dose for acute myocardial infarction and massive PE: 1.5×10^6 U over 60 min, for DVT: 250,000 U (30 min), maintenance dose 100,000 U/h, duration 24–72 h; alternative dose schedule (in Europe) 9×10^6 U/6 h, to be repeated every 24 h two to five times. Pyrogenic reactions are the main side effect of streptokinase.

3.8.2. UROKINASE

Direct plasminogen activator; for acute myocardial infarction 1.5 to 3×10^6 U over 60 to 90 min; for PE and DVT 4000 U/(kg · h), 12–48 h, with loading dose (30 min); for severe PE also 1.5 to 3×10^6 U over 60–90 min.

3.8.3. rt-PA (ALTEPLASE)

Has particularly high affinity for fibrin, less systemic activation of fibrinolysis. In acute myocardial infarction as in severe PE, 100 mg over 90 min; "frontloaded" regime (GUSTO Study): 15 mg 1–3 min, 50 mg over 30 min, 35 mg over 60 min. At present, rt-PA can not be recommended for the treatment of DVT (high costs, no advantage).

3.9. Antiplatelet Drugs

The antiplatelet drugs, such as aspirin, ticlopidine, and GP IIb/IIIa antagonists, are discussed under "Arterial Thrombosis."

REFERENCES

1. Dahlbäck B, Carlsson M, Svensson PJ. Familial thrombophilia due to a previously unrecognized mechanism characterized by poor anticoagulant response to activated protein C: prediction of a cofactor to activated protein C. *Proc Natl Acad Sci USA* 1993;90(3):1004–1008.
2. Ryan DH, Crowther MA, Ginsberg JS, Francis CW. Relation of factor V Leiden genotype to risk for acute deep venous thrombosis after joint replacement surgery. *Ann Intern Med* 1998;128(4):270–276.
3. Kraaijenhagen RA, Anker PS, Koopman MMW, et al. High plasma concentrations of factor VIIIc is a major risk factor for venous thromboembolism. *Thromb Haemost* 2000;83: 5–9.
4. Baglin T, Luddington R, Brown K, Baglin C. Incidence of recurrent venous thromboembolism in relation to clinical and thrombophilic risk factors: prospective cohort study. *Lancet* 2003;362:523–526.
5. Ridker PM, Goldhaber SZ, Danielson E, et al. Long-term, low intensity warfarin therapy for the prevention of recurrent venous thromboembolism. *N Engl J Med* 2003;348:1425–1434.

SUGGESTED READING

Ansell J, Hirsh J, Poller L, Bussey H, Jacobson A, Hylek E. The pharmacology and management of the vitamin K antagonists: the Seventh ACCP Conference on Antithrombotic and Thrombolytic Therapy. *Chest* 2004;126:204S–233S.

Bates SM, Ginsberg JS. Treatment of deep-vein thrombosis. *N Engl J Med* 2004;351:268–277.

Bauer KA. Management of thrombophilia. *J Thromb Haemost* 2003; 1(7):1429–1434.

Büller HM, Agnelli G, Hull RD, et al. Antithrombotic therapy for venous thromboembolic disease. *Chest* 2004;401S–428S.

Crowther MA, Weitz JI. Ximelagatran: the first oral direct thrombin inhibitor. *Expert Opin Investig Drugs* 2004;13:403–413.

Den Heijer M, Rosendaal FR, Blom HJ, Gerrits WBJ, Bos GMJ. Hyperhomocysteinemia and venous thrombosis: a meta-analysis. *Thromb Haemost* 1998;80:874–877.

Goldhaber SZ. Thrombolysis in pulmonary embolism: a debatable indication. *Thromb Haemost* 2001;86:444–451.

Hillarp A, Zöller B, Svensson P, Dahlbäck B. The 20210 A allele of the prothrombin gene is a common risk factor among Swedish outpatients with verified deep vein thrombosis. *Thromb Haemost* 1997;78:990–992.

Hirsh J, Raschke R. Heparin and low-molecular-weight heparin: The Seventh ACCP Conference on Antithrombotic and Thrombolytic Therapy.2004;126:188S–203S.

Iorio A, Guercini F, Pini M. Low-molecular-weight heparin for the long-term treatment of symptomatic venous thromboembolism: meta-analysis of the randomized comparisons with oral anticoagulants. *J Thromb Haemost* 2003;1:1906–1913.

Levine JS, Branch DW, Rauch J. The antiphospholipid syndrome. *N Engl J Med* 2002;346:752–763.

Simoni P, Prandoni P, Lensing AWA, et al. The risk of recurrent venous thromboembolism in patients with an Arg[506]–Gln mutation in the gene for factor V (factor V Leiden) *N Engl J Med* 1997;336:399–403.

Turpie AGG, Norris TM. Thromboprophylaxis in medical patients. The role of low-molecular-weight heparin. *Thromb Haemost* 2004;92:3–12.

Wells PS, Forster AJ. Thrombolysis in deep vein thrombosis. Is there still an indication? *Thromb Haemost* 2001;86:499–508.

22 Transfusion Medicine and Immunohematology

Grace C. Tenorio, MD, Snehalata C. Gupte, PhD, and Reinhold Munker, MD

CONTENTS

INTRODUCTION
RED CELL SEROLOGY
LEUKOCYTE ANTIGENS
BLOOD PRODUCTS AND INDICATIONS FOR BLOOD
    TRANSFUSION
ADVERSE REACTIONS TO BLOOD TRANSFUSION
DISEASES TRANSMITTED BY BLOOD TRANSFUSION
OTHER ADVERSE EFFECTS OF BLOOD TRANSFUSION
AUTOLOGOUS BLOOD TRANSFUSION
SUGGESTED READING

1. INTRODUCTION

Blood transfusion is essential and vital in the successful treatment of many malignant and nonmalignant hematological disorders. Children with thalassemia, adults with myelodysplastic syndromes, and patients with autoimmune hemolytic anemias, leukemias, or aplastic anemias become chronically dependent on blood transfusions. Modern treatment procedures such as high-dose chemotherapy and progenitor cell transplantation require intensive support with blood components and products. The serological basis of blood transfusion, the available blood

From: *Contemporary Hematology: Modern Hematology, Second Edition*
Edited by: R. Munker, E. Hiller, J. Glass, and R. Paquette © Humana Press Inc., Totowa, NJ

components and products, and adverse effects of blood transfusion with special emphasis on infectious disease transmission are discussed in this chapter.

2. RED CELL SEROLOGY

2.1. The ABO, Hh, and Sese Systems

Genes for three different blood group systems (ABO, Hh, and Sese) indirectly control the expression of the A, B, and O antigens because antigenic activity is determined by sugars linked to either polypeptides (forming glycoproteins) or lipids (forming glycolipids). Each of the A, B, and H genes code for a specific enzyme (glycosyltransferase) that adds a different sugar on a polypeptide or lipid to form the ABH antigens.

The ABO system is the most important system in red cell serology and involves three allelic genes (A, B, and O) in chromosome a. The A and B genes encode glycosyltransferases (enzymes) that produce the A and B antigens, respectively. The O gene is considered to be nonfunctional because it determines no detectable blood group antigen. The expression of the O gene results in loss of production of a functional protein or enzyme; consequently, no product is formed. The red cells of a group O individual lack A and B antigens, but have an abundant amount of H antigen. The precursor H enzyme (fucosyltransferase) specifically adds fucose to a terminal galactose, thus giving H antigenic expression. If the glycosyltransferase adds N-acetyl-D-galactosamine to the terminal D-galactose of an H antigen, then the red cells will have the A antigen on their surface. Correspondingly, if the glycosyltransferase adds D-galactose, a B antigen is formed. ABO specificity is dependent on both ABO and Hh genes. Table 1 shows the incidence of the four main phenotypes of the ABO system.

The A blood group has two main subgroups: A_1 and A_2, which could be distinguished using the *Dolichos biflorus* lectin reagent. A_1 individuals have more A antigen sites than A_2 individuals. The A_2 gene differs from the A_1 gene by one base pair. Variability in genes causes variable reactivity as well add after "as well." Subgroups of B are very rare and less frequent than A subgroups.

In the ABO system, naturally occurring antibodies (isoagglutins) are present against A or B antigens. Individuals with the blood group A have isoagglutinins against B red cells and vice versa (*see* Table 1). These antibodies invariably are immunoglobulin (Ig)M that activate complement and cause immediate intravascular hemolysis resulting in severe acute hemolytic transfusion reactions (HTR). They are absent at birth and develop within 3–6 mo of age, when the immune system is exposed to ABH antigenic determinants present in our environment (i.e., bacteria, plants, dust, and food). Antibodies are naturally developed against the ABH antigens absent in the individual. Generally, the antibody titer increases until the age of 10 yr and progressively falls with increasing age in adults. In

Table 1
ABO Antigens and Antibodies (Isoagglutinins)

enotype	*Genotype*	*Antigens*	*Antibodies*	*Incidence (%)[a]*	
				Whites	*Blacks*
	OO	(H)	Anti-A Anti-B	45	49
(A$_1$ or A$_2$)	AA or AO	A (A$_1$ or A$_2$) and (H)	Anti-B	40	27
	BB or BO	B and (H)	Anti-A	11	20
B (A$_1$B or A$_2$B)	AB	A, B, and (H)	None	4	4

[a]Incidence (%) in the United States among whites and blacks.
From Brecher ME, ed. *American Association of Blood Banks Technical Manual* (14th. ed.). Bethesda,
D: AABB Publications, 2002:p. 272.

acquired immunodeficiency states (e.g., leukemias and lymphomas) the levels
may be significantly low.

The ABH antigens present in red cells have been demonstrated in most tissues
of the body, including platelets and leukocytes. The ability to secrete soluble
ABH antigens is controlled by the secretor (*Se*) gene that is separate from the
ABH system. About 80% of the population have the dominant secretor (*Se*) gene
that controls one's ability to secrete soluble ABH antigens. These individuals
(secretors) distinctly have soluble ABH substances in their plasma and secretions (i.e., saliva, semen, and sweat).

2.2. The Rhesus System

The Rhesus (Rh) system is the second most clinically important and complex
blood group system. It consists of some 50 different antigens, but only 5 antigens—D, C, c, E, and e—are inherited in various combinations and account for
most of the Rh-related problems encountered in practice. The Rh antigen with the
strongest antigenicity is the Rh (D) antigen. As a simple rule, it can be noted that
persons whose red cells express the D antigen are Rh (D) positive and individuals
whose red cells lack the D antigen are Rh (D) negative. The different genotypes,
their Rh status, and the frequency of these genotypes in Caucasians are shown in
Table 2. About 85% of North American Caucasians are Rh (D) positive.

After the discovery of the Rh system in 1940, various theories were postulated
to explain the mode of inheritance and different nomenclatures were proposed.
The Wiener system proposed that the gene product was a single entity with
multiple serological specificities. The Fisher-Race system postulated three sets
of closely linked genes and gene products (C and c, D and d, and E and e).
Rosenfield proposed a third nomenclature system based on serological reactions,
which assigns a number for each Rh antigen. The World Health Organization in

Table 2
Rhesus Genotype Frequencies and Their Rh Status

Genotype	Rhesus status	Frequency[a]
CDe/cde or $R^1 r$	Positive	32%
CDe/CDe or $R^1 R^1$	Positive	16%
CDe/cDE or $R^1 R^2$	Positive	11%
cDE/cde or $R^2 r$	Positive	11%
Other genotypes with D	Positive	<13%
cde/ cde or rr	Negative	15%
Weaker variants of D or C	Positive for donors, negative for recipients	<1%
Rh-null	Null	Extremely rare

[a]In Caucasians.

1977 recommended the CDE nomenclature of Fisher-Race as it easily fits with the serological reactions. Cde or [R1] and cde or [r] are the most common haplotypes in Caucasians. cDe or [R^0] is most common in blacks.

Genomic studies have revealed the presence of two closely linked genes (*RHD* and *RHCE*) with considerable homology that refutes both Wiener and Fisher-Race postulates. The *RHD* gene controls the production of the D antigen and is absent in Rh (D)-negative individuals and explains the absence of the "d" antigen. The *RHCE* gene encodes for Cc and Ee antigens. The D and CE polypeptides differ in only 36 amino acids, the C and c polypeptides differ in four amino acids, and E and e differ in only one amino acid. The approximate molecular weight of a nonglycosylated Rh protein is 30 kDa. Recently, a D protein (a mixture of Rh [c] and [e]) has been isolated from Rh (D)-negative red cells that differ from the D protein of Rh (D)-positive cells. Genetic polymorphism may account for the difference.

Individuals whose red cells give weaker reactions with anti-D reagents are classified as *quantitative weak D* (red cells that require additional steps to demonstrate D were formerly classified as *D variant or D*^{u}). The D antigen has more than 37 epitopes, and if a significant number of epitopes are absent, then the individual is known to have *partial D* antigen (formerly classified "*D mosaic*" or "*D variant*") and can produce an antibody to the portion of the D antigen they lack. *Partial D* phenotypes arise from nucleotide interchange between the *RHCE* and the *RHD* genes or from single mutations. Gene interaction also depends on the position of the genes that ultimately affect the expression of the D antigen. A *weak D* antigen can also result from the suppressive effect of *C in trans position to a **D** on the opposite chromosome* exemplified by *CDe/Cde*. A *weak D* individual because of gene interaction has the entire D antigen and can receive D-positive blood. In contrast, *weak D* individuals who have partial absence of the D should only be transfused with D-negative blood because they can produce anti-D antibodies. The American Association of Blood Banks (AABB) requires that blood donors be screened for weak expression of the D antigen and to be labeled as Rh (D)-positive if the test is positive; however, recipients need not be tested for weak D.

On very rare occasions, red cells may lack the expected Rh antigens (e.g., –D–, –De, cD–). In Rh-null individuals, the Rh antigens are completely absent. This can arise from the absence of the gene that regulates Rh antigen expression or the presence of an amorphic gene at the Rh locus. Rh-null individuals have a compensated hemolytic anemia and abnormal red cell morphology (stomatocytosis). If transfused, they will produce antibodies against the different Rh antigens; therefore, Rh null individuals should be transfused only with Rh-null cells from the rare donor registry or with autologous red cells.

Rh antibodies can be acquired during pregnancy or a blood transfusion. The most common Rh antibody is anti-D. Rhesus immunization during pregnancy or delivery may occur when an Rh (D)-negative woman has an Rh (D)-positive child. This can be prevented by the prophylactic injection of anti-D Igs (RhIg). Rh antibodies are predominantly IgG and react at 37°C. They do not fix complement effectively, but can cause hemolytic disease of newborn (HDN; *see* Chapter 6) and hemolytic transfusion reaction (HTR). Extravascular hemolysis occurs through the mononuclear phagocyte system.

2.3. Other Red Cell Systems

Red cells bear antigens of many other blood group systems besides the ABO and Rh systems (Kell, Duffy, Lewis, I, P, MN, Lutheran, Kidd, and others). These red cell antigens are not routinely typed and generally are rare causes of HDN. The Kell and Duffy systems are briefly discussed. For more comprehensive information on the other red cell antigen systems, the reader is referred to reference texts. (*see* "suggested reading").

The Kell blood group system is clinically important, as the K antigen follows the D antigen in immunogenicity and its antibodies can cause HDN and HTR. Currently, this system includes 24 alloantigens, the most common being the K, k, Kp(a), Kp(b), Js(a), and Js(b) antigens. A defective and weak expression of Kell antigens (also lack Kx) is observed in individuals with the McLeod phenotype. These individuals have a chronic compensated hemolytic anemia and abnormal red cell morphology (acanthocytosis). Individuals with McLeod red cells also have neuromuscular and cardiovascular abnormalities (myopathy, areflexia, and cardiomyopathy). Rarely, the McLeod phenotype is associated with chronic granulomatous disease and arises from the deletion of the X chromosome that includes both XK and X-CGD loci.

The Duffy system is unusual in that the antigen frequency varies in different racial groups. The Duffy glycoprotein is the receptor for the malarial parasite and serves as an erythrocyte receptor for a number of cytokines, notably interleukin (IL)-8. Duffy glycoproteins also serve as a sponge for excess chemokines without any adverse effect on the red cell. This system has six antigens; two of these are important and deserve mention. Both Fy^a and Fy^b antigens have low incidence in Africans. In West Africa, most probably by natural selection, both antigens are absent in the majority of blacks [Fy (a–b–)]. Their red cells exhibit resistance to infection by *Plasmodium vivax* and *P. knowlesi*. Anti-Fy^a antibody may cause mild HDN and rare but severe HTR. Infrequently, Anti-Fy^b is associated with either HDN or HTR; other antibodies of this system have not been implicated at all.

2.4. Diagnostic Methods in Blood Group Serology

Prior to any blood transfusion, the red cell ABO and Rh(D) blood group (blood type) of the recipient is determined, and the serum is screened for any unexpected red cell antibodies (usually IgM and IgG antibodies). Thereafter, a cross-match is carried out between the donor's red cells and the recipient's serum. Blood group antigens or antibodies are determined with agglutination methods. The IgM antibodies (i.e., anti-A or anti-B) are usually detected by saline techniques, whereas enzyme, albumin, or antiglobulin methods are employed for the IgG antibody detection. Low ionic strength solution (LISS) is widely used in blood group serology as it shortens the incubation period and is helpful with emergency blood requests. The antiglobulin (Coombs') test detects antibodies coated on the red cells. The direct antiglobulin test (DAT) detects antibodies that are already bound to red cells in vivo, whereas the indirect antiglobulin test (IAT) detects antibodies present in the serum. The direct antiglobulin test may be positive in: (1) autoimmune hemolytic anemias (seen in lymphomas, system lupus erythematosus, cold agglutinin syndrome, and paroxysmal cold hemoglobinuria); (2) alloimmune hemolytic anemias (HDN and HTR); and (3) drug-induced hemolytic anemia. Figure 22.1 schematically outlines the determination of the ABO blood group with agglutination methods, whereas Fig. 22.2 shows the principles of both DAT and IAT.

3. LEUKOCYTE ANTIGENS

Human leukocytes bear two types of surface antigens: the human tissue or cell-specific antigens and individual type-specific antigens.

The first group is described in the cluster designation (CD) nomenclature. These antigens characterize the lineage, function, or activation state of the individual type of leukocyte (e.g., CD3 for mature T-cells). A list of the most current

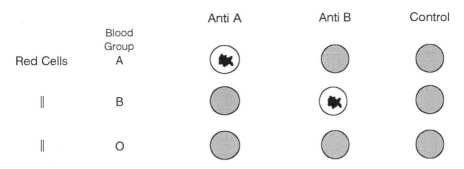

Fig. 22.1. Agglutination of red cells.

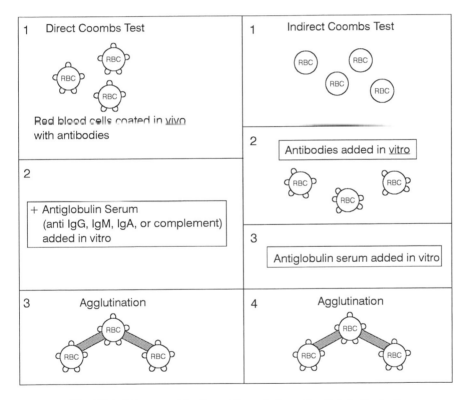

Fig. 22.2. Direct and indirect Coombs' test (antiglobulin test).

CD markers is given in Appendix 2. The second group, the family of human
leukocyte antigens (HLAs) (Class I, II, and III antigens), is encoded by the major
histocompatibility complex (MHC) genes on the short arm of chromosome 6.
Class I and II antigens are the classic transplantation antigens that define tissue

tolerance or rejection and are important for organ transplantation, but their primary role is in immune response regulation. Class III antigens (i.e., complement C2 and C4 or tumor necrosis factor [TNF]-α) may be directly or indirectly involved with MHC function.

The HLA system is expressed on many tissues. The Class I antigens (HLA-A, -B, and -C molecules) are present on all nucleated cells and platelets. Class II antigens (HLA-D molecules) are expressed on B-lymphocytes, antigen-presenting cells (monocytes, macrophages, and dendritic and Langerhans cells), and activated T-lymphocytes. HLA Class I and Class II antigens differ in immunological function. Class I antigens interact with CD8$^+$ lymphocytes, which recognize endogenous antigens. Class II molecules on the surface of antigen-presenting cells bring exogenous antigens in contact with CD4$^+$ lymphocytes.

Class I molecules consist of two glycosylated heavy chains of 44–45 kDa and a noncovalently bound 12 kDa molecule (β_2-microglobulin). The class I heavy chain has three extracellular domains, a transmembrane region, and an intracytoplasmic domain. Each of the class II molecules (HLA-DR, DQ, and DP) consists of two transmembrane noncovalently associated glycosylated polypeptide chains. The α-chain has a molecular weight of about 30–34 kDa; the β-chain has a molecular weight of about 26–29 kDa.

The inheritance of the HLA genes is closely linked, and the entire MHC is inherited as an HLA haplotype (half of the genotype) in a Mendelian fashion from each parent. For example, a haplotype of *A3, B7, Cw7, and DR2* may come from the father and the other haplotype of *A9, B27, Cw1, and DR7* may come from the mother. Distances between loci may permit some chance of recombination within the HLA system, but this occurs only infrequently (<1%) and usually between DP and DQ loci. Statistically, siblings have a 25% chance of inheriting the same pairs of HLA molecules from the parents (i.e., being HLA identical).

The HLA system is the most polymorphic human antigen system, thereby showing an enormous number of different HLA haplotype combinations. The HLA antigen pattern varies among different ethnic groups. Because of linkage disequilibrium, some haplotypes occur more frequently in certain populations. For example, HLA-*A1, B8, DR3* is the most common HLA haplotype among Caucasians with a 5% frequency.

The HLA complex is divided into three regions indicating the locations of loci. Serological and DNA techniques differ in the number of alleles that they can identify for each locus. HLA-A, HLA-C, and HLA-B loci have 20, 8, and 30 serologically defined alleles but have 309, 167, and 563 alleles detected by DNA analysis. Among the Class II antigens, the HLA-DR, HLA-DP, and HLA-DQ molecules expressed on the cell membranes are most important with 442, 81, and

127 alleles defined by DNA techniques. The allelic variations of DQ-A, DP-A, and DP-B can only be defined by DNA methods.

Two HLA nomenclatures are currently in use. The older list of specificities is based on detection of epitopes by immunological techniques (serology or mixed leukocyte culture reactions) and the newer molecular nomenclature is based on specific nucleotide sequences of alleles using DNA-based methods, now a commonly used technique in HLA-typing laboratories. Peripheral blood lymphocytes express class I antigens and are used for the serological typing of HLA-A, HLA-B, and HLA-C. Class II antigens are typed using B-lymphocytes. Classic serology uses lymphocyte microcytotoxicity tests (by Terasaki) utilizing sera from multiparous women who have been immunized against certain HLA antigens. Clinical molecular techniques have revealed the complexities of both class I and II antigens. For example, the identities of class II antigens can be shown by the mixed lymphocyte reaction but HLA–D identical pairs remain nonreactive using this method. However, molecular typing is able to distinguish serologically indistinguishable but functionally discrete HLA alleles.

All current DNA-based HLA typing assays utilize PCR to amplify the genes of interest. There are three commonly used procedures: sequence–specific primers (PCR–SSP), sequence specific oligonucleotide probes (PCR SSOP), and sequence-based typing (PCR–SBT). DNA typing is specific (no batch-to-batch variation in specificity) and flexible (new reagents can be designed as new alleles or new nucleotide sequences are identified). It is highly reproducible (with SSOP) and more robust than other techniques because it does not require viable lymphocytes nor is it influenced by the patient's health. DNA based methods have the added advantage of HLA-typing large numbers of volunteers for donor registries. Furthermore, it can detect the full range of HLA diversity. HLA alleles can specify the HLA proteins that are indistinguishable by serology. For example, *DRB1*0401* and *DRB1*0412* are allele splits identified by DNA typing that belong to the broad specificity *DR4* serological type.

In addition to the major histocompatibility antigens just described, minor histocompatibility antigens (mHags) have been defined by both Class I and II MHC-restricted T-cells and may affect the outcome of progenitor stem cell and solid organ transplantation. The mHags are immunogenetic peptides bound to Class I molecules that stimulate T-cell responses. They are also inherited and the number of minor histocompatibility loci is probably high. To date, the range of polymorphism of these antigens is not well characterized. The disparity of mHags can be associated with graft-vs-host disease (GVHD) in HLA-identical transplants (i.e., H–Y antigen in a male recipient and a female donor immunized by pregnancy). The frequency of allelic forms, immunogenicity of peptides and tissue-specific expression of proteins will determine the role of mHag disparity in either GVHD or graft rejection.

3.1. Applications of HLA Testing

HLA testing is used in progenitor stem cell and organ transplantation, disease susceptibility studies, and parentage testing. HLA identity is the *sine qua non* of allogeneic bone marrow transplantation. Despite full HLA-identical progenitor cell grafts, a substantial number of patients develop graft-vs-host mHag reactivity (details about allogeneic progenitor stem cell and bone marrow transplantation are described in Chapter 4). The HLA antigens are also important for solid organ transplantation (i.e., kidney or liver). HLA-A, HLA-B, and HLA-DR are considered to be the major transplantation antigens, whereas HLA-C, HLA-DP, and HLA-DQ are generally of minor importance. In kidney transplantation, HLA matching between donor and recipient is done routinely. HLA-matched kidney grafts have better outcomes than unmatched grafts. In contrast to bone marrow transplantation, solid organ transplantation requires ABO-compatible grafts. For logistic reasons, other solid organs (heart, liver, lung, and pancreas) are not routinely matched for HLA-antigens. HLA antibodies play a major role in graft survival and chronic rejection. The presence of cytotoxic HLA antibodies in the serum of transplant recipients reactive against a panel of cells (expressed as panel reactive antibodies or [PRA]) lowers the graft survival rates and may be a contraindication for kidney transplantation. The PRA effect is greater among recipients of a second transplant.

Multiparous women and patients who receive multiple blood transfusions are frequently alloimmunized to HLA antigens. These HLA antibodies are broadly reactive. Post-transfusion HLA alloimmunization is variable and dependent on the patient's diagnosis and therapy. Patients with leukemia have lower detectable antibodies (25 to 30%) than patients with aplastic anemia (80%) because they are usually immunosuppressed from intensive chemotherapy when the transfusions are given. Leukocyte reduction of blood components to less than 5×10^6 has significantly reduced the development of primary HLA alloimmunization. This can be achieved by the use of third-generation leukocyte filters for red blood cells (RBCs) and platelets or by inline leukoreduction systems of blood cell separators used to collect pheresis blood components. As will be discussed later in the chapter, HLA antibodies have been implicated in febrile nonhemolytic transfusion reactions and transfusion-related acute lung injury.

Immunological refractoriness to platelet transfusions results from immune destruction of transfused platelets more often by HLA antibodies (Class I antigens are expressed on platelets) than by platelet-specific antibodies. Nonimmune causes of platelet refractoriness need to be ruled out such as splenomegaly, disseminated intravascular coagulation (DIC), bleeding, infection, marrow transplantation, and antibiotics (amphotericin B, vancomycin, ciprofloxacin). Detection of HLA- or platelet-specific antibodies is usually done by solid phase red cell adherence assay

(SPRCA), flow cytometry, ELISA, monoclonal antibody specific immobilization of platelet antigen assay, or mixed passive hemagglutination assay.

Once immune refractoriness is established, special platelet products are indicated. These patients can receive HLA-matched platelets, or platelet crossmatching can be done using SPRCA or flow cytometry. Both methods of crossmatching will detect platelet antibodies against Class I and platelet-specific antigens. The efficacy of crossmatched platelets may be as good as HLA-matched platelets. Platelet-crossmatched units have the additional advantage of being readily available for transfusion. Crossmatching is not always practical because alloimmunized patients may have HLA antibodies that react to more than 90% of the random population. These patients may also have few broadly reactive antibodies against public epitopes of Class I molecules, which will make it harder for a blood center to provide a product because the best HLA-matched platelet unit can still have some incompatibility.

Numerous diseases have a more or less strong association with certain HLA antigens. Well-known examples are ankylosing spondylitis associated with HLA-B27, narcolepsy associated with HLA-DR2, hemochromatosis associated with HLA-A3, celiac disease with HLA-*DQB1*02,* and type I diabetes mellitus with DR-3 and -4 heterozygotes. The *HLA-A1, B8, DR3* haplotype is frequently involved in autoimmune disorders. These disease associations indicate the central role of the major histocompatibility complex in determining the susceptibility to disease and immune responsiveness.

The HLA system is used in parentage testing because of its polymorphism with a low recombination rate and Mendelian inheritance. There is a decreasing use of HLA typing because it does not provide a high exclusion probability when a case involves a paternal haplotype common in one particular ethnic group. Thus, molecular techniques using non-HLA genetic systems are widely favored.

4. BLOOD PRODUCTS AND INDICATIONS FOR BLOOD TRANSFUSION

4.1. Whole Blood

The use of whole blood is limited and is indicated in massive blood loss to replace the loss of both RBC mass and blood volume. Many trauma centers have abandoned the transfusion of whole blood in favor of intravenous solutions in conjunction with RBCs and other blood components. Currently, whole blood units serve as source material for blood components and plasma products.

4.2. Red Blood Cells

RBCs are indicated for replacement of red cell mass in patients who require increased oxygen-carrying capacity to prevent tissue hypoxia. The hemoglobin or hematocrit value, at which a transfusion is given, depends on the clinical circumstances. Current information supports a "restrictive strategy." Transfusions are indicated when hemoglobin concentration falls below 7 g/dL. The hemoglobin concentration should be maintained between 7 and 9 g/dL. **Note:** In younger patients, it may be necessary to transfuse if the hemoglobin concentration drops below 6 g/dL. In elderly anemic patients with cardiovascular disease (acute myocardial infarction and unstable ischemic syndromes), the threshold for transfusion may be 9 or 10 g/dL. To avoid volume overload, transfusions should be given slowly. In recent years, the recommended hemoglobin value for transfusion during surgery has been lowered from 10 to 7 g/dL. In a typical 70-kg (155-lb) patient, each unit of transfused RBCs is expected to raise the hemoglobin 1 to 1.5 g/dL and the hematocrit by 3 to 5%.

4.3. Platelets

Two types of platelet components are available for transfusion: "Pheresed Platelets," derived from single donors using an automated cell separator, and "Pooled Platelets," derived from whole blood donation and multiple donors. Automated cell separators effectively collect platelets (3 to 4×10^{11}/U) from donors.

The major goal of prescribing platelet transfusions is to effectively and safely prevent and/or treat bleeding in thrombocytopenic patients. Platelets may be given prophylactically in severely thrombocytopenic patients who have a hemorrhagic tendency or to patients on intensive myelosuppressive chemotherapy to keep the platelet count above 10×10^9/L. The success of modern chemotherapy in patients with hematological disorders (i.e., acute leukemias and myelodysplastic syndromes) and progenitor cell transplantation (bone marrow or stem cell transplantation) is largely dependent on effective platelet transfusions. Platelet counts for those at risk for spontaneous bleeding (patients with fever, infection, impaired platelet function from drugs, or hepatic or renal failure) should be kept above 15 to 20×10^9/L. Platelets are also indicated in other thrombocytopenic states: consumption coagulopathy, massive transfusion, GVHD, von Willebrand disease, and congenital and acquired platelet defects. Invasive procedures (i.e., lumbar puncture and liver biopsy) can be performed safely when the platelet count is at least 50×10^9/L. Counts of 100×10^9/L should be maintained if excessive bleeding cannot be tolerated (i.e., CNS or retinal procedures). In autoimmune thrombocytopenia, hypertransfusions of platelets are only indicated in cases of major hemorrhage. Platelets are not useful in most other instances, as the autoantibody shortens the survival of both transfused and patient's own platelets.

To investigate the mechanism of a poor response to a platelet transfusion, a platelet count is usually obtained within 1 h of the transfusion and the corrected count increment (CCI) or percent recovery is calculated. Patients who are refractory to platelet transfusions (CCI < 7.5×10^9/L or percent recovery of <15 or 20%) may have a better response if transfused with a sufficient dose of apheresis platelets. For those who become immunologically refractory, HLA-matched or crossmatched compatible platelets may offer satisfactory results. However, patients refractory to all available platelet concentrates may benefit from intravenous immunoglobulin (IVIg), plasma exchange, massive ABO-identical platelet transfusions, and acid-treated platelets (stripped of HLA antigens).

Platelets are stored at 20–22°C (room temperature) with agitation for no more than 5 d. More recently (April 2005), the Food and Drug Administration (FDA) extended the shelf-life of apheresis platelets to 7 d only if collected by the Trima® COBE Spectra™ blood separator in conjunction with 100% testing by bacterial culture system, bioMerieux BactT/ALERT Microbial Detection System Release Test®, to monitor for any bacterial contamination.

4.4. Granulocytes

Current blood separators can collect granulocytes at high yields (20 to 30×10^9 granulocytes) from donors stimulated with recombinant granulocyte colony-stimulating factor (G-CSF) and steroids, however, granulocyte transfusions lost popularity between 1985 and 1995 because of reported adverse pulmonary reactions and marginal clinical results. The unimpressive clinical efficacy may be attributed to rapid postcollection neutrophil apoptosis and inadequate doses (because previous donors did not undergo any stimulation/mobilization). Renewed interest in granulocyte transfusion stems from the availability of G-CSF that not only increases the yield of granulocyte collections but also inhibits neutrophil apoptosis. Currently, granulocyte transfusion has limited indications that include refractory fungal or bacterial infections in neutropenic patients and those with qualitative neutrophil defects. Granulocyte transfusions may also be beneficial to newborns with sepsis, neutrophil counts of less than 3000/μL or a defective marrow response. Granulocytes have no defined regulatory specifications because the FDA does not license them. However, the American Association of Blood Banks (AABB) requires that each unit contain at least 1.0×10^{10} granulocytes (**Note:** value intended as a goal for adequate collection but not as an adequate clinical dose). At least four consecutive transfusions of 1.0×10^{10} granulocytes are recommended. The use of additional transfusions is based on the patient's response or clinical course and the clinician's judgment. Granulocyte units are suspended in 200 to 400 mL plasma and contain significant numbers of platelets (1 to 6×10^{11} platelets, equivalent to an apheresis platelet unit), RBCs, and viable lymphocytes. Thus, they must be ABO and Rh compatible with the recipient and irradiated to prevent transfusion-associated (TA)-GVHD.

Granulocytes have to be transfused as soon as possible and, if necessary, stored without agitation at 20–24°C for no more than 24 h.

4.5. Fresh-Frozen Plasma

Fresh-frozen plasma (FFP) is a single-donor unit of plasma that has been separated from one unit of whole blood or collected by apheresis and frozen at −18°C or lower within 6 to 8 h of collection. It contains coagulation factor levels at 1 U/mL (or 100% activity) and is indicated to treat global or multiple coagulation factor deficiencies (i.e., liver failure and dilutional coagulopathy in massively transfused patients). Other uses for FFP include emergent reversal of warfarin therapy (when time does not allow the use of vitamin K) and plasma exchanges in thrombotic thrombocytopenic purpura and hemolytic uremic syndrome. The timing and dose are important. Correction of a markedly abnormal prothrombin time and activated partial thromboplastin time requires FFP transfusions immediately before surgery because several of the coagulation factors have very short half-lives (particularly factor VII with a biological half-life of 3 to 6 h). The dose is based on the patient's weight at 10 to 20 mL/kg. FFP contains ABO antibodies and therefore must be compatible with the recipient's red cells.

4.6. Cryoprecipitated Antihemophilic Factor

Cryoprecipitated antihemophilic factor (CRYO) is the cold insoluble portion of plasma processed from FFP by cold precipitation. The precipitate is formed as FFP is thawed at 1 to 6°C. The stability of the coagulation factors is maintained for up to 1 yr at −18°C storage. It is a plasma-derived product that contains the highest concentration of fibrinogen (250 mg, primarily used in acquired hypofibrinogenemia of DIC), factor VIII (80–120 U/concentrate), and a variable percentage of the original plasma concentration of von Willebrand factor (40–70%) and factor XIII (30%). It is indicated for the treatment of hemorrhagic disorders resulting from either quantitative or qualitative defects of these factors. However, the availability of factor concentrates and recombinant factors have contributed to its diminished usage. CRYO is also used as a source of fibrinogen to form a fibrin glue or sealant (when added to thrombin) and is also indicated to ameliorate the platelet dysfunction in uremia. Like FFP, it contains ABO antibodies, requiring consideration of recipient red cell compatibility.

4.7. Immunoglobulins

Parenteral Igs are manufactured from pooled human plasma and are used in primary or acquired hypogammaglobulinemia to protect against viral and bacterial infections. They consist of all subclasses and allotypes of IgG with only trace amounts of IgM and IgA. Polyvalent/multispecific immunoglobulins offer protection against many infections, whereas hyperimmune/specific immunoglobulins are obtained from actively immunized donors and contain high titers of disease-specific antibodies (i.e., hepatitis B virus [HBV]), *Varicella zoster*, rabies, or cell-specific [RhIg]). Rigorous donor screening and modified Cohn fractionation have made immunoglobulin preparations relatively safe.

Immunoglobulins can either be administered intravenously (IVIg) or intramuscularly (immune serum globulins) and are generally well tolerated. Adverse effects are rare (<1%) and include headache, nausea, vomiting, chills, volume overload, and allergic and pulmonary reactions that can be prevented by slow infusion and pretreating with diphenhydramine and/or hydrocortisone. True anaphylactic reactions are very rare and are seen in common variable immune deficiency and IgA deficiency. IgA deficient products are recommended in these cases.

Polyvalent immunoglobulins are indicated in hypogammaglobulinemias (congenital or acquired) and for immunomodulation in certain disorders. **Note:** the plasma half-life of IgG (the major human immune globulin) is 21–23 d, but longer in hypogammaglobulinemia. In hypogammaglobulinemia, a dose of 0.4–0.6 g/kg body weight is given every month to maintain serum IgG levels. In acquired hypogammaglobulinemia (e.g., multiple myeloma), immunoglobulins are recommended in patients with frequent infections. Established indications for immunoglobulin replacement or prophylaxis are parvovirus B19 infections (among immunosuppressed patients) and recurrent life-threatening infections (among HIV-infected children). The use of prophylactic IVIg in adults with advanced HIV infection has shown equivocal results.

High-dose polyvalent immunoglobulins achieve immunomodulatory effects through multiple mechanisms: (1) by suppressing antibody production directly through its effect on B-lymphocytes, (2) by interfering in the interaction between autoantibodies and cellular targets through its anti-idiotypic antibodies, and (3) by blocking the Fc-receptors on macrophages. Higher doses of IVIg (e.g., 0.4 g/kg × 5 d) are recommended for immunomodulation in Kawasaki syndrome (a mucocutaneous lymph node syndrome in children) and idiopathic thrombocytopenic purpura.

5. ADVERSE REACTIONS TO BLOOD TRANSFUSION

5.1. Acute Hemolytic Transfusion Reactions

Acute hemolytic transfusion reactions (AHTR) involves rapid destruction of blood cells immediately or within 24 h of a transfusion, commonly of RBCs or whole blood. It has a low rate of occurrence but is the most dangerous complication with a high mortality. Mortality depends on the amount of incompatible blood infused (25 to 44 % with infusion of less than or more than 1000 mL, respectively). ABO incompatibility is the most common cause of immune AHTR and accounts for 74% of all fatal reactions. AHTR is due to preformed antibodies, often IgM (commonly anti-A), that bind complement and cause red cell lysis. Nonimmune causes of hemolysis mimic immune mediated hemolysis and have to be excluded. Chemical, mechanical, thermal, and physical damage of red cells may result from bacterial contamination, mechanical trauma during infusion, thermal hemolysis (from overheating or freezing a unit), and osmotic hemolysis (use of hypotonic reconstituting solutions and co-administration of drugs during transfusions)

The patients commonly experience fever and chills, hypotension, and chest pain. Other signs and symptoms include low back pain, flushing, dyspnea, hemoglobinuria, gastrointestinal symptoms (abdominal pain, diarrhea, and vomiting), and unexpected bleeding from DIC. In patients under anesthesia, no immediate reactions may be recognized. Changes in blood pressure, diffuse bleeding, and hemoglobinuria may be the only signs. AHTR may cause oliguria and acute renal failure.

The classic laboratory changes include a drop in hemoglobin and hematocrit, hemoglobinemia (free hemoglobin can be demonstrated in serum or plasma), hemoglobinuria, reduced serum haptoglobin, and positive DAT. Elevations of unconjugated bilirubin, methemalbumin, and lactate dehydrogenase, and an unexpected red cell antibody may be present.

The signs and symptoms of an IgM-type acute hemolysis result from complement-mediated lysis of red cells and the release of cytokines. Binding of complement to the red cell surface is a major factor in cytokine production. The symptoms of IgG-type hemolysis also involve several cytokines (IL-1, IL-6, IL-8, and TNF). Coagulopathy, frequently seen in hemolytic transfusion reactions, especially due to IgM antibodies, results from several mechanisms. The coagulation cascade is activated by (1) antigen–antibody complexes (activates Hageman factor); (2) thromboplastic substances of the red cell stroma; (3) platelet factor 3 released by activated platelets; and (4) tissue factor release secondary to hypotension.

In order to minimize AHTRs, all transfusions should have clearly defined indications. If an AHTR is suspected, the transfusion must be stopped and immediate steps taken to confirm or exclude this possibility. Management of AHTR is dependent on the clinical status of the patient and may include cardiopulmonary support, prevention of renal failure (i.e., fluid resuscitation, vasopressors, and diuretics), and treatment of DIC. Severe bleeding in DIC requires platelets, replacement of procoagulant factors and fibrinogen (FFP and CRYO transfusions), and administration of low-dose heparin. Heparin limits both hemolysis (by its direct anticomplement activity) and inappropriate activation of procoagulant activity (by enhancing antithrombin III-neutralizing serine proteases).

5.2. Delayed Hemolytic Transfusion Reaction

Delayed hemolytic transfusion reaction (DHTR) represents an anamnestic response to a red cell antigen to which the patient has been previously sensitized by pregnancy or previous transfusions. It occurs in patients without identifiable antibody detected in the pretransfusion compatibility testing who experience accelerated red cell destruction of the transfused red cells after an interval of 3 to 10 d from transfusion. Such reactions are due to weaker antigen–antibody reactions and may develop over days. Because of the low titer of reactivity, the implicated antibody is not detectable at the time of screening or compatibility testing. The sensitivity of the antibody-screening test is important in preventing DHTRs because insensitive tests will miss weak-reacting antibodies. **Note:** these weak-reacting antibodies commonly include Rh antibodies (against CEce) and other antibodies in the Kell (anti-K), Kidd (anti-JK^a), and Duffy (anti-Fy^a) blood group systems.

DHTRs often remain asymptomatic and have milder symptoms than AHTRs, including unexplained anemia, jaundice, and fever. In patients with sickle cell disease, DHTRs may precipitate a sickle cell crisis. Laboratory findings are similar to those of AHTR, except for the identification of a new alloantibody in the patient's RBC eluate or serum or both. The degree of hyperbilirubinemia will depend on the rate and amount of hemolysis and the patient's liver function. Hemolysis is usually extravascular but intravascular hemolysis can occur. Both AHTRs and DHTRs can demonstrate a positive, mixed-field, or negative DAT. A mixed-field reaction will show a mixture of agglutinated transfused donor cells along with unagglutinated patient's cells. The DAT can be negative if all the incompatible transfused donor cells are immediately destroyed.

There is a need to differentiate DHTR from delayed serological transfusion reactions (DSTRs), in which only serological incompatibility is evident without clinical evidence of hemolysis. DSTRs are more common than DHTRs in the multiply transfused patient as more sensitive screening methods are employed and the length of stay for in-patients increases.

DHTRs are tolerated well by many patients and may only require close monitoring. Typically, fluid loading and diuresis are not indicated unless active intravascular hemolysis is present. Complications, such as renal failure and sickle cell crisis, should be treated accordingly. A red cell exchange is indicated if there is a large burden of antigen-positive cells. IVIg may be useful because extravascular hemolysis is similar to acute immune hemolytic anemia. Transfusion should be avoided until the causative antibody is identified and antigen-negative units are available. Withholding transfusions because of the lack of serologically compatible blood in patients with severe anemia is associated with significant morbidity. This can be avoided by good communication between the clinician and transfusion service.

5.3. Febrile Nonhemolytic Transfusion Reactions

Febrile nonhemolytic transfusion reactions (FNHTR) are defined as a temperature rise of at least 1°C in association with a transfusion or up to 4 h after that may be accompanied by chills or rigors. Such reactions are due to acquired antibodies to donor leukocyte antigens or pyrogenic cytokines (IL-1, IL-6, IL-8, and TNF-α) elaborated by leukocytes present in the blood components or products. FNHTRs are less frequent with prestorage leukocyte-depleted blood components. They occur in 0.5–1.4% of all transfusions. The fever is self-limited and resolves after 4–6 h. Antipyretics are effective as symptomatic treatment. Meperidine can be useful for treating rigors. Among patients who have experienced a FNHTR, there is a 15% recurrence rate.

5.4. Allergic Reactions

Allergic reactions are probably the most frequent, occurring in 1–2% of all transfusion reactions. The symptoms range from local or diffuse pruritus, urticaria, erythema, and cutaneous flushing to anaphylactic allergic reactions occurring within minutes of the transfusion. Anaphylactoid reactions fall in between the two ends of the spectrum.

Allergic disorders afflict 30% of donors, and passive transfer of IgE antibodies may be involved. Uncomplicated allergic reactions are associated with increased histamine (increased during storage), cytokines, mast cell activators (i.e., leukotrienes), and other vasoactive substances ($C3_a$ and $C5_a$) produced by donor leukocytes during storage. Some allergic reactions only have pulmonary signs and symptoms without cutaneous involvement (10%).

Severe anaphylactic reactions may occur after infusion of a very small volume (<10 mL) in patients with IgA deficiency and are due to preformed, class specific, recipient anti-IgA antibodies against infused donor IgA proteins. Additionally, they may be due to antibodies against complement C_4 and haptoglobin. Patients with Chido (Ch) and Rogers (Rg) antibodies (against the Ch/Rg blood group antigens carried by complement C4d of the classic complement pathway) also exhibit anaphylactoid reactions following plasma product transfusions. Haptoglobin deficiency is rare in North American populations but more common than IgA deficiency among Japanese patients experiencing anaphylactic reactions.

Anaphylactoid reactions are typically associated with subclass, allotypic, or specific anti-IgA in patients with normal or demonstrable levels of IgA. These reactions may be seen in other transfused products, such as peanut allergen transfused to patients with peanut allergy.

Mild uncomplicated allergic reactions involving hives (without other symptoms) respond to antihistamines (such as diphenhydramine). The transfusion may be restarted after treatment if there is no recurrence or progression of symptoms. Restarting a transfusion is not advisable with more serious reactions; in particular, pulmonary symptoms with airway involvement. Treatment of severe anaphylactic reactions is the same as for any anaphylactic reaction and requires immediate cessation of the transfusion, epinephrine, and other supportive care. Prevention of anaphylaxis in IgA-deficient individuals requires avoidance of all plasma containing products unless collected from a known IgA-deficient donor and washing of all red cell and platelet products.

6. DISEASES TRANSMITTED BY BLOOD TRANSFUSION

The major concern is to make all blood transfusions as safe and effective as possible. Several infectious agents, viruses, bacteria, and parasites are transmissible by transfusion of whole blood, blood components, or products. Attention will focus on those transfusion-transmissible diseases (TTD) that present risks of chronic infection in the recipient.

Major strategies available to reduce transmission include: stringent donor selection and laboratory testing; use of autologous blood, pharmacological substitutes, or new transfusion strategies; inactivation of residual infectious agents in the units to be transfused, and limiting the number of donor exposures and allogeneic transfusions.

Blood donor screening is one of the more important steps in protecting the safety of the blood supply. Nonremunerated, voluntary donors with low infectious risks are encouraged and recruited to become blood donors. The scarcity of the blood supply in many countries has spurred the use of paid donors. Direct interviews, miniphysical examinations and laboratory testing of all blood collections help to exclude donors who have exposure to transmissible infections or who have the risk factors for TTD.

The blood supply is screened or tested for bacterial and viral infections (including tick borne infections), parasites (i.e., malaria, babesia, Chagas' disease, and microfilariasis).

Blood intended for autologous (only if transfused outside the collection facility) and allogeneic use require tests for syphilis (STS), HBV (HBV surface antigen [HBsAg] and antibodies to the hepatitis core antigen [anti-HBc]), hepatitis C virus (HCV, anti-HCV, and HCV RNA), HIV (antibodies to HIV-1/HIV-2 and HIV-1 RNA), and human T-cell lymphotropic virus (anti-HTLV-I and II). Other infectious agents can be tested or excluded based on the epidemiology of the infectious agent, geographic area, and intended use of the blood product. In

Table 3
Risk Estimates of Transfusion-Transmitted
Infections in the United States[a]

Infection	Risk estimate (per unit transfused)
Hepatitis B	1/205,000
Hepatitis C	1/1,935,000
HTLV	1/2,993,000
HIV	1/2,135,000

[a]Estimates of residual risk in donations from repeat donors of the American Red Cross blood donor population from 1995 to 2001 (after NAT testing for HIV and HCV).

From Dodd RY, Notari EP 4th, Stramer SL.Current prevalence and incidence of infectious disease markers and estimated window-period risk in the American Red Cross blood donor population. *Transfusion* 2002;42(8):975–979.

countries with endemic malaria, testing for malaria parasites is mandatory. The general safety of the blood supply will be enhanced if these concerns are addressed; however, minimal risks still remain because very recent infections are not detected by recommended/standard laboratory tests (*see* Table 3).

6.1. Bacterial Infections Transmitted by Blood Transfusion

Bacterial contamination resulting in transfusion-associated bacterial sepsis is now believed to be the most common infectious source of morbidity and the most frequently reported cause of transfusion-related fatalities in the United States (accounting for 16% of transfusion fatalities). Bacteria are believed to originate from the donor either from the venipuncture site or unsuspected bacteremia. Excluding donors with chronic diseases or recent febrile infections and scrupulous disinfection of the skin reduces the risk of bacterial transmission. Both Gram-positive and -negative bacteria have been implicated.

Bacterial multiplication is more likely in components stored at room temperature (i.e., platelets) than refrigerated components (i.e., RBCs) or frozen components (FFP and CRYO). Bacterial contamination of platelet transfusion is one of the most common infectious risks of transfusion, causing life-threatening sepsis in 1 in 100,000 recipients and immediate fatal outcome in 1 in 500,000 recipients. Despite limiting platelet storage to 5 d, various pathogens have been implicated (*Staphylococcus*, *Enterobacteriaceae*, *Streptococcus*, *Bacillus*, and *Pseudomonas*).

The low incidence of platelet-associated sepsis may be due to underreporting because (1) they typically occur several hours after transfusion and are not as catastrophic as RBC-associated sepsis; and (2) sepsis is attributed to other causes because platelets are commonly transfused to immunocompromised patients with other complex problems.

Psychrophilic Gram-negative bacteria can multiply in refrigerated blood and components. RBC contamination is primarily from *Yersinia enterocolitica* and *Serratia liquifaciens*. *Y. enterocolitica* proliferates and produces an endotoxin in refrigerated anticoagulated blood because it can grow at temperatures below 37°C in a calcium-free medium even after a long lag period. Any bacterial contamination of blood products is potentially serious.

P. cepacia and *P. aeruginosa* are environmental organisms that grow optimally at 30°C and have been isolated from cryoprecipitate and plasma thawed in contaminated water baths.

Syphilis transmission by blood transfusion is possible but its occurrence is extremely rare because the phase of spirochetemia is short and the infective organism, *Treponema pallidum*, does not survive refrigerated storage for more than 96–120 h. Seroconversion occurs after the phase of spirochetemia so testing donor blood by standard STS does not effectively prevent transmission. However, most positive STS results are demonstrated by donors with inadequately treated noninfectious syphilis, or are biological false positives (may be positive for hepatitis, mononucleosis, measles, chickenpox, immunizations, rheumatoid arthritis, and pregnancy). There have only been two cases of transfusion-transmitted syphilis reported in the English literature. Another spirochete, *Borrelia burgdorferi*, causing Lyme disease (transmitted by the Ixodes deer tick) can survive routine storage of RBCs and FFP. However, transfusion-related transmission has not been reported at this time. The phase of spirochetemia is associated with clinical symptoms that would render potential donors ineligible for donation. Donors diagnosed with Lyme disease are accepted provided they have completed antibiotic therapy and are completely asymptomatic.

6.2. Viral Diseases Transmitted by Blood Transfusion

6.2.1. HEPATITIS

Before the 1980s, the transmission of hepatitis was the major transfusion-related viral infection. The absolute number of hepatitis infections post-transfusion has decreased significantly, because reliable tests for HBV and HCV were introduced. In the past, donors having elevated alanine aminotransferases were rejected. This surrogate marker is no longer used with the availability of more specific tests for anti-HCV and HCV RNA. Anti-HBc testing has been retained because it may still detect a few donors with infectious HBV who are negative for HBsAg.

Hepatitis A (HAV), an RNA virus, is generally transmitted by the oral-fecal route and very rarely transmitted by transfusion. The main concern of HAV (and parvovirus B19 as well) is transmission by plasma derivatives (particularly human source factor VIII concentrates) because it does not have a lipid envelope and is not inactivated during the manufacturing process. Nucleic acid testing (NAT) is available and is done only for *source plasma* (plasma intended for manufacture of blood derivatives/products). NAT testing for this virus is currently considered an "in-process control" by the FDA so donor notification (for positive tests) is not required. In contrast to persons infected with HBV, persons who are exposed to HAV do not develop a chronic carrier state. Blood donors are not routinely screened for HAV because of the rarity of transfusion transmissible HAV and the absence of HAV antibody at the time of viremia. The risk for HAV is estimated at 1 per 10 million units.

HBV, a DNA virus, is primarily transmitted by the parenteral route. It can be transmitted within the first 100 d after infection when viremia is present and no protective immunity has yet developed, or in the chronic carrier state. Donor screening to detect HBV infection includes assays for the HBsAg and for anti-HBc. Most infections are asymptomatic and HBsAg positivity occurs 2 to 6 wk before the onset of symptoms; thus, an apparently healthy but infectious donor will be eligible for donation.

A "window period" for any transfusion-transmissible agent is defined as the period of time that an individual is potentially infectious but demonstrates negative serological tests (without detectable antibodies). A licensed NAT test is not available for HBV because of low levels of viremia during the "window phase" resulting from a slow viral doubling time. However, a recent publication reported that the "window period" can be reduced by 25–36 d using single donor NAT (SDNAT), further reduced by 9–11 d using minipool NAT (MPNAT) and reduced by 2–9 d using a new and more sensitive HBsAg assay. Disagreement exists as to whether HBV-NAT will be cost effective to further reduce the risk of transfusion-transmissible HBV.

HCV, an RNA virus, was discovered in 1989 and was linked with most cases of non-A, non-B hepatitis in the past. HCV infections are mild and generally (80%) asymptomatic. The long-term effects are far more serious in that the majority of HCV infected patients develop chronic liver disease with 20% developing cirrhosis. In addition, those with HCV cirrhosis develop hepatocellular carcinoma. It was estimated that the elimination of hepatitis C by anti-HCV antibody testing prevented 40,000–50,000 new cases of post-transfusion hepatitis per year (an additional 10,000–13,000 cases may have been prevented by newer versions of the test). The risks of transfusion-transmissible HCV has further been reduced by HCV-NAT. Prior to HCV-NAT, the window period because of a slower doubling time was 70 d. The newly developed HCV-NAT (MPNAT/SDNAT) has further closed the window phase to 10 d, so that the transfusion-transmissible risk for HCV is reduced to 1:1,935,000 per unit transfused from 1:276,000 in the past (*see* Table 3).

Hepatitis D (or δ), another RNA virus, exists as a co-infection in patients chronically infected with HBV because the "delta agent" cannot multiply in the absence of HBV. Testing for HBV markers eliminates hepatitis D-positive donors.

The hepatitis G virus (HGV, also known as GBV-C), a newly discovered RNA virus, is potentially transmitted by blood products. Among normal donors, the reactivity is 1–4% by PCR techniques. Currently, HGV has not been associated with a specific disease entity and its designation as a "hepatitis" virus may have been premature. Thus, no routine donor testing is performed.

Two other hepatitis viruses, hepatitis E virus (HEV) and SEN virus, are apparently transmitted by transfusion. HEV does not occur in the United States but is endemic in other parts of the world, although its true incidence remains unknown. SEN virus is the latest virus postulated to cause the remaining non A–E transfusion-transmitted hepatitis. At present, the biological role of SEN virus has not been clearly defined.

Lastly, TT virus, a DNA virus, first described by a Japanese group was originally postulated to cause non-A–E hepatitis. This virus is prevalent in many countries and is currently not associated with hepatitis.

6.2.2. Retroviruses

Retroviral infections transmitted by blood transfusion include HIV-1 and HIV-2 and human lymphotropic virus (HTLV-I and HTLV-II). HIV is transmitted by both cellular blood components and plasma; however, both types of HTLV are highly cell-associated and require viable lymphocytes for transfusion transmission.

HIV is a cytopathic retrovirus that preferentially infects CD4-positive T-lymphocytes. The infection begins as a viremia of cell-free virions that may be clinically manifested by an acute nonspecific flu-like illness. Viremia is detectable in the plasma 10 d to 3 wk after infection. As HIV antibodies appear, the disease enters a clinically latent phase. Viral replication and dissemination continues and the virus can be transmitted by blood or genital secretions.

HIV-2 causes endemic infection in West Africa and has apparently spread with population movements. It is indistinguishable from HIV-1 in disease spectrum although HIV-2 has a longer incubation period and is less efficiently transmitted than HIV-1.

The AIDS epidemic in the early 1980s had a catastrophic impact on the safety of blood transfusions but triggered a major impetus for improvement in blood safety. The risk of HIV transmission through blood components/products dramatically decreased with more stringent donor history screening and improvement of donor testing (*see* Table 3). Combination HIV-1/HIV-2 tests implemented in the United States in 1992 have identified to date three HIV-2 infected donors, none appear to have been infected in the United States.

Prior to 1992, the window period for HIV averaged 45 d. More sensitive HIV-antibody screening tests closed this window to 22 d. In 1996, HIV antigen (p24 antigen) testing reduced this infectious window by an estimated 6 d; such that circulating cell-free virions could be detected as early as 16 d following infection. With the newly developed PCR-based NAT, this window period was further reduced to about 10 d. Although SDNAT has a detection sensitivity of less than 50 viral copies/mL, its higher cost prompted many blood centers into using MPNAT with 14–16 donors per pool. An estimate of residual risk of HIV infection from repeat donors after NAT is 1 per 2,135,000 (per unit transfused). Currently, many blood centers have implemented NAT and discontinued p24 antigen testing following the FDA's licensure of the HIV-NAT assay.

HTLV-I and II are human retroviruses that can be transmitted by blood, sexual contact (predominantly male-to-female), and through breast milk. It circulates as a provirus that is incorporated into the DNA of lymphocytes. No cases of transfusion-transmitted HTLV have been reported with noncellular blood components. Prolonged storage for more than 10 to 14 d (refrigeration inactivates the lymphocytes) also reduces transmission risk. Compared to other viruses, HTLV-I and -II transfusion transmission is less efficient because exposure invariably does not result in infection. Look-back studies have shown that one in three HTLV-contaminated units transmitted the virus.

Risk factors for HTLV-1 infection are birth or sexual contact in areas where the disease is endemic (Japan and certain Pacific Islands, Caribbean basin, sub-Saharan Africa, Central and South America). The natural epidemiology of HTLV-II is not fully known, although a high prevalence is seen in some Native American populations. HTLV-II is presumably associated with parenteral transmission with risk factors of intravenous drug use (1 to 20% seroprevalence) and sexual contact with an IV drug user.

An excess of infectious syndromes (i.e., bronchitis, pneumonia, and urinary infections) is seen among blood donors infected with HTLV-I or -II. However, most HTLV-1-positive individuals remain asymptomatic donors with an extremely long latency period (decades) and a 2–5% life-long risk of developing adult T-cell lymphoma/leukemia or HTLV-associated myelopathy/tropical spastic paresis in areas of high endemicity. Enzyme immunoassay (EIA) for both HTLV-I and -II is used to screen donors, and EIA-reactive donors are indefinitely deferred regardless of investigational supplemental tests since there is no licensed confirmatory test.

The risk of transfusion-transmissible HTLV with the same "51-d window period" has decreased from 1:514,000 (in 1998–1999) to 1:2,993,000 (in 2000–2001). Such a dramatic risk reduction may be partly attributed to the implementation of universal leukocyte reduction. Viral load reduction by removal of infected leukocytes remains controversial.

6.2.3. Human Herpesviruses

Leukocytotropic human herpesvirus (HHV) may contaminate blood components. Cytomegalovirus (CMV or HHV-5) and Epstein-Barr virus (EBV or HHV-4) have the greatest clinical relevance to transfusion medicine.

CMV is transmitted by transfusion in the latent, noninfectious state in the genome of leukocytes present in cellular blood components. Seropositivity in the general population, United States ranges from 20 to 80%, but only a small fraction of these individuals have circulating virion. Exposure and host factors determine symptomatology. Among immunocompetent individuals, CMV causes a mononucleosis-like syndrome or an asymptomatic infection and remains latent in tissues and leukocytes.

Symptomatic CMV infections develop in immunosuppressed, seronegative hosts. Human progenitor cell transplant (HPCT) recipients (develop CMV pneumonitis), low birth weight neonates (<1500 g) of seronegative/seropositive mothers and HIV-infected patients (develop CMV chorioretinitis, encephalitis, and enteritis) are particularly at risk. Among seropositive HPCT recipients, viral reactivation is the most common cause of CMV infection (up to 69% in one study). Generally, the donor organ is the source among transplant recipients. Additionally, the risk of transfusion-transmitted CMV is high in heavily transfused recipients (liver, heart-lung, and pancreas transplants).

"CMV-reduced-risk blood components" are recommended to reduce CMV transmission. Leukoreduced cellular blood components are comparable to seronegative cellular blood components. Nonetheless, there remains a small risk of transmission with either type of component. Most centers in the United States, Canada, Australia, and Europe recommend transfusion of CMV-negative blood components to CMV-negative pregnant women and for intrauterine transfusions (to prevent transplacental infection), and to CMV-negative immunosuppressed individuals (i.e., HPCT recipients, HIV-positive with AIDS, and other immunosuppressed individuals). It is also prudent to extend this consideration to CMV-negative candidates for HPCT. Despite transfusions of "CMV-reduced-risk blood components," a few marrow transplant patients (1 to 4%) still develop primary CMV infection.

EBV targets B-lymphocytes causing polyclonal proliferation with T-lymphocyte response and demonstration of "atypical lymphocytes." It causes infectious mononucleosis, the endemic form of Burkitt's lymphoma in Africa and nasopharyngeal carcinoma. EBV can be transmitted by blood transfusion, but is a rare cause of significant disease in immunocompetent individuals. Transfusion-transmitted EBV is usually asymptomatic. Rarely, EBV causes posttransfusion hepatitis and "postperfusion syndrome." The latter is characterized as a viral-like illness following massive transfusion of fresh blood during cardiac surgery.

EBV contributes to the development of lymphoproliferative disorders among immunosuppressed HPCT and organ transplant recipients from a reactivation of a latent infection. The high seropositivity rate (90%) among blood donors and the low risk of acquiring clinical disease among immunocompetent recipients make blood donor screening and laboratory testing less beneficial.

6.2.4. OTHER VIRUSES AND UNCONVENTIONAL INFECTIOUS AGENTS (PRIONS)

Parvovirus B19 is the etiological agent of erythema infectiosum ("fifth disease") in children, arthritis in adults, and hypoplastic anemias in HIV-infected individuals. More ominously, it causes an aplastic crisis among patients with chronic hemolytic anemias who rely on active erythropoiesis to offset the shortened red cell survival. The red cell P antigen is the cellular receptor for parvovirus B19 so those who do not possess the antigen are naturally resistant to infection. The presence of parvovirus B19 antibodies (30 to 60% prevalence) and the brief viremia in blood donors make viral transmission uncommon (ranging from 1 in 3300 to 1 in 50,000). The rarity of clinically significant disease or viral transmission has not made donor screening and testing imperative. There are reports of parvovirus B19 transmission by solvent-detergent plasma (solvent detergent viral inactivation is ineffective because the virus lacks a lipid envelop), cellular blood components, and clotting factor concentrates. There are no reports of transmission from IVIg and albumin. NAT screening has been implemented only for in-process manufacturing control of plasma derivatives.

West Nile virus (WNV), a flavivirus, is transmitted through mosquito bites (an arthropod-borne-virus), blood transfusions (first reported during the 2002 epidemic), and organ transplants to humans causing encephalitis, meningitis, and very rarely asymmetrical flaccid paralysis. Immunocompromised and elderly individuals are at risk of developing severe disease. Viremia occurs 1 to 3 d following an infecting mosquito bite and lasts from 1 to 11 d.

WNV transfusion-transmission risk (per 10,000 donations) ranges from 1.46 to 12.33 for selected metropolitan areas and from 2.12 to 4.76 for six high-incidence states. Serological tests are ineffective in donor screening as viremia disappears by the time IgM antibodies are detected by ELISA tests. The seasonal increase in 2003 prompted MPNAT under a clinical protocol in the United States. Likewise, donor history questionnaires have been implemented to reduce the risk of WNV transmission. During periods of high endemicity, frozen products have been withdrawn voluntarily from the supply, as cessation of donor collection is not feasible. Other blood derivatives do not appear to be at risk for transmission as the WNV is inactivated by heat or solvent-detergent treatment.

The severe acute respiratory syndrome (SARS) virus that first appeared in Guangdong, China is spread by close person-to-person contact and is believed caused by a *corona virus* that causes the common cold and/or probably a *paramyxovirus*. Its spread to other countries was linked to airline travel, often by health care workers in contact with SARS patients. The virus has been isolated from the blood of an infected individual but its risk of transmission through blood transfusion remains unknown. However, because of its highly contagious nature, transfusion transmission is possible if blood collection coincides with the viremic phase of the disease. The FDA recommends deferral of at-risk donors for 14 d after a possible exposure and at least a 28-d deferral after resolution of symptoms. Likewise, deferral is extended to donors with a history of travel or residence in SARS-affected areas.

Transmissible spongiform encephalopathies (TSEs) are rare, fatal degenerative neurological disorders caused by infectious agents classified as prions or proteinaceous infectious particles that lack nucleic acid. A prion is an abnormal isoform (PrP^{SC}) of a normal cellular protein (PrP^C) that is resistant to inactivation by alcohol, formalin, ionizing radiation, proteases, and nucleases; but is disrupted by autoclaving, phenols, detergents, and extremes in pH. TSEs have long incubation periods (years to decades).

Two such TSEs, classic Creutzfeld-Jakob disease (CJD) and variant Creutzfeld-Jakob disease (vCJD) are important from the transfusion medicine perspective. Unlike classic CJD, which presents in older patients, vCJD is observed in young adults and has an acute course with rapid progression to death in 2 yr.

The majority of classic CJD is sporadic (80%). Familial cases (10–15%) are caused by mutations and the rest (10%) arise from iatrogenic transmission (administration of growth hormone and gonadotropic hormone derived from pooled human pituitary tissue, allografts of dura mater and cornea, and reuse of intracerebral electroencephalographic electrodes from such patients). To date, transfusion transmission of CJD has been reported in experimental rodent models, but not in humans. Although theoretically possible, there is growing consensus that CJD transmission by blood or its components is unlikely.

Variant CJD (vCJD), first reported in the United Kingdom in 1996, is caused by the same prion responsible for bovine spongiform encephalopathy (BSE) but might be entirely different. Its potential for transmission by blood and blood components is heightened by the fact that vCJD can spread from cattle to humans (presumably by ingestion) and from human to humans (a recipient developed symptoms 6.5 yr after a red cell transfusion). In December of 2003, a potential case of vCJD associated with blood transfusion was reported in the United Kingdom. Its presence in lymphoreticular tissue of vCJD patients, determined by animal studies and its association with B-lymphocytes, suggests possible transmission through blood transfusions. As a safety measure, several European countries and Canada implemented universal leukocyte reduction for all blood products to prevent lymphocytes from transmitting vCJD. However, the efficacy of such intervention remains uncertain.

Expanded donor deferral criteria have been implemented to reduce the risk of transmission of both TSEs. This includes deferral of donors at risk of exposure due to travel or residency in areas with BSE epidemics, deferral of donors who received bovine insulin and pituitary-derived human growth hormone or dura transplants since 1980, and deferral of donors with blood relatives diagnosed with CJD.

6.3. Parasites Transmitted by Blood Transfusion

Malaria is caused by several species of the intraerythrocytic protozoan *Plasmodium* and can be transmitted by transfusion of parasitemic blood. Malarial parasites survive for at least 1 wk in blood components stored at room temperature (i.e., platelets) or at 4°C. They can survive cryopreservation with glycerol. Any blood component that contains red cells can transmit infection via the asexual form of the parasite. It is frequently transmitted by red cell transfusions, rarely by platelet transfusions, and is absent in plasma products. It is recognized as a global health problem, but is very rare in the United States. However, it is the most commonly recognized parasitic complication of transfusion and occurs as at an estimated rate of 0.25 cases per 1 million blood units collected. Asymptomatic carriers are the general source of transfusion acquired infections. At present, there are no practical serological tests to screen asymptomatic carriers. Prevention of malaria transmission is possible by deferral of prospective donors with increased risk of infectivity based on medical and travel history. In Western Europe and the United States, blood donors are deferred for 12 mo after travel to malaria-endemic areas. Individuals born in areas endemic for malaria generally are excluded from blood donation for 3 yr after leaving the area.

Chagas' disease (American Trypanosomiasis) endemic in South and Central America is caused by another protozoan parasite, *Trypanosoma cruzi,* transmitted by reduviid bugs (cone-nosed or "kissing" bugs). Infection occurs from fecal contamination of the reduviid bug bite wound by the infectious trypomastigote. Acute infections are mild to asymptomatic and 20–40% of infected individuals enter a chronic phase of intermittent parasitemia manifested by "megasyndromes" (cardiomegaly, megaesophagus, and megacolon). Blood transfusion is a major source of infection in South America, where parasite reduction using chemicals (like gentian violet) on donated blood pose additional risks. Six cases of transfusion-transmitted Chagas' disease have been reported in the United States (New York, Los Angeles, Texas, and Florida) and Canada, involving platelet concentrates in at least four cases. Currently, there is a 0.1 to 0.2% seroprevalence in areas with high immigrant populations from Central and South America. To date, no tests are licensed by the FDA for screening, but highly specific confirmatory tests (i.e., Western blot assays) are available. Close monitoring is needed to define the risk of transfusion transmitted Chagas' disease.

7. OTHER ADVERSE EFFECTS OF BLOOD TRANSFUSION

7.1. Iron Overload

Patients who are transfusion-dependent for aplastic anemias or chronic hemolytic anemias (sickle cell anemia and thalassemias) such as genetic hemochromatosis may develop iron overload (hemosiderosis), which may result in organ failure, primarily of the heart, liver, and pancreas. Every milliliter of transfused RBCs contains approx 1 mg of elemental iron. Signs of clinical toxicity become evident when total body iron reaches 400 to 1000 mg/kg of body weight. Patients who develop iron overload on chronic transfusion are candidates for chelation therapy with parenteral deferoxamine or oral iron chelators (see Chapter 23). Transfusion of RBC units enriched with a younger cell population or "neocytes" (reticulocytes), advocated by some investigators, potentially increases transfusion intervals and intravascular survival of RBCs (41%). However, its value in reducing hemosiderosis has not yet been established.

7.2. Transfusion-Associated GVHD

A transfusion recipient's ability to mount an immune response and inability to reject transfused (donor) T-lymphocytes in cellular blood components is fundamental to the pathogenesis of TA-GVHD. Only whole blood and its cellular components (RBCs, granulocytes, and platelets) containing sufficient, viable, cytotoxic T-lymphocytes can mediate TA-GVHD. No cases have been reported following FFP transfusions. This disease has been reported in immunosuppressed patients with hematological and solid malignancies. Rarely, it occurs after organ and HPCT and in patients receiving myeloablative therapy. Immunocompetent transfusion recipients at risk of TA-GVHD share a haplotype with related or unrelated HLA homozygous donors (HLA haploidentical). TA-GVHD typically appears 2 to 50 d after transfusion. The development of marrow aplasia and progressive pancytopenia distinguishes TA-GVHD from GVHD following

HPCT. These patients may develop a skin rash, diarrhea, fever, and abnormal liver function accompanied by extensive hepatocellular damage.

Most cases (>90%) of TA-GVHD are fatal. Treatment with immunosuppressive regimens (steroids, cytoxan, and antithymocyte globulin, including OKT3) has been ineffective. As a consequence, immunosuppressed patients (with congenital immunodeficiency syndromes, hematological malignancies undergoing myeloablative therapy, allogeneic or autologous HPCT) premature neonates (<1200 g), intrauterine transfusions, recipients of blood from biological relatives and HLA-matched platelets should receive only irradiated blood. Solid organ transplant recipients receiving immunosuppressive therapy or those undergoing chemotherapy/radiation therapy for solid tumors do not require irradiated blood componenets. Interestingly, TA-GVHD has not been reported in patients with AIDS. Gamma irradiation with 25–30 gy inactivates all immunoreactive lymphoid cells and prevents TA-GVHD. Leukocyte reduction is insufficient to prevent TA-GVHD.

7.3. Transfusion-Related Acute Lung Injury

The transfusion-related acute lung injury (TRALI) reaction is rare (1:2000 to 1:5000 units) and occurs during or within the 4–6 h after a transfusion. Patients suddenly develop shortness of breath with severe hypoxemia, chills, fever, cough, and tachycardia. Noncardiogenic pulmonary edema recognized on chest X-ray as bilateral diffuse interstitial infiltrates results from leukocytic activation and aggregation in the pulmonary bed causing "capillary leak." The pathophysiology of this reaction is thought to be immune-mediated, typically resulting from (1) donor antibodies (granulocytic or lymphocytotoxic antibodies) directed against white blood cell antigens, (2) HLA Class I and II antibodies, and (3) lipid activators of neutrophils in donor plasma. In very rare cases, these antibodies may be present in the recipient.

Most donors associated with TRALI are multiparous females or donors with multiple exposures to varying HLA types. Treatment is supportive; however, ventilatory and pressor support may be necessary. Resolution occurs within 3 to 7 d in 81% of cases but is fatal in a small proportion of cases. TRALI is the third leading cause of transfusion-related deaths, accounting for 13% of all transfusion fatalities.

8. AUTOLOGOUS BLOOD TRANSFUSION

An autologous donor donates blood for his or her own future use. For practical reasons, the transfusion of autologous RBCs is an attractive option for patients undergoing elective surgery. Autologous blood can be collected from a patient in advance of anticipated need (preoperative collection) or at the start of surgery (acute normovolemic hemodilution); additionally, shed blood can be recovered for reinfusion during surgery (intraoperative collection) or during the postoperative period from drainage devices (postoperative collection). Clinicians should be aware that recovered blood does not provide platelets or coagulation factors.

Autologous blood transfusion avoids the small risk of transfusion-transmitted infectious agents, red cell alloimmunization, adverse reactions resulting from antibody-mediated hemolysis, and leukocyte-associated febrile reactions. In a larger perspective, autologous transfusion supplements and preserves the blood supply for other patients who acutely or chronically need allogeneic transfusions.

Autologous donors undergoing preoperative collection should be in satisfactory or good health without major cardiac problems or anemia. The predonation hemoglobin requirement is lower (11 g/dL) for autologous donation than for allogeneic donation (12.5 g/dL). Autologous donors can donate as often as every 72 h before the scheduled surgery. Ideally, supplemental iron is prescribed before the first collection because iron-restricted erythropoiesis is one of the limiting factors in collecting multiple units of blood over a short period of time. Oral or parenteral iron supplement enhances recovery of hematopoiesis. Rarely, recombinant human erythropoietin must be administered to donors who have insufficient erythropoietic response.

In order to justify the cost effectiveness of autologous collections, there should be a high likelihood that at least two units of blood will be used during surgery. Hospitals must establish guidelines regarding indications for autologous blood. During a 4–5 wk collection period, 2–4 units of RBCs can be collected. The storage time of autologous blood is comparable to blood from other donors (up to 42 d with additive solutions). Unused autologous blood may be discarded or may be used for allogeneic transfusions in facilities that allow "crossover" only after infectious disease testing. Only 30% of collections are typically eligible for allogeneic use. Many institutions choose not to "crossover" autologous units because of the cost, complexity, and error risks associated with the process. Freezing and long-term storage of RBCs is indicated for patients with rare blood group antibodies, making it difficult to find compatible blood (*see* p.439).

SUGGESTED READING

Anderson KC and Ness PM, eds. Scientific Basis of Transfusion Medicine, 2nd ed. Philadelphia: WB Saunders, 2000.

Biggerstaff BJ and Petersen LR. Estimated risk of transmission of the West Nile virus through blood transfusion in the US, 2002. Transfusion 2003; 43: 1007-1017.

Brecher ME, ed. American Association of Blood Banks, Technical Manual (15th ed.). Bethesda, MD: AABB Press, 2005.

Busch PB, Kleinman SH, and Nemo GJ. Current and emerging infectious risks of blood transfusions. JAMA 2003; 289 (8): 959-962.

Dodd RY, Notari EP, Stramer SL. Current prevalence and incidence of infectious disease markers and estimated window-period risk in the American Red Cross blood donor population. Transfusion 2002;42:975-979.

Harmening DM: Modern Blood Banking and Transfusion Medicine, 5th ed.: Philadelphia: F.A. Davis Company, 2005.

Hillyer CD, Silberstein LE, Ness PM, Anderson KA, eds. Blood Banking and Transfusion Medicine. Philadelphia: Churchill Livingstone, 2003.

Klein, HG (Chair), Standards for Blood Banks and Transfusion Services. 23rd ed. Bethesda, MD: AABB Press, 2005.

McCullough JM. Transfusion Medicine, 2nd ed. New York: McGraw-Hill, 2005.

Mintz PD, ed. Transfusion Therapy: Clinical Principles and Practice, 2nd ed. Bethesda, MD: AABB Press, 2005.

Murphy S, ed. The HLA System: Basic Biology and Clinical Applications. Bethesda, MD: AABB Press, 1999.

Petz LD, Swisher SN, Kleinman S, Spence RK, and Strauss RG, eds. Clinical Practice of Transfusion Medicine, 3rd ed. New York: Churchill Livingstone, 1996.

Pomper GJ, Wu YY, Snyder EL. Risks of transfusion-transmitted infection: 2003. Curr Opin Hematol 2003; 10:412-418.

Simon TL, Dzik WH, Snyder EL, Stowell CP and Strauss RG, eds. Rossi's Principles of Transfusion Medicine, 3rd ed. Philadelphia, PA: Lippincott Williams & Wilkins, 2002.

Rossi EC, Simon TL, Moss GS, Gould SA, eds. Principles of Transfusion Medicine, 2nd Baltimore, MD: Williams & Wilkins, 1996.

U.S. Food and Drug Administration Center for Biologic Evaluation and Research. Request for an exception under 21 CFR (Code of Federal Regulation) 640.120, Alternative Procedures, to 610.53 (d), Dating Periods, to use the Gambro 7-day ELP Platelet Storage System Using Apheresis Platelets Collected with the Cobe Spectra Apheresis System and Gambro Trima Automated Blood Component Collection System.

US Food and Drug Administration approves Gambro BCT's 7-day platelet Post-Market Surveillance Plan. GAMBRO.BCT March 2005 Press Release (http://www.gambrobct.com)

23 Storage Disorders in Hematology

Reinhold Munker, MD

CONTENTS

1. GAUCHER DISEASE

1.1. Definition

Gaucher disease is characterized by the accumulation of glycosphingolipids (glycosylceramide) in lysosomes due to a defect in acid-β-glucosidase. The gene for acid-β-glucosidase is located on the long arm of chromosome 1. More than 200 mutations of the gene are known to date. Gaucher disease is inherited in an autosomal-recessive pattern. Three types of Gaucher disease have been described based on clinical characteristics. Type 1 is the most common variant and will be described in detail in this chapter. Type 1 Gaucher disease results in hepatosplenomegaly, cytopenias, and progressive bone disease and has a highly variable clinical course. Type 2 Gaucher disease is rare and leads to death early in life as a result of severe CNS disease. Type 3 Gaucher disease also is rare, has a variable course, and combines CNS disease with visceral manifestations. The incidence of Gaucher disease varies between 1:40,000 in Western countries and 1:2000 in Israel.

1.2. Etiology and Pathogenesis

Because of defective acid-β-glucosidase, lipid-laden macrophages accumulate in the reticuloendothelial system of various organs like liver, spleen, bone marrow, and the CNS and lead to an enlargement of these organs and/or functional disturbances.

From: *Contemporary Hematology: Modern Hematology, Second Edition*
Edited by: R. Munker, E. Hiller, J. Glass, and R. Paquette © Humana Press Inc., Totowa, NJ

1.3. Diagnosis

The diagnosis of Gaucher disease is established by measuring acid-β-glucosidase in leukocytes (0–15% of normal values is considered as pathological). A bone marrow biopsy (which is rarely necessary for the diagnosis of Gaucher disease) shows the presence of lipid-laden macrophages (Gaucher cells). The diagnosis should be supported by a molecular analysis of the *acid-β-glucosidase* gene. If the mutation is known, heterozygotes can be detected by PCR. Certain mutations have ethnic and clinical correlations. Data from the Gaucher registry show that the most common alleles are N370S (53%), L444P (18%), 84 GG (7%), and IVS2+1 (2%). Homozygotes for N370S often have a more benign clinical course than other genotypes and never develop CNS disease. Homozygotism for L444P is associated with early symptomatic disease and CNS manifestations (types 2 and 3). Biochemical markers for active Gaucher disease are increases in chitotriosidase (which can be used to monitor enzyme replacement), angiotensin-converting enzyme, tartrate-resistant acid phosphatase, lysozyme, and the chemokine CCL18. Typical radiological manifestations are Erlenmeyer flask deformity, osteolytic lesions, osteopenia, and avascular necrosis. Most patients with bone disease have multiple manifestations. The extent of marrow infiltration can best be quantitated by magnetic resonance imaging (MRI).

1.4. Clinical Manifestations

A common manifestation of type 1 Gaucher disease is hepatosplenomegaly and anemia, thrombocytopenia, and/or leukopenia. Thrombocytopenia may result in bleeding. The disease becomes symptomatic around 10 to 25 yr; however, in some cases the diagnosis is made earlier or much later in adulthood. Children with Gaucher disease have growth retardation. Adults with Gaucher disease are commonly fatigued. Bone disease manifests itself often later in life with bone pain or frank fractures including collapse of vertebrae. The degree of hepatosplenomegaly is variable. Liver failure develops rarely. Splenic infarcts may occur in massively enlarged spleens. All bones of the axial skeleton and extremities can be involved. Patients with bone disease often experience pain crises. Rarely, other organs are involved in Gaucher disease: skin, kidneys, and lungs. Patients with CNS manifestations may have a supranuclear gaze palsy, myoclonus, and often develop progressive dementia.

1.5. Treatment

The treatment of choice in symptomatic patients with type 1 Gaucher disease is enzyme replacement. Acid-β-glucosidase is available in two forms. Alglucerase (Ceredase®) is isolated from placenta. Imiglucerase (Cerezyme®) is recombinant mannose-terminated (macrophage-targeted) acid-β-glucosidase. The initial recommended dose is 60 IU/kg for children and for adults with severe bone disease or massive hepatosplenomegaly. Both forms are given by intravenous infusion over 2 h at 2-wk intervals and are generally well tolerated. In adults with less severe disease manifestations or in children after clinical improvement, a lower dose (20–40 IU/kg) may be given. This treatment has to be continued indefinitely as maintenance. Enzyme replacement is expensive, but effectively reduces hepatosplenomegaly, and improves cytopenias and bone or bone marrow involvement by Gaucher disease. Cytopenias and pain generally improve within a few months. It may take several years before radiological improvement can be seen. Supportive treatment (e.g., joint replacement) or treatment of severe cytopenias is necessary in patients with long-standing Gaucher disease. Splenectomy, for example for the treatment of hypersplenism, is rarely necessary since enzyme replacement became available and may actually worsen bone disease. In Gaucher disease, the proof of principle for an effective somatic gene transfer has been made, but has not found clinical application. For patients with less severe forms of Gaucher disease (type 1) who cannot tolerate enzyme replacement, recently miglustat (Zavesca®) has become available. Miglustat is taken orally, inhibits glucosyl ceramide synthase and thereby reduces the accumulation of glucocerebrosides. This "substrate reduction therapy" also leads to clinical improvement but the follow-up is shorter than for enzyme replacement. Common side effects of miglustat are diarrhea and weight loss.

2. HEREDITARY HEMOCHROMATOSIS

2.1. Definition

Hereditary hemochromatosis is a common genetic disease in Caucasians characterized by acquired iron overload, autosomal recessive inheritance, and (in the vast majority of cases) by the presence of two mutated copies of the *HFE* gene (type 1 hemochromatosis).

2.2. Etiology and Pathogenesis

In classic hereditary hemochromatosis, the *HFE* gene located on chromosome 6 is mutated. The most common mutation is an amino acid substitution at position 282 (C282Y). Homozygosity for this mutation is observed in up to 0.5% of persons of Scandinavian descent. Less common mutations are H63D and S65C. Most homozygotes for C282Y develop a progressive expansion of the plasma iron compartment, which is subsequent to increased intestinal iron absorption. This is explained by two models. In the crypt-programming model, the presence of mutated *HFE*, which is unable to interact with transferrin receptor-1, leads to iron-deficient crypt cells, which give rise to iron-deficient daughter cells. These cells are programmed to absorb iron continuously from the intestinal lumen, even if all iron stores are saturated. In the hepcidin model, macrophages and their interaction with enterocytes play a major role. In the normal state, high iron levels lead to a diminished production of hepcidin, thereby modulating the release of iron into the circulation. In hereditary hemochromatosis, a mutant *HFE* gene interacts with the signaling pathway for hepcidin and leads to uncontrolled release of iron from macrophages and enterocytes.

2.3. Diagnosis

The diagnosis of hereditary hemochromatosis today is often made at an asymptomatic or presymptomatic stage. Suggestive evidence is elevated ferritin and an elevated transferrin saturation (>45%). The diagnosis is established by the presence of an *HFE* mutation. A liver biopsy is no longer mandatory, but is helpful to rule out or confirm liver cirrhosis. The typical *HFE* mutations are not present in all patients with hereditary hemochromatosis. Especially, in persons of southern European origin, other mutations may be observed. In certain patients (negative for *HFE* mutations but having a typical presentation) a liver biopsy can be used to calculate the hepatic iron index (hepatic iron concentration divided by age). Values of 1.9 or higher are considered as pathognomonic for hereditary hemochromatosis. The extent of iron deposition in the liver can be estimated semiquantitatively by MRI.

2.4. Clinical Manifestations

Patients with hemochromatosis may be asymptomatic, but the classical manifestations are cutaneous hyperpigmentation, diabetes mellitus, and hepatomegaly. As a result of iron loss from menstruation and other factors, women develop symptomatic hemochromatosis less frequently and later than men. Patients with symptomatic disease often feel weak, lose weight, and are lethargic. Patients with hepatomegaly commonly have abnormal liver function tests and experience pain in the right upper quadrant. Liver cirrhosis develops in long-standing hemochromatosis and up to 30% of patients with liver cirrhosis develop hepatocellular carcinoma. Endocrine disturbances (due to iron deposition) are common in symptomatic patients: diabetes mellitus, hypogonadism (in men loss of libido, testicular atrophy, in women amenorrhea), hypothyroidism. Joint disease is common (arthralgias, arthritis, often beginning in metacarpophalangeal joints). Congestive heart failure is common, as well as ventricular and supraventricular atopias, as well as different degrees of heart block.

2.5. Treatment

The treatment of hereditary hemochromatosis consists of regular phlebotomies removing the excess iron stored in the body. Phlebotomies can prevent or ameliorate most complications of the disease, including endocrine dysfunction and liver function abnormalities. Advanced hypogonadism, arthralgias, and liver cirrhosis (including the risk of hepatocellular carcinoma) are not influenced by phlebotomies. Therefore, the diagnosis and the treatment of hereditary hemochromatosis should be made as early as possible. A common regimen of phlebotomy is to remove one unit of blood weekly until the serum ferritin drops to 50 ng/mL. The serum transferrin saturation should drop below 30%. Then, maintenance phlebotomy should be started to keep serum in the range of 50–100 ng/mL. This is generally accomplished by phlebotomizing once every 3–4 mo.

2.6. Other Forms of Hereditary Iron Overload

Rarely, other genetic diseases cause iron overload. In juvenile hereditary hemochromatosis (type 2 of hereditary hemochromatosis), severe disease manifestations occur at an early age. Juvenile hereditary hemochromatosis is caused by mutated hemojuvelin or hepcidin genes. In type 3 hereditary hemochromatosis, a mutated transferrin receptor 2 was found. Both type 2 and 3 hereditary hemochromatosis have autosomal recessive inheritance and have an excellent response to phlebotomy. Type 4 hereditary hemochromatosis has autosomal dominant inheritance and is caused by a mutation of ferroportin. In type 4 hemochromatosis, iron is mainly deposited in reticuloendothelial tissues of liver and spleen. The response to phlebotomy is only partial and patients often develop anemia during aggressive phlebotomy.

3. SECONDARY IRON OVERLOAD

Secondary hemochromatosis can arise in many hematological disorders when chronic blood transfusions are needed. These disorders may be acquired or congenital. Examples for hereditary disorders are the hemoglobinopathies, red cell enzyme deficiencies, membrane defects, and sideroblastic or dyserythropoietic anemias. Any hematological disorder, for example acute leukemias and myelodysplastic syndromes, necessitating frequent blood transfusions will result, over time, in iron overload. Diseases with ineffective erythropoiesis and a prolonged clinical course, for example sideroblastic anemias, are especially prone to develop iron overload. As a rule of thumb, one unit of red blood cells contains 200 to 250 mg of iron. Clinical symptoms of iron overload often develop after the transfusion of 50 units and, in most cases, after the transfusion of 100 units of red blood cell concentrates. For the diagnosis of secondary iron overload, a liver biopsy is rarely necessary. The hepatic iron content can be estimated by MRI. A simple measurement for the estimation of transfusion-related hemochromatosis is serum ferritin. Serum ferritin correlates more with reticuloendothelial iron than with hepatic iron storage, but was found useful for the diagnosis and follow-up of secondary iron overload. Because patients with secondary iron overload are almost always anemic, phlebotomy is rarely feasible for the treatment of secondary iron overload. Instead, iron chelation therapy should be instituted in all patients who need chronic blood transfusions or have developed iron overload as a result of ineffective erythropoiesis. The longest clinical experience is available for the iron chelator deferoxamine, which has to be administered by subcutaneous infusion. More recently, oral chelators (deferiprone and deferasirox [ICL 670]) were introduced.

- Deferoxamine (DFO) is hexadentate (one molecule binding one atom of iron). DFO prevents most symptoms of iron overload (liver disease, heart failure, endocrine disturbances). It is administered by subcutaneous infusion over 8–12 h, 5–7 d per week. The standard dose is 20–40 mg/kg in children and 2 g in adults. Early treatment is recommended, in children after 10–20 blood transfusions, and in adults when long-term transfusions are needed and organ complications can be foreseen. A serum ferritin level greater than 900 µg/L is sometimes used as indicator of iron overload. Vitamin C, 200 mg given orally with DFO, increases the urinary excretion of iron. Side effects are observed in 5–10% of patients on intensive chelation therapy (high-tone hearing loss, growth delay, cartilage damage, retinal changes). Continued monitoring is required.
- Deferiprone is bidentate, is rapidly absorbed and has a peak plasma level after 45–60 min. The standard oral dose 75 mg/kg fractionated in three doses per day. Arthropathy, agranulocytosis, gastrointestinal disturbances, and zinc deficiencies were described as side effects. At present, the indication for deferiprone is the intolerance of or the inability to receive deferoxamine. Several studies compared both chelators. DFO may be equivalent or superior to mobilize hepatic iron. Deferiprone may be superior to prevent cardiac hemosiderosis. More recently, combination studies of both drugs (2 d of DFO with 7 d of deferiprone) were published. If the positive effects of the combination treatment are confirmed, the side effects of either drug will be reduced and the compliance of patients with chelation will increase.
- Deferasirox (ICL 670 or tridentate) is also rapidly absorbed and is highly selective for iron. The therapeutic dose is 20 mg/kg given once daily orally.

SUGGESTED READING

Balicki D, Beutler E. Gene therapy of human disease. *Medicine* 2002;81:69–86.
Beutler E, Hoffbrand AV, Cook JD. Iron deficiency and overload. *Hematology (Am Soc Hematol Educ Program)* 2003:40–61.
Charrow J, Andersson HC, Kaplan P, et al. The Gaucher registry. *Arch Int Med* 2000;160:2835–2843.
Germain DP. Gaucher's disease: a paradigm for interventional genetics. *Clin Genet* 2004;65:77–86.

Limdi JK, Crampton JR. Hereditary haemochromatosis. *Q J Med* 2004;97:315–324.
Pietrangelo A. Hereditary hemochromatosis—a new look at an old disease. *N Engl J Med* 2004;350:2383–2397.

---

*Deferasirox was approved by the US Food and Drug Administration in November 2005 for chronic iron overload due to multiple blood transfusions in patients 2 yr of age or older. Deferasirox also received orphan drug designation. Common side effects are nausea or abdominal pain; less frequent or rare side effects are increases in liver enzymes, creatinine, hearing loss, visual disturbances, or rashes.

APPENDIX 1

Glossary of Cytostatic Drugs and Targeted Therapies

Michael Cockerham, PharmD
and Reinhold Munker, MD

A number of antimetabolites or cytostatic agents are employed in treating leukemias and lymphomas. These drugs act through different mechanisms and their correct use requires special knowledge and expertise. We have listed them as follows in alphabetical order. Brief descriptions of the various routes of administration, the mechanisms of action, and the common side effects are provided. Details about the dosage of the cytostatic drugs are given in the treatment protocols and product information.

Arsenic Trioxide (Trisonex)

ROUTE OF ADMINISTRATION: Intravenous injection

DRUG CLASS: Antineoplastic and antiangiogenic

MECHANISM OF ACTION: Causes morphological changes and DNA fragmentation characteristic of apoptosis in NB4 human promyelocytic leukemia cells in vitro. Arsenic trioxide also causes damage or degradation of the fusion protein PML-RARα

INDICATIONS: Induction of remission and consolidation in patients with acute promyelocytic leukemia (APL) who are refractory to, or have relapsed from, retinoid and anthracycline chemotherapy, and whose APL is characterized by the presence of the t(15;17) translocation or *PML/RAR a* gene expression.

From: *Contemporary Hematology: Modern Hematology, Second Edition*
Edited by: R. Munker, E. Hiller, J. Glass, and R. Paquette © Humana Press Inc., Totowa, NJ

SIDE EFFECTS: Leukocytosis (up to 50%), tachycardia (55%), nausea/vomiting/ diarrhea, abdominal pain (58%), fatigue, edema, hyperglycemia, dyspnea, cough, rash or itching, headaches, dizziness, QT prolongation

COMMENT: In clinical trials these side effects did not always require interruption of therapy, nor have they been observed to be permanent or irreversible. Electrocardiograph (EKG) monitoring recommended, electrolyte abnormalities should be corrected

---

Asparaginase (Elspar, Erwinar)

Route of administration: Intravenous injection

DRUG CLASS: Enzyme

MECHANISM OF ACTION: Depletes cells of L-asparagine

INDICATIONS: Acute lymphoblastic leukemia

SIDE EFFECTS: Hypersensitivity and anaphylactic reactions, fever, bronchospasm, reduced synthesis of coagulation factors, increase in liver enzymes, hyperglycemia, rarely pancreatitis, CNS toxicity (25–50%)

COMMENT: During treatment, a substitution of fresh frozen plasma or fibrinogen and antithrombin III may become necessary. Because of anaphylactic reactions, a test dose should be given first. In case of intolerance, an alternative preparation of asparaginase should be used (e.g., erwinia asparaginase).

Azacitidine (Vidaza)

ROUTE OF ADMINISTRATION: Subcutaneous injection

DRUG CLASS: Antimetabolite, pyrimidine nucleoside analog

MECHANISM OF ACTION: Hypomethylation of DNA and exerting direct cytotoxic in abnormal hematopoietic cells in the bone marrow

INDICATIONS: Myelodysplastic syndromes

SIDE EFFECTS: Thrombocytopenia, neutropenia, nausea/vomiting, anorexia, arthralgias, injection site erythema, injection site pain

---

Bleomycin (Blenoxane)

ROUTE OF ADMINISTRATION: Intravenous injection, in some cases also intracavitary, topical, intra-arterial

DRUG CLASS: Antibiotic

MECHANISM OF ACTION: Intercalates DNA, induces DNA breaks

INDICATIONS: Lymphomas, other malignant tumors

SIDE EFFECTS: Fever, myalgias, anorexia, skin pigmentation, rash, mucositis, alopecia, pneumonitis (may progress to lung fibrosis), occasionally hypersensitivity reactions, minor myelosuppression

COMMENT: Pulmonary toxicity may be severe in older patients, in patients with chronic lung disorders, or after thoracic irradiation. If higher dose therapy is planned, lung function should be controlled regularly.

Bortezomib (Velcade)

ROUTE OF ADMINISTRATION: Intravenous injection
DRUG CLASS: Proteasome inhibitor
MECHANISM OF ACTION: Reversibly inhibits chymotrypsin-like activity at the 26S proteasome leading to cell-cycle arrest and apoptosis.
INDICATIONS: Multiple myeloma patients who have received at least one prior therapy, some non-Hodgkin's lymphomas (NHLs)
SIDE EFFECTS: Asthenia, nausea/vomiting/diarrhea, appetite decreased, constipation, thrombocytopenia, peripheral neuropathy, pyrexia, anemia, headache, insomnia, edema

---

Busulfan (Myleran, Busulfex)

ROUTE OF ADMINISTRATION: Intravenous injection, oral
DRUG CLASS: Alkylating agent
MECHANISM OF ACTION: Alkylates DNA, RNA, induces DNA breaks
INDICATIONS: Chronic myelogenous leukemia (CML), transplantation
SIDE EFFECTS: Severe pancytopenia, skin hyperpigmentation, nausea/vomiting/ diarrhea

---

Carmustine (BCNU)

ROUTE OF ADMINISTRATION: Intravenous injection
DRUG CLASS: Nitrosurea alkylating agent
MECHANISM OF ACTION: Bifunctional alkylating agent, induces DNA breaks
INDICATIONS: Lymphomas, solid tumors
SIDE EFFECTS: Prolonged myelosuppression, cumulative lung toxicity, nausea, vomiting, in some cases hepatic and renal toxicity, in some cases neurotoxicity

---

Chlorambucil (Leukeran)

ROUTE OF ADMINISTRATION: Oral
DRUG CLASS: Alkylating agent
MECHANISM OF ACTION: Alkylates DNA, RNA, induces DNA breaks
INDICATIONS: Chronic lymphocytic leukemia (CLL), other low-grade lymphomas
SIDE EFFECTS: Leukopenia, minor gastrointestinal discomfort, rarely neurotoxicity, sterility at high doses, pulmonary toxicity

Cladribine (Leustatin, 2-CDA)

ROUTE OF ADMINISTRATION: Intravenous injection
DRUG CLASS: Antimetabolite
MECHANISM OF ACTION: Purine nucleoside analogue, DNA strand breaks
INDICATIONS: Hairy cell leukemia, CLL, CML, other low-grade lymphomas
SIDE EFFECTS: Fever (70%), leukopenia, anemia, fatigue, edema, rash

Clofarabine (Clolar)

ROUTE OF ADMINISTRATION: Intravenous injection
DRUG CLASS: Antimetabolite
MECHANISM OF ACTION: Purine nucleoside analog, interfering with DNA replication, disrupts the integrity of the mitochondrial membrane, releasing proapoptotic mitochondrial proteins, cytochrome C, and apoptosis-inducing factor, activating pathways of programmed cell death
INDICATIONS: Acute lymphoblastic leukemia (pediatric)
SIDE EFFECTS: Febrile neutropenia, Systemic Inflammatory Response Syndrome (SIRS), nausea/vomiting/diarrhea, pyrexia, rigors, abdominal pain, fatigue, tachycardia, anorexia

Cyclophosphamide (Cytoxan, CTX)

ROUTE OF ADMINISTRATION: Intravenous injection, oral
DRUG CLASS: Alkylating agent
MECHANISM OF ACTION: Alkylates DNA and RNA, induces DNA breaks
INDICATIONS: Lymphomas, leukemias, solid tumors, immunosuppression, conditioning for bone marrow transplantation
SIDE EFFECTS: Myelosuppression, thrombocytopenia, nausea, vomiting, mucositis, fever, hemorrhagic cystitis, tubular nephropathy
COMMENT: Hemorrhagic cystitis can be prevented if adequate hydration (>200 mL/h) and Mesna are given. Mesna should always be given when cyclophosphamide is administered at greater than 400 mg/($m^2 \cdot$ d). If renal function is compromised, the dosage of cyclophosphamide has to be adapted accordingly,

Cytosine-Arabinoside (Cytarabine, ARA-C)

ROUTE OF ADMINISTRATION: Intravenous, subcutaneous, intrathecal injection
DRUG CLASS: Antimetabolite, analogue of deoxycytidine
MECHANISM OF ACTION: Incorporates into DNA, inhibits DNA polymerases, S-phase-specific
INDICATIONS: Acute and chronic leukemias, malignant lymphomas

SIDE EFFECTS: Myelosuppression, gastrointestinal toxicity (nausea, vomiting, rarely pancreatitis), pulmonary toxicity at high doses, alopecia, keratoconjunctivitis, rash, neurotoxicity (at higher doses and in older patients' severe cerebellar syndrome, other neurologic disturbances)

COMMENTS: Also available as a liposomal preparation (DepoCyt) for lymphomatous meningitis.

Dacarbazine (DTIC-Dome, DTIC)

ROUTE OF ADMINISTRATION: Intravenous injection
DRUG CLASS: Alkylating agent
MECHANISM OF ACTION: Methylates DNA causing cross-linking
INDICATIONS: Lymphomas, other malignancies
SIDE EFFECTS: Severe nausea/vomiting, myelosuppression, alopecia, less frequent: hepatotoxicity, diarrhea, and thrombophlebitis

---

Daunorubicin (Cerubidine)

ROUTE OF ADMINISTRATION: Intravenous injection
DRUG CLASS: Anthracycline antibiotic
MECHANISM OF ACTION: Intercalates DNA, forms free oxygen radicals, inhibits topoisomerase II
INDICATIONS: Acute leukemias, lymphomas, solid tumors
SIDE EFFECTS: Myelosuppression, acute and chronic cardiotoxicity, mucositis, nausea, alopecia, severe tissue necrosis in case of extravasation
COMMENT: The cumulative cardiotoxicity (dilative cardiomyopathy) limits the total dose to 450–550 mg/m^2. Risk factors are mediastinal irradiation, previous cardiac disease. Do not administer if left ventricular ejection fraction is less than 40–45%.

Decitabine (Dacogen)

ROUTE OF ADMINISTRATION: Intravenous injection
DRUG CLASS: Antimetabolite
MECHANISM OF ACTION: Hypomethylating agent
INDICATIONS: Myelodysplastic syndromes
SIDE EFFECTS: nausea, vomiting, neutropenia, headaches
COMMENTS: Investigational

Denileukin Diftitox (Ontak)

ROUTE OF ADMINISTRATION: Intravenous injection

DRUG CLASS: Fusion protein

MECHANISM OF ACTION: Fusion protein of interleukin-2 and diphtheria toxin delivers diphtheria toxin to targeted cells inhibiting intracellular protein synthesis.

INDICATIONS: Lymphomas

SIDE EFFECTS: Infusion related hypersensitivity (69%), vascular leak syndrome, fever/chills (81%), asthenia, infection, nausea/vomiting, edema, hypotension, rash, hypoalbuminemia, increased transaminases, and lymphopenia.

COMMENTS: Side effects diminish after first two treatment courses.

Doxorubicin (Adriamycin)

ROUTE OF ADMINISTRATION: Intravenous injection

DRUG CLASS: Anthracycline antibiotic

MECHANISM OF ACTION: Intercalates DNA, forms free oxygen radicals, inhibits topoisomerase II

INDICATIONS: Lymphomas, solid tumors

SIDE EFFECTS: Myelosuppression, acute and chronic cardiotoxicity, mucositis, nausea, alopecia, severe tissue necrosis in case of extravasation

COMMENT: The cumulative cardiotoxicity (dilative cardiomyopathy) limits the total dose to 450–550 mg/m^2. Risk factors are mediastinal irradiation, previous cardiac disease. Do not administer if left ventricular ejection fraction is less than 40–45%.

Epirubicin (Ellence)

ROUTE OF ADMINISTRATION: Intravenous injection

DRUG CLASS: Anthracycline antibiotic

MECHANISM OF ACTION: Intercalates DNA, forms free oxygen radicals, inhibits topoisomerase II

INDICATIONS: Lymphomas, solid tumors

SIDE EFFECTS: Myelosuppression, acute and chronic cardiotoxicity, mucositis, nausea, alopecia, severe tissue necrosis in case of extravasation

COMMENT: Risk of cardiotoxicity increases sharply above 900 mg/m^2.

Etoposide (VePesid, VP-16)

ROUTE OF ADMINISTRATION: Intravenous injection, oral

DRUG CLASS: Mitotic inhibitor

MECHANISM OF ACTION: Complexes with topoisomerase II induces DNA breaks

INDICATIONS: Leukemias, lymphomas, solid tumors

SIDE EFFECTS: Bone marrow depression, especially neutropenia, alopecia, some nausea, some patients experience allergic or anaphylactic reactions, hypotension

Fludarabine (Fludara)

ROUTE OF ADMINISTRATION: Intravenous injection
DRUG CLASS: Antimetabolite (purine analogue)
MECHANISM OF ACTION: inhibits enzymes of DNA synthesis
INDICATIONS: B-cell CLL, lymphomas, leukemias
SIDE EFFECTS: Myelosuppression, some nausea, neurotoxicity (encephalopathy at high doses), protracted immunosuppression, fatigue, and somnolence.

Gemtuzumab ozogamicin (Mylotarg)

ROUTE OF ADMINISTRATION: Intravenous injection
DRUG CLASS: Monoclonal antibody
MECHANISM OF ACTION: Binding to CD33 antigen results in the formation of a complex that is internalized, the calicheamicin derivative is released inside the lysosomes of the myeloid cell, calicheamicin derivative binds to DNA resulting in DNA double strand breaks and cell death.
INDICATIONS: Treatment of CD33-positive AML in first relapse in patients 60 yr of age or older
SIDE EFFECTS: Peripheral edema, chills, fever, nausea/vomiting, headache, rash, hypotension, hypertension, hypoxia, dyspnea, hyperglycemia

Hydroxyurea (Hydrea, Droxia)

ROUTE OF ADMINISTRATION: Oral
DRUG CLASS: Antimetabolite
MECHANISM OF ACTION: Inhibits ribonucleotide reductase
INDICATIONS: CML, other myeloproliferative syndromes, sickle cell anemia
SIDE EFFECTS: Short-acting myelosuppression; some gastrointestinal toxicity; rarely pigmentation; renal, hepatic, and neurologic side effects (dose adjustment in renal failure necessary)

Idarubicin (Idamycin)

ROUTE OF ADMINISTRATION: Intravenous injection
DRUG CLASS: Anthracycline antibiotic
MECHANISM OF ACTION: Intercalates DNA, forms free oxygen radicals, inhibits topoisomerase II
INDICATIONS: Acute leukemias, lymphomas
SIDE EFFECTS: Myelosuppression, acute and chronic cardiotoxicity, mucositis, nausea, alopecia, severe tissue necrosis in case of extravasation

Ifosfamide (Ifex)

ROUTE OF ADMINISTRATION: Intravenous injection
DRUG CLASS: Alkylating agent (derivative of cyclophosphamide with a particular toxicity profile)
MECHANISM OF ACTION: Alkylates DNA and RNA, induces DNA breaks
INDICATIONS: Lymphomas, other malignancies
SIDE EFFECTS: Myelosuppression, nausea/vomiting/diarrhea, mucositis, hemorrhagic cystitis, alopecia, acute CNS toxicity (encephalopathy, cerebellar syndrome, ataxia, seizures; especially in older patients and higher dosage)
COMMENT: Hemorrhagic cystitis can be prevented if adequate hydration (>200 mL/h) and Mesna are given. If renal function is compromised, the dosage of ifosfamide has to be adapted accordingly. The infusion of Na bicarbonate is recommended for the prophylaxis of CNS toxicity.

Imatinib (Gleevec)

ROUTE OF ADMINISTRATION: Oral
DRUG CLASS: Tyrosine kinase inhibitor
MECHANISM OF ACTION: Inhibition of BCR-ABL tyrosine kinase induces apoptosis
INDICATIONS: CML, gastrointestinal stromal tumors (GIST)
SIDE EFFECTS: Nausea/vomiting/diarrhea, fluid retention, muscle cramps, hemorrhage, musculoskeletal pain, skin rash, headache, fatigue.

Ibritumomab tiuxetan (Zevalin)

ROUTE OF ADMINISTRATION: Intravenous injection
DRUG CLASS: Monoclonal antibody/radioisotope
MECHANISM OF ACTION: Antibody linked to the radioactive isotope yttrium-90, monoclonal antibody targets the CD20 antigen, and cytotoxic radiation is delivered directly to malignant cells.
INDICATIONS: Relapsed or refractory low-grade, follicular, or transformed B-cell NHL
SIDE EFFECTS: Nausea/vomiting/diarrhea, anorexia, thrombocytopenia, neutropenia, anemia, arthralgias, dizziness, dyspnea, increased cough

Lenalidomide (Revlimid)

ROUTE OF ADMINISTRATION: Oral
DRUG CLASS: Immunomodulatory agent
MECHANISM OF ACTION: Inhibits secretion of pro-inflammatory cytokines, inhibits expression of Cox-2

INDICATIONS: Myelodysplastic syndromes (MDS) with 5q deletion
SIDE EFFECTS: Neutropenia, thrombocytopenia, pruritus, nausea, diarrhea, fatigue
COMMENT: Due to teratogenic risk, patient must be registered in distribution monitoring program

---

Lomustine (CeeNU, CCNU)

ROUTE OF ADMINISTRATION: Oral
DRUG CLASS: Alkylating agent (nitrosurea derivative)
MECHANISM OF ACTION: Alkylates DNA and RNA
INDICATIONS: Hodgkin's lymphoma, solid tumors
SIDE EFFECTS: Nausea, stomatitis, alopecia, delayed myelotoxicity, less frequent renal and hepatic toxicity

---

Mechlorethamine (Mustargen, Nitrogen Mustard)

ROUTE OF ADMINISTRATION: Intravenous injection
DRUG CLASS: Alkylating agent (nitrogen mustard)
MECHANISM OF ACTION: Bifunctional alkylating agent, induces DNA breaks
INDICATIONS: Lymphomas, solid tumors
SIDE EFFECTS: Alopecia, nausea/vomiting, myelosuppression, vesicant

---

Melphalan (Alkeran)

ROUTE OF ADMINISTRATION: Intravenous, oral
DRUG CLASS: Alkylating agent
MECHANISM OF ACTION: Crosslinks DNA
INDICATIONS: Multiple myeloma, solid tumors
SIDE EFFECTS: Nausea, protracted myelosuppression, rarely skin rash, pulmonary toxicity, alopecia

---

6-Mercaptopurine (Purinethol, 6-MP)

ROUTE OF ADMINISTRATION: Oral
DRUG CLASS: Antimetabolite
MECHANISM OF ACTION: Inhibits purine synthesis
INDICATIONS: Acute leukemias, NHL
SIDE EFFECTS: Nausea, myelosuppression, liver toxicity (cholestasis), fever, skin rash
COMMENT: If concomitant allopurinol is given, the dose has to be reduced by 65–75%.

Methotrexate (Folex, Abitrexate, MTX)

ROUTE OF ADMINISTRATION: Intravenous injection, oral, intrathecal
DRUG CLASS: Antimetabolite
MECHANISM OF ACTION: Inhibits dihydrofolate reductase, inhibiting purine synthesis
INDICATIONS: Leukemias, lymphomas, other malignancies
SIDE EFFECTS: Myelosuppression, severe mucositis (dose dependent), nausea, diarrhea, hepatic, renal and pulmonary toxicity, skin rash, acute encephalopathy, arachnoiditis with intrathecal administration,
COMMENT: At high doses of methotrexate, measurement of plasma levels and "rescue" with folinic acid (leucovorin) are important.

Mitoxantrone (Novantrone)

ROUTE OF ADMINISTRATION: Intravenous injection
DRUG CLASS: Anthracycline antibiotic (Anthracenedione)
MECHANISM OF ACTION: Intercalates DNA, forms free oxygen radicals, inhibits topoisomerase II
INDICATIONS: Acute leukemia, NHL
SIDE EFFECTS: Myelosuppression, acute and chronic cardiotoxicity, mucositis, nausea, alopecia, severe tissue necrosis in case of extravasation, discoloration of urine
COMMENTS: Cumulative dose greater than 160 mg/m^2 may cause congestive heart failure.

Nelarabine (Arranon)

ROUTE OF ADMINISTRATION: Intravenous injection
DRUG CLASS: Antimetabolite, deoxyguanosine analog
MECHANISM OF ACTION: Disrupts DNA synthesis, induces apoptosis
INDICATION: Relapsed or refractory T-cell acute lymphoblastic leukemia and lymphoma
SIDE EFFECTS: Pancytopenia, anemia, hepatic enzyme elevations, nausea, vomiting, electrolyte disturbance, infection, cough, fatigue, dyspnea, headache, somnolence, neuropathy, leukencephalopathy

Pentostatin (Nipent, Desoxycoformine)

ROUTE OF ADMINISTRATION: Intravenous injection
DRUG CLASS: Antimetabolite
MECHANISM OF ACTION: Purine analogue, inhibits adenosine deaminase

INDICATIONS: Hairy cell leukemia, other low-grade NHLs

SIDE EFFECTS: Myelosuppression, infection, nausea, hepatic and renal toxicity, rash

---

Procarbazine (Matulane)

ROUTE OF ADMINISTRATION: Oral

DRUG CLASS: Alkylating agent

MECHANISM OF ACTION: Alkylates DNA, methylates nucleic acids

INDICATIONS: Lymphomas, multiple myeloma

SIDE EFFECTS: Myelosuppression, nausea, vomiting, skin toxicity, secondary malignancies, CNS depression (synergistic with other depressants)

Rituximab (Rituxan)

ROUTE OF ADMINISTRATION: Intravenous injection

DRUG CLASS: Monoclonal antibody

MECHANISM OF ACTION: Antibody directed against CD20 antigen, which arrests cell cycle initiation, compliment dependent cytotoxicity.

INDICATIONS: Refractory B-cell lymphoma, in combination for other CD20-positive NHLs

SIDE EFFECTS: Headache, chills, rigors, nausea, hypotension, rash

---

Teniposide (Vumon)

ROUTE OF ADMINISTRATION: Intravenous injection

DRUG CLASS: Mitotic inhibitor

MECHANISM OF ACTION: Topoisomerase II inhibitor, DNA strand breaks

INDICATIONS: Acute lymphoblastic leukemia, lymphoma

SIDE EFFECTS: Mucositis, nausea/vomiting/diarrhea, myelosuppression

---

Thalidomide (Thalomid)

ROUTE OF ADMINISTRATION: Oral

DRUG CLASS: Immunomodulatory agent

MECHANISM OF ACTION: Suppress excess tumor necrosis factor-α and vascular endothelial growth factor-inhibiting angiogenesis.

INDICATIONS: Multiple myeloma, myelodysplastic syndrome

SIDE EFFECTS: Somnolence, rash, headache, neutropenia

COMMENT: Because of teratogenic risk, patient must be registered in distribution monitoring program.

Thioguanine (6-Thioguanine, 6-TG)

ROUTE OF ADMINISTRATION: Oral
DRUG CLASS: Antimetabolite
MECHANISM OF ACTION: Inhibits purine synthesis, incorporated into DNA
INDICATIONS: AML
SIDE EFFECTS: Myelosuppression, some nausea, diarrhea, cholestasis

Thiotepa (Thioplex)

ROUTE OF ADMINISTRATION: Intravenous and intrathecal injection
DRUG CLASS: Alkylating agent
MECHANISM OF ACTION: Polyfunctional agent, DNA crosslinking
INDICATIONS: Lymphomas, CNS leukemias (intrathecal), solid tumors
SIDE EFFECTS: Myelosuppression, pain at injection site

Tositumomab (Bexxar)

ROUTE OF ADMINISTRATION: Intravenous injection
DRUG CLASS: Monoclonal antibody/radioisotope
MECHANISM OF ACTION: Antibody linked to the radioactive isotope iodine 131, monoclonal antibody targets the CD20 antigen, and cytotoxic radiation is delivered directly to malignant cells.
INDICATIONS: CD20-positive, follicular NHL, with and without transformation, whose disease is refractory to rituximab and has relapsed following chemotherapy
SIDE EFFECTS: Infection, myelosuppression, allergic reaction, anaphylactoid reaction, gastrointestinal symptoms, fever, nausea, sweating, hypotension, asthenia

Tretinoin (Vesanoid, all-trans retinoic acid, ATRA)

ROUTE OF ADMINISTRATION: Oral
DRUG CLASS: Vitamin A derivative
MECHANISM OF ACTION: Inhibits clonal proliferation and/or granulocyte differentiation
INDICATIONS: APL
SIDE EFFECTS: Arrhythmia, hypotension, peripheral edema, headache, fever, rash, nausea/vomiting, abdominal pain, retinoic acid syndrome, myelosuppression, diaphoresis

Vinblastine (Velban, Velsar)

ROUTE OF ADMINISTRATION: Intravenous injection
DRUG CLASS: Vinca alkaloids
MECHANISM OF ACTION: Inhibit function of microtubules, inhibit DNA-dependent RNA polymerases
INDICATIONS: Lymphomas, leukemias, other malignancies
SIDE EFFECTS: Nausea/vomiting, myelosuppression, diarrhea, constipation, stomatitis, mouth ulcers, neurotoxicity (cumulative, dose limiting: peripheral neuropathy, paresthesias, autonomous neuropathy, rarely ataxia, seizures)
COMMENTS: Vinblastine less likely to produce severe neurotoxicity compared to other
vinca alkaloids

Vincristine (Oncovin, Vincasar)

ROUTE OF ADMINISTRATION: Intravenous injection
DRUG CLASS: Vinca alkaloids
MECHANISM OF ACTION: Inhibit function of microtubules, inhibit DNA-dependent RNA polymerases
INDICATIONS: Lymphomas, leukemias, other malignancies
SIDE EFFECTS: Mild nausea/vomiting, pulmonary toxicity, diarrhea, constipation, stomatitis, mouth ulcers, major neurotoxicity (cumulative, dose limiting: peripheral neuropathy, paresthesias, autonomous neuropathy, rarely ataxia, seizures), alopecia, syndrome of inappropriate antidiuretic hormone secretion
COMMENTS: Myelosuppression minor with vincristine

APPENDIX 2

CD Nomenclature
for Human Leukocyte Antigens

Reinhold Munker, MD

Designation	Cellular distribution	Function, comments
CD1	Cortical thymocytes, dendritic cells	Role in antigen presentation (four subtypes)
CD2	Pan T-cell, NK cells	Receptor for sheep red blood cells, interaction with CD48 and CD58
CD3	Pan T-cell	Signal transduction from T-cell receptor
CD4	T-helper subset	Binds to class II MHC antigen
CD5	Pan T-, B-cell subset	Marker for B-CLL
CD6	T-cell subset	Binds to CD166
CD7	Early T-cell marker	Expressed on T-ALL
CD8	T suppressor cells	Co-receptor in antigen recognition
CD9	Broad (platelets, lymphoid progenitors, activated active lymphocytes)	Belongs to tetraspanin family of proteins
CD10	Immature, some mature B-cells	CALLA-antigen, expressed in pre-B-ALL, some lymphomas, kidney, intestine, brain
CD11a	Leukocytes	Adhesion
CD11b	Granulocytes, monocytes, NK cells	Adhesion
CD11c	Granulocytes, monocytes, macrophages, NK cells	Adhesion
CD12	Monocytes, granulocytes	

(continued)

From: *Contemporary Hematology: Modern Hematology, Second Edition*
Edited by: R. Munker, E. Hiller, J. Glass, and R. Paquette © Humana Press Inc., Totowa, NJ

CD Nomenclature for HLA *(continued)*

Designation	Cellular distribution	Function, comments
CD13	Monocytes, granulocytes	Membrane metalloprotease
CD14	Monocytes	Receptor for lipopolysaccharide
CD15	Granulocytes, monocytes	Lewis x antigen
CD16	NK cells, granulocytes, mast cells	Fc gamma receptor type III
CD17	Granulocytes, monocytes, platelets	Lactosylceramide
CD18	Leukocytes	Integrin β2 subunit (adhesion)
CD19	B-cells	Regulates B-cell antigen receptor signal transduction
CD20	B-cells	
CD21	Mature B-cells	Receptor for EBV, complement type 2, C3d
CD22	B-cells	
CD23	Activated B-cells, macrophages, follicular dendritic cells	Regulates IgE synthesis
CD24	B-cells, granulocytes, some tumors	Mucin-like adhesion molecule
CD25	Activated T-cells, B-cells, macrophages	Receptor for interleukin-2 (α-chain)
CD26	Thymocytes, activated T-cells, tumors, other cells	Membrane-bound protease
CD27	T-cells, other cells	Member of TNF receptor superfamily
CD28	T-cells, plasma cells	T-cell, B-cell interactions
CD29	Most cells	Adhesion (integrin β1 subunit)
CD30	Activated T- and B-cells	Member of TNF receptor superfamily (present on anaplastic large lymphomas, Reed-Sternberg cells)
CD31	Monocytes, platelets, granulocyte, lymphocyte subset, endothelial cells	PECAM-1, mediates adhesion
CD32	Monocytes, platelets, other cells	Fc γRII (Fc receptor for aggregated IgG)
CD33	Monocytes, immature myeloid cells	Member of sialoadhesin family
CD34	Hematopoietic progenitors, endothelial cells	
CD35	Red cells, B-cells, subset of T-cells, granulocytes, other cells	Complement receptor type I (binds C3b, C4b)

CD36	Platelets, monocytes, other cells	Multifunctional glycoprotein
CD37	Mature B-cells, some other cells	
CD38	Immature B- and T-cells, plasma cells, some other cells	Multifunctional
CD39	Activated B-cells, some other cells	
CD40	Mature B-cells	Member of TNF receptor superfamily, interacts with CD 154
CD41	Platelets, megakaryocytes	Integrin αIIb subunit, interacts with glycoprotein IIIa. Defect in Glanzmann thrombasthenia
CD42a,b	Platelets, megakaryocytes	Platelet adhesion, binds to VWF, defect in Bernard-Soulier syndrome
CD43	Leukocytes, mast cells	Leukosialin
CD44	Widely expressed on hematopoietic and nonhematopoietic cells	Several isoforms, adhesion of leukocytes to endothelial cells, stroma, and extracellular matrix
CD45	Leukocytes	Leukocyte common antigen, several epitopes with differential expression
CD46	Leukocytes, endothelial, epithelial cells	Regulates complement activation
CD47	Broad tissue expression	Integrin-associated protein, absent on Rh_{null} erythrocytes
CD48	Hematopoietic cells	
CD49a	Monocytes, activated T-cells	Subunit of α1-integrin (VLA-1α)
CD49b	Monocytes, platelets, T- and B-cells	Subunit of integrin-α2
CD49c	Cultured adherent cell lines	Subunit of integrin-α3
CD49d	Most leukocytes	Subunit of integrin-α4
CD49e	T cells, monocytes, platelets, activated B-cells	Subunit of integrin-α5
CD49f	T-cells, monocytes, nonlymphoid tissues	Subunit of integrin-α6
CD50	Leukocytes	ICAM-3, mediates adhesion
CD51	Platelets, endothelial and other cells	Alpha subunit of vitronectin receptor
CD52	Lymphocytes, monocytes	
CD53	Leukocytes and other cells	
CD54	Hematopoietic and nonhematopoietic cells	ICAM-1, mediates adhesion, T-cell activation
CD55	Broad expression	Decay-accelerating factor
CD56	NK cells, T-cell subpopulation, neural tissue	Isoform of NCAM, cell–cell interactions
CD57	Subset of NK cells and T-cells	
CD58	Most hematopoietic cells, other cells	LFA-3 adhesion ligand for CD2

(continued)

CD Nomenclature for HLA *(continued)*

Designation	Cellular distribution	Function, comments
CD59	Many cells	Complement protectin (via GPI anchor)
CD60	T-cell subset, platelets	
CD61	Platelets, monocytes, megakaryocytes, endothelial cells	Integrin β subunit (combines with CD41 and with CD51)
CD62E	Endothelial cells	E-selectin (adhesion of leukocytes)
CD62L	Most hematopoietic cells	L-selectin (homing of lymphocytes)
CD62P	Megakaryocytes, activated endothelial cells and platelets	P-selectin (adhesion)
CD63	Widely distributed	
CD64	Monocytes, macrophages	High-affinity Fc γ-receptor
CD65	Granulocytes	
CD66	Granulocytes	Cell adhesion (belongs to CEA family
CD68	Monocytes, macrophages, other cells	Belongs to family of lysosomal-associated membrane proteins
CD69	Activated T-cells, B-cells. NK cells	Signal transduction
CD70	Activated B-cells, some activated T-cells	Member of TNF receptor superfamily co-stimulation of T-cell proliferation
CD71	Proliferating cells	Transferrin receptor
CD72	B-cells	B-cell co-receptor
CD73	Subsets of mature lymphocytes	Ecto-5'-nucleotidase
CD74	B-cells, monocytes	MHC class II-associated invariant chain
Cdw75	Mature B-cells	
CD76	Mature peripheral B-cells, mantle zone B-cells, activated cells	
CD77	Subset of germinal center B-cells	Marker for Burkitt's lymphomas
CD79 *(a,b)*	B-lymphocytes, B-cell neoplasms	B-cell antigen receptor complex
CD80	Activated T-cells, B-cells, monocytes	Co-stimulatory signal for T-cells (B7-1)
CD81 (TAPA1)	Broad expression	Receptor for hepatitis C virus envelope E2 glycoprotein
CD82	Broad expression	Suppresses metastasis in tumor cells (KAI-1)
CD83	Dendritic cells	
Cdw84	Macrophages and platelets	
CD85	Plasma cells, monocytes, other cells	
CD86	Monocytes, dendritic cells, activated cells	Co-stimulatory signal for T-cells (B7-2)

CD87	Monocytes, granulocytes, large granular lymphocytes	Receptor for urokinase plasminogen activator
CD88	Myeloid and other cells	Receptor for C5a (G protein-coupled receptor)
CD89	Most phagocytic cells, other cells	Receptor for IgA
CD90	Prothymocytes, brain	Thy-1
CD91	Phagocytes of liver, lung, lymphoid tissues	Binds protease-inhibitor complexes
CDw92	Myeloid cells	
CD93	Granulocytes, monocytes, endothelial cells	
CD94	NK cells, subset of T-cells	Receptor for HLA-E
CD95	Activated lymphocytes, monocytes, fibroblasts, cell lines	Member of TNF receptor superfamily (induces apoptosis)
CD96	Activated T-cells, NK cells, T-cell lines	NK cell recognition
CD97	Granulocytes, monocytes, activated T- and B-cells	
CD98	Monocytes, some other cells	
CD99	Pan leukocyte	
CD100	B-cells, T-cells, NK cells, most myeloid cells, neurons	Class 4 semaphorin
CD101	Monocytes, granulocytes, mucosal T-cells	
CD102	Most leukocytes, vascular endothelium	ICAM-2, major LFA-1 ligand on endothelial cells
CD103	Intraepithelial lymphocytes	Integrin αE subunit
CD104	Desmosomes of epithelia	Integrin $\beta 4$ subunit
CD105	Endothelial cells	Endoglin (receptor for TGFβ)
CD106	Vascular endothelium, dendritic cells, some other cells	VCAM-1
CD107	Granulocytes, T-cells, other cells	Lysosome-associated membrane protein
CDw108	Some lymphoid and other cells	
CD109	Platelets, activated T-cells, umbilical vein endothelial cells	Gov$^{a/b}$ alloantigen
CD116	Myeloid cells	Receptor for granulocyte/macrophage colony-stimulating factor
CD117	Hematopoietic progenitors, mast cells, some AMLs, some solid tumors	c-kit
CD120a,b	Low-level expression on many cells	TNF receptors (type I and II)
CD133	Early hematopoietic cells, endothelial cells	

(continued)

CD Nomenclature for HLA *(continued)*

Designation	Cellular distribution	Function, comments
CD134	Activated T-cells	Member of TNF receptor family, co-stimulates T-cell proliferation
CD135	Hematopoietic stem cells	FLT-3, receptor for FLT-3/flk-2 ligan
Cdw137	Activated T-, B-cells, monocytes	Co-stimulation of T-cell growth
CD138	Immature B-cells, plasma cells	Syndecan- I
CD147	Activated cells, tumor cells	Extracellular matrix metalloproteinas inducer
CD148	Broad expression	Transmembrane tyrosine phosphatas
Cdw150	Immature thymocytes, some B-cells	Signaling lymphocyte activation molecule, receptor for measles virus
CD151	Platelets, megakaryocytes, monocytes, keratinocytes	Member of tetraspanin family
CD152	Activated T-lymphocytes	Binds CD80, CD86
CD153	Activated T-cells	CD30 ligand
CD 154	Activated T-cells	CD40 ligand
CD155	Various types of cells	Receptor for polio virus
CD157	Neutrophils	GPI-anchored protein
CD158	NK cells	Killer cell Ig-like receptor
CD160	NK cells	Receptor for HLA-C
CD161	Natural killer cells, some T-cells	
CD162	Granulocytes, monocytes, most lymphocytes	Ligand for selectins
CD163	Monocytes, macrophages	Hemoglobin scavenger
CD164	Early hematopoietic progenitors	Sialomucin
CD166	Broad expression	Activated leukocyte cell adhesion molecule
CD170	Myeloid cells	Siglec-5
CD171	Neurons, certain tumors	L1 adhesion molecule
CD172	Monocytes, dendritic cells	Signal regulatory phosphatase
CD177	Neutrophils	Polymorphic
CD178	Various cell types	Ligand for CD95
CD180	B-cells	Belongs to toll-like receptor family
CD184	Various cell types	Chemokine receptor CXCR-4
CD200	Broad distribution	OX2 (interacts with CD200R on myeloid cells)
CD204	Macrophages	Class A scavenger receptor
CD206	Macrophages, dendritic cells	Mannose receptor
CD208	Activated dendritic cells	Member of LAMP family
CD209	Dendritic cells	DC-SIGN

CD222	Many cells	Multifunctional receptor
CD226	Hematopoietic cells, epithelial cells, tumors	MUC1
CD229	B- and T-lymphocytes	Ly9 (cell surface receptor)
CD244	NK cells, monocytes, basophils, some T-cells	2B4 (NK receptor)

The list is not complete, and additional surface markers do not yet have a CD designation.

REFERENCES

Barclay A.N., Brown M.H. Alex Law S.K. et al., *The Leucocyte Antigen Facts Book*, 2nd ed. San Diego: Academic, 1997.

Zola H, Swart B, Nicholson I, et al. CD molecules 2005:human cell differentiation molecules. *Blood* 2005;106:3123–3126.

APPENDIX 3

Laboratory Values

Parameter	Normal range
Hemoglobin	Males: 13.5–17.5 g/dL
	Females: 11.5–15.5 g/dL
Red cell number	Males: $4.5–6.5 \times 10^9$/L
	Females: $3.9–5.6 \times 10^9$/L
Hematocrit	Males: 40–52%
	Females: 36–48%
MCV	80–95 fL
MCHC	30–35 g/dL
Reticulocytes	0.5–2.5% or $50–100,000 \times 10^9$/L
Leukocytes (white cells)	4000–10,500/μL
Neutrophils	2500–7500/μL
Lymphocytes	1500–4000/μL
Monocytes	200–800/μL
Eosinophils	40–500/μL
Basophils	0–100/μL
Platelets	150,000–440,000/μL
LDH (lactate dehydrogenase)	100–240 IU/L
Haptoglobin	0.3–2 g/L
Serum alkaline phosphatase	30–120 U/L
Serum bilirubin (total)	<10 mg/L or 17 μmol/L
Serum bilirubin (indirect)	<7 mg/L or 7 μmol/L
Serum transferrin receptors	4–9 μg/L
Serum iron	Males: 80–150 μg/dL or 14–27 μmol/L
	Females: 60–140 μg/dL or 11–25 μmol/L
Serum ferritin	Males: 40–350 μg/L
	Females: 20–250 μg/L

(continued)

From: *Contemporary Hematology: Modern Hematology, Second Edition*
Edited by: R. Munker, E. Hiller, J. Glass, and R. Paquette © Humana Press Inc., Totowa, NJ

Laboratory Values *(continued)*

Parameter	*Normal range*
Serum vitamin B_{12}	160–900 ng/L
Serum folate	3.1–15 µg/L
C-reactive protein	0.08–3.1 mg/L
Serum β_2-microglobulin	1.2–2.8 mg/L
Total protein	60–80 g/L
IgG (adults)	6–16.0 g/L
IgA (adults)	0.8–4.0 g/L
IgM (adults)	0.5–3.3 g/L
IgD (adults)	<0.14 g/L
Serum viscosity	1.4–1.8 relative units
IgE	20–150 U/mL
Fibrinogen	2–4 g/L
Activated PTT	22.1–35.1 s
Prothrombin time	11.1–13.1 s
Thrombin time	± 3 s of control
D-dimer	<0.5 mg/L

All laboratory values depend on the methods used and may vary in different age and ethnic groups. The values in the table can only he considered as an approximate range.

APPENDIX 4

Program Requirements for Residency Education in Hematology

Reinhold Munker, MD

RECOMMENDATIONS OF THE ACCREDITATION COUNCIL FOR GRADUATE MEDICAL EDUCATION (ACGME)

The ACGME has published the requirements for graduate specialty training in the United States in hematology/oncology (duration 3 yr) and hematology (duration 2 yr). Details are available at www.acgme.org.

In these guidelines (version of July 2005) specific program contents, and requirements for faculty, facilities, resources, and procedures are described.

The Hematology and Oncology and the Hematology Curriculum list a variety of topics (specific program content).

The subspecialty examination in Hematology is administered by the American Board of Internal Medicine (ABIM). Details are available at www.abim.org.

The minimum training required for the examination is 24 mo in an accredited program, 12 of which have to be clinical training. The special procedures required are:

Participation for a minimum one-half day per week in a continuity outpatient clinic; bone marrow aspiration and biopsy, including preparation, staining, examination, and interpretation of blood smears, bone marrow aspirates, and touch preparations of bone marrow biopsies; measurement of complete blood count, including platelets and white cell differential, using automated or manual techniques with appropriate quality control; administration of chemotherapeutic agents and biological products through all therapeutic routes; and management and care of indwelling venous access catheters.

From: *Contemporary Hematology: Modern Hematology, Second Edition*
Edited by: R. Munker, E. Hiller, J. Glass, and R. Paquette © Humana Press Inc., Totowa, NJ

RECOMMENDATIONS FOR TRAINING BY ASH AND ASCO

The American Society of Hematology (ASH) has developed a "Hematology Curriculum". Details can be found at www.hematology.org/training. This curriculum gives a detailed description of the knowledge and skills expected from a trainee in hematology. The "Hematology Curriculum" is accompanied by a reading list with 54 chapters.

The American Society of Oncology (ASCO) has developed a subspecialty curriculum in Medical Oncology, which includes all hematologic malignancies. An updated version of the ASCO Core Curriculum was published in JCO in March 2005 and can be accessed at www.asco.org.

APPENDIX 5

Databases in Hematology

Reinhold Munker, MD *and Vishwas Sakhalkar,* MD

The expansion of knowledge in the area of blood diseases and in the basic sciences related to hematology makes the use of databases mandatory. In this section, we list and review English-language data bases (both electronic and print media). This list is far from complete, but an effort was made to include the most important and readily available databases. The databases, books, and journals are shown in alphabetical order. Textbooks of Internal Medicine and Oncology also include sections on hematologic disorders, but are excluded from this collection of databases. Also excluded are databases devoted to pure basic research.

I. TEXTBOOKS OF HEMATOLOGY AND RELATED DISCIPLINES

A. MAJOR TEXTBOOKS (>1000 PAGES)

BLOOD: Principles and Practice of Hematology, 2nd Edition, 2304 pp.
Ed.: Handin RI, Lux SE, Stossel TP.
Publ.: Lippincott Williams & Wilkins, 2003
Comment: Multi-author textbook on hematology

CLINICAL BONE MARROW AND BLOOD STEM CELL TRANSPLANTA-TION, 3rd Edition, 1968 pp.
Ed.: Atkinson K, Champlin R, Ritz J, et al.
Publ.: Cambridge University Press, 2004
Comment: Standard textbook of clinical bone marrow and stem cell transplantation

From: *Contemporary Hematology: Modern Hematology, Second Edition*
Edited by: R. Munker, E. Hiller, J. Glass, and R. Paquette © Humana Press Inc., Totowa, NJ

HEMATOLOGY BASIC PRINCIPLES AND PRACTICE, 4th Edition, 282 pp.
Ed.: Hoffman R, Benz EJ, Shattil SJ, et al.
Publ.: Elsevier Churchill Livingstone, 2005
Comment: Standard textbook of modern hematology including basic and clinical sciences, available as electronic version

HEMATOLOGY OF INFANCY AND CHILDHOOD, 6th Edition, 2060 pp.
Ed.: Nathan DG, Orkin SH, Look AT, et al.
Publ.: WB Saunders, 2003
Comment: Standard textbook of pediatric hematology

HEMOSTASIS AND THROMBOSIS: BASIC PRINCIPLES AND CLINICAL PRACTICE, 4th Edition, 1600 pp.
Ed.: Colman RW, Hirsh J, Marder VJ, et al.
Publ.: Lippincott Williams & Wilkins, 2001
Comment: Standard textbook of thrombosis and hemostasis

POSTGRADUATE HAEMATOLOGY, 5th Edition, 1080 pp.
Ed.: Hoffbrand AV, Tuddenham T, Catovsky D.
Publ.: Blackwell, 2005
Comment: Compendium for fellowship education and practicing physicians, recently updated

THOMAS' HEMATOPOIETIC CELL TRANSPLANTATION, 3rd Edition, 1563 pp.
Ed. Blume KG, Forman SJ, Appelbaum FR.
Publ. Blackwell, 2004
Comment: Standard textbook of bone marrow and stem cell transplantation

WILLIAMS HEMATOLOGY, 6th Edition, 1941 pp.
Ed.: Beutler E, Lichtman MA, Coller BS, et al.
Publ. McGraw Hill Professional, 2001
Comment: Standard textbook of hematology

WINTROBE'S CLINICAL HEMATOLOGY, 11th Edition, 2719 pp.
Ed.: Greer JP, Foerster J, Lukens JN, et al.
Publ. Lippincott Williams & Wilkins, 2004
Comment: Standard textbook of hematology

B. SMALLER COMPENDIA

AMERICAN SOCIETY OF HEMATOLOGY SELF-ASSESSMENT PROGRAM, 2nd Edition, 451 pp.
Ed.: Williams ME, Kahn MJ.
Publ.: Blackwell, 2005

Comment: Intended for fellowship education in hematology, published with a series of board-type questions (sold separately)

BETHESDA HANDBOOK OF CLINICAL HEMATOLOGY, 1st Edition, 494 pp.
Ed.: Rodgers GP, Young NS.
Publ.: Lippincott Williams & Wilkins, 2005
Comment: Short textbook, multiple authors from one institution

BONE MARROW PATHOLOGY, 2nd Edition, 704 pp.
Ed.: Foucar K.
Publ.: ASCP, 2001
Comment: Standard text of bone marrow pathology

ESSENTIAL HAEMATOLOGY, 4th Edition, 349 pp.
Ed.: Hoffbrand AV, Pettit J, Moss P.
Publ.: Blackwell, 2001
Comment: Essential facts in hematology

HEMATOLOGY FOR MEDICAL STUDENTS, 1st Edition, 270 pp.
Ed.: Schmaier AH, Petruzzelli LM.
Publ.: Lippincott Williams & Wilkins, 2003
Comment: Introduction for students

HEMATOLOGY FOR STUDENTS, 1st Edition, 341 pp.
Ed.: MacKinney AA.
Publ.: Martin Dunitz, 2002
Comment: Introduction for students

HEMATOLOGY IN CLINICAL PRACTICE, 3rd Edition, 429 pp.
Ed.: Hillman RS, Ault KA.
Publ.: McGraw-Hill, 2002
Comment: Short clinical text of hematology

OXFORD HANDBOOK OF CLINICAL HAEMATOLOGY, 2nd Edition, 736 pp.
Ed.: Provan D, Singer CRJ, Baglin T, et al.
Publ.: Oxford University Press, 2004
Comment: Pocket text of clinical hematology, many tables and protocols

TEXTBOOK OF MALIGNANT HEMATOLOGY, 2nd Edition, 876 pp.
Ed.: Degos L, Linch DC, Löwenberg B.
Publ.: Taylor & Francis, 2005
Comment: Covers many topics in leukemia and other hematologic malignancies

*TRANSFUSION THERAPY: CLINICAL PRINCIPLES
AND PRACTICE*, 2nd Edition, 690 pp.
Ed. Mintz PD.
Publ. AABB, 2005
Comment: Standard text of blood transfusion

II) PERIODICALS SPECIALIZING IN HEMATOLOGY
OR PUBLISHING MAJOR HEMATOLOGIC ARTICLES
(IMPACT FACTOR GIVEN FOR 2004)

AMERICAN JOURNAL OF CLINICAL PATHOLOGY	2.716
AMERICAN JOURNAL OF HEMATOLOGY	1.701
ANNALS OF HEMATOLOGY	1.292
ANNALS OF INTERNAL MEDICINE	13.114
BIOLOGY OF BLOOD AND MARROW TRANSPLANTATION	3.278
BLOOD	9.782
BLOOD CELLS, MOLECULES & DISEASES	2.549
BLOOD REVIEWS	2.838
BONE MARROW TRANSPLANTATION	2.101
BRITISH JOURNAL OF HAEMATOLOGY	3.195
CURRENT OPINION IN HEMATOLOGY	4.513
EUROPEAN JOURNAL OF HAEMATOLOGY	1.729
EXPERIMENTAL HEMATOLOGY	4.681
HAEMATOLOGICA	4.192
HUMAN PATHOLOGY	3.369
JOURNAL OF CLINICAL ONCOLOGY	9.835
JOURNAL OF PEDIATRIC HEMATOLOGY/ ONCOLOGY	1.161
LANCET	21.713
LEUKEMIA	5.810
LEUKEMIA RESEARCH	2.244
MODERN PATHOLOGY	3.643
NEW ENGLAND JOURNAL OF MEDICINE	38.570
THROMBOSIS AND HAEMOSTASIS	3.413
TRANSFUSION	3.708

III. ELECTRONIC DATABASES AND SOURCES
OF INFORMATION

BLOODLINE
Website: www.bloodline.net
Has multiple resources, book reviews, teaching cases, news, and links to educational resources (organized by a publisher)

BLOODMED
Website: www.bloodmed.com
Organized into several sections with section editors (mainly British hematologists), provides news (both scientific and clinical aspects of hematology), experts answer questions, original reviews (organized by a publisher, registration required)

CLINICAL PRACTICE GUIDELINES IN ONCOLOGY
Website: www.nccn.org
Panel of experts gives recommendations for diagnosis and treatment. This includes most hematologic malignancies

MDCONSULT
Website: www.mdconsult.com
Offers news, online books, databases, including some hematologic resources

MEDLINE
Website: www.ncbi.nlm.nih.gov/entrez
Database of the National Library of Medicine, complete listing of medical and biomedical journal articles

MEDSCAPE HEMATOLOGY-ONCOLOGY
Website: www.medscape.com/hematology-oncologyhome
News in clinical hematology and oncology with some basic science content, some full-text articles, educational resources, conference coverage, and case discussions

ONCOLOGY & HEMATOLOGY 2003 (Available in print and online, edited by Abeloff MD, gives review and ratings of 1600 web sites, focus on oncology, but gives information about most hematology sites). Internet access via: www.eMedguides.com

UPTODATE
Website: www.uptodate.com
Database for internists and subspecialists, comprehensive reviews, written and updated by experts, has multiple references and cross-references

IV. SPECIALIZED WEBSITES AND ORGANIZATIONS

APLASTIC ANEMIA & MDS INTERNATIONAL FOUNDATION
Website: www.aamds.org or www.aplastic.org
Patient-oriented resources and information about bone marrow failure syndromes, offers research grants

COOLEY'S ANEMIA FOUNDATION
Website: www.cooleysanemia.org
Patient-oriented resources and information about thalassemias

FANCONI ANEMIA RESEARCH FUND
Website: www.fanconi.org
Patient-oriented information about Fanconi anemia, offers research support

INTERNATIONAL BONE MARROW TRANSPLANT REGISTRY
Website: www.ibmtr.org
International database on autologous and allogeneic bone marrow and stem cell transplantation, performs outcomes research

INTERNATIONAL MYELOMA FOUNDATION
Website: www.myeloma.org
Patient-oriented resources and information about multiple myeloma and related conditions, promotes research and offers research support

LEUKEMIA & LYMPHOMA SOCIETY
Website: www.leukemia.org or www.lls.org
Patient oriented resources, support and information about different types of leukemias and lymphomas, has several types of research grants

NATIONAL HEMOPHILIA FOUNDATION
Website: www.hemophilia.org
Information about bleeding disorders for patients and health professionals, gives recommendations for treatment, has research grants

NATIONAL MARROW DONOR PROGRAM
Website: www.marrow.org
Information about the activities of the National Marrow Donor Program (NMDP) facilitating matched unrelated transplantation. This information is directed to potential donors, patients, and physicians. The NMDP maintains the world's largest volunteer donor database and performs accreditation of transplant centers and outcomes research

NATIONAL ORGANIZATION FOR RARE DISORDERS
Website: www.rarediseases.org
Systematic catalog of diseases, organizations, information, and support for many rare disorders including many hematologic disorders. Fee-based direct access to relevant publications and journals.

SICKLE CELL DISEASE ASSOCIATION OF AMERICA
Website: www.sicklecelldisease.org
Patient-oriented resources and information about sickle cell disease

V. PROFESSIONAL ASSOCIATIONS OF HEMATOLOGISTS AND RELATED SPECIALISTS OR SCIENTISTS

AMERICAN ASSOCIATION FOR CANCER RESEARCH
Website: www.aacr.org

Largest scientific association for basic and translational cancer research. Publishes research journals and organizes meetings and workshops. Has both physicians and scientists as members.

AMERICAN CANCER SOCIETY
Website: www.cancer.org

Association of cancer professionals, has local chapters, publishes journals for clinical research in the different types of cancer

AMERICAN SOCIETY FOR BLOOD AND MARROW TRANSPLANTATION
Website: www.asbmt.org

Association of North American transplant physicians and scientists. Promotes research and issues guidelines for blood and marrow transplantation. Website has links to other transplant-related organizations.

AMERICAN SOCIETY OF CLINICAL ONCOLOGY
Website: www.asco.org

Association of American oncologists with many international members. Issues practice guidelines and patient information including hematologic malignancies. Promotes education and clinical and translational research

AMERICAN SOCIETY OF HEMATOLOGY
Website: www.hematology.org

The American Society of Hematology (ASH) is the world's largest professional society concerned with causes and treatments of blood disorders. ASH has both physicians and pure scientists as members and merges the clinical and scientific aspects of hematology. Membership is very broad and includes hematologists in the United States and virtually every country of the world. The website has a host of information both for members, non-members and patients. There are educational materials, grant opportunities, news releases and information about past and future annual meetings.

AMERICAN SOCIETY OF PEDIATRIC HEMATOLOGY/ ONCOLOGY
Website: www.aspho.org

Association of pediatric hematologists and oncologists

BRITISH SOCIETY FOR HAEMATOLOGY
Website: www.b-s-h.org.uk
Association of British hematologists

EUROPEAN GROUP FOR BLOOD AND MARROW TRANSPLANTATION
Website: www.ebmt.org
European association for research and clinical practice in bone marrow and stem cell transplantation. Issues guidelines for transplantation. Has members in many countries and promotes clinical research in 11 working parties

EUROPEAN HEMATOLOGY ASSOCIATION
Website : www.ehaweb.org
European organization for research and education in hematology

INTERNATIONAL SOCIETY FOR EXPERIMENTAL HEMATOLOGY
Website : www.iseh.org
International organization of basic, clinical, and translational scientists in the area of hematology

INTERNATIONAL SOCIETY FOR HAEMATOLOGY
Website: www.ish-world.org
World organization of hematologists (organized in several divisions)

SOUTH AFRICAN SOCIETY OF HAEMATOLOGY
Website : www.sash.org.za
Organization of South African hematologists

VI. PATIENT-ORIENTED DATABASES AND SOURCES OF INFORMATION

- List of clinical trials compiled by the U.S. National Institutes of Health and the National Library of Medicine
  Internet Address: http:// clinicaltrials.gov
- MedlinePLUS
  Website: www.medlineplus.gov
  Information about over 700 health-related topics (database maintained by the U.S. National Library of Medicine and the National Institutes of Health)
- UPTODATE® Patient Information
  Website: http://patients.uptodate.com
  Useful information for patients, written by experts, includes some hematologic topics

Index